HANDBOOK OF
CARDIOVASCULAR
CLINICAL TRIALS

SHILPESH S. PATEL, M.D.
Clinical Fellow
Division of Cardiology
Clinical Instructor
Department of Internal Medicine
University of Texas Medical School at Houston
Houston, Texas

JAY N. COHN, M.D.
Professor
Cardiovascular Division
Department of Medicine
University of Minnesota Medical School
Minneapolis, Minnesota

JAMES T. WILLERSON, M.D.
Edward Randall III Professor and Chairman
Department of Internal Medicine
University of Texas Medical School at Houston
Medical Director and Director
Cardiology Research
Texas Heart Institute
St. Luke's Episcopal Hospital

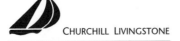
CHURCHILL LIVINGSTONE

New York, Edinburgh, London, Madrid, Melbourne, San Francisco, Tokyo

1352663

Library of Congress Cataloging-in-Publication Data

Patel, Shilpesh S.
    Handbook of cardiovascular clinical trials / Shilpesh S. Patel,
  Jay N. Cohn, James T. Willerson.
        p.   cm.
    Includes bibliographical references and index.
    ISBN 0-443-07925-0 (alk. paper)
    1. Cardiovascular system—Diseases—Treatment—Handbooks, manuals,
  etc. 2. Cardiology, Experimental—Handbooks, manuals, etc.
  3. Clinical trials—Handbooks, manuals, etc. I. Cohn, Jay N.
  II. Willerson, James T., date. III. Title.
    [DNLM: 1. Cardiovascular Diseases—prevention & control—handbooks.
  2. Clinical Trials—handbooks. 3. Research Design—handbooks   WG 39 P295h 1997]
  RC683.8.P38   1997
  616.1′06—dc21
  DNLM/DLC
  for Library of Congress

                                                              96-43506
                                                                   CIP

© Churchill Livingstone Inc. 1997

Distributed in the United Kingdom by Churchill Livingstone, Robert Stevenson House, 1-3 Baxter's Place, Leith Walk, Edinburgh EH1 3AF, and by associated companies, branches, and representatives throughout the world.

Medical knowledge is constantly changing. As new information becomes available, changes in treatment, procedures, equipment and the use of drugs become necessary. The editors/authors/contributors and the publishers have, as far as it is possible, taken care to ensure that the information given in this text is accurate and up to date. However, readers are strongly advised to confirm that the information, especially with regard to drug usage, complies with the latest legislation and standards of practice.

The Publishers have made every effort to trace the copyright holders for borrowed material. If they have inadvertently overlooked any, they will be pleased to make the necessary arrangements at the first opportunity.

Acquisitions Editor: *Allan Ross*
Assistant Editor: *Jennifer Hardy*
Production Editor: *David Terry*
Desktop Coordinator: *Jo-Ann Demas*
Production Supervisor: *Sharon Tuder*
Cover Design: *Jeannette Jacobs*

Printed in the United States of America

To my wife, Nikita,
and my children, Akash and Juhi,
for their patience, support, and love

S.P.

To our families, with our gratitude
for their patience and support

J.C.
J.W.

Preface

Cardiology is a relatively unique field in which many clinical trials have been performed to determine benefits and limitations of various treatments. These trials have offered vital information to clinicians taking care of cardiac patients. However, due to the large volume of completed trials and ongoing investigations, it has become increasingly difficult to remain familiar with these important results.

We have therefore prepared this detailed compilation of the major completed clinical cardiovascular trials since 1981. The trials selected are large, randomized, prospective studies or series that establish the benefit and limitations of a treatment modality in a particular disease process. Each trial is succinctly summarized in a uniform format describing purpose, study design, results, and conclusions. Figures from the original papers have been included when applicable to provide visual representation of the major finding of the study.

This handbook is divided into twelve sections according to the subspecialty of the studies. In addition, a summary table that lists the name of the study and the major conclusions has been included in the Introduction, thereby providing quick reference for the reader. We have also summarized and analyzed the key points of each section in the Overview portion of each chapter.

We hope this handbook will prove useful to the medical community caring for patients with cardiovascular diseases, including technical personnel, nurses, medical students, house staff, cardiology fellows, and practicing physicians. We are committed to updating this handbook frequently with the most recently published major clinical trials, and we welcome the reader's comments and suggestions for improving future editions.

Shilpesh S. Patel, M.D.
Jay N. Cohn, M.D.
James T. Willerson, M.D.

Contents

Introduction

SUMMARY OF CONCLUSIONS

Myocardial Infarction Trials (Ch. 1)

CONSENSUS 2
In patients receiving standard therapy for acute myocardial infarction, the administration of enalapril within 24 hours of onset of chest pain did not improve 6-month survival compared to placebo.

GISSI 1
Intravenous infusion of 1.5 million U of streptokinase (SK) over 45 to 60 minutes produced a significant 18% reduction in overall in-hospital mortality compared to no thrombolytic therapy in patients with acute myocardial infarction. The reduction in mortality was persistent up to 12-month follow-up and was limited to patients who received SK within 6 hours of onset of symptoms.

GISSI 2
Streptokinase and tissue plasminogen activator (t-PA) are equally effective in reducing in-hospital mortality and preserving left ventricular function when administered with aspirin and atenolol in the setting of acute myocardial infarction. The addition of subcutaneous heparin started 12 hours after thrombolytic therapy offered no significant benefit.

GISSI 3
In the setting of acute myocardial infarction, lisinopril alone and in combination with transdermal glyceryl trinitrate significantly reduced 6-week mortality by 11% and 17%, respectively, and also significantly reduced 6-week combined end point events (deaths, congestive heart failure, and left ventricular ejection fraction less than 35%) by 8% and 13%, respectively, compared to control. Transdermal glyceryl trinitrate alone provided no significant benefit.

1

GUSTO 1

In the setting of acute myocardial infarction, accelerated dose t-PA and intravenous heparin resulted in a significant 14% reduction in total 30-day mortality compared with SK and intravenous or subcutaneous heparin. Accelerated t-PA was associated with a significantly higher incidence of hemorrhagic stroke compared to SK. Overall benefit, as assessed by the combined end point of total mortality and disabling stroke, was significantly better with accelerated t-PA. Accelerated t-PA led to an actual survival benefit of 10 additional lives saved per 1,000 patients treated when compared with SK.

GUSTO ANGIOGRAPHIC

Accelerated t-PA provided more rapid and complete flow in the infarct-related artery at 90 minutes compared with SK in patients with acute myocardial infarction. Patency rates by 180 minutes and later were not significantly different among the four treatment groups. No significant difference in left ventricular ejection fraction was found at 90 minutes or 5 to 7 days among the four treatment groups, although other indicators of ventricular function were better in the accelerated t-PA group.

GUSTO 2A

The use of heparin and hirudin in acute coronary syndromes in the doses used in the GUSTO 2A study resulted in a significantly higher rate of intracranial hemorrhage compared to the results of GUSTO 1. The trial has been reinitiated, as GUSTO 2B, at lower doses of heparin and hirudin.

ISIS 1

The use of atenolol, administered immediately and continued for 1 week, in the setting of acute myocardial infarction reduced 1-week vascular mortality by 15% compared to placebo with most of the benefit occurring during days 0 to 1. There was no significant difference in vascular mortality at 20-month follow-up.

ISIS 2

In the setting of acute myocardial infarction, SK alone, aspirin alone, and the combination of SK/aspirin significantly reduced 5-week vascular mortality by 23%, 21%, and 40%, respectively, over control. This survival benefit remained statistically significant during the 15-month follow-up. Treatment with SK significantly reduced vascular mortality even for patients treated 13 to 24 hours after symptom onset, but the benefit was greatest when SK was given early. Streptokinase therapy was also associated with a small but significant excess of major bleeds and cerebral hemorrhage compared to control.

ISIS 3

In patients with acute myocardial infarction, no significant difference in 5-week or 6-month mortality was observed between treatment with SK, t-PA, or acylated plasminogen streptokinase activator complex (APSAC). The addition of subcutaneous heparin to thrombolytic/aspirin therapy resulted in no significant difference in 5-week or 6-month mortality but did result in a significant increase in major bleeds and hemorrhagic strokes compared to thrombolytic/aspirin alone. Tissue plasminogen activator and APSAC, both with aspirin alone or with aspirin and heparin, were associated with significantly higher incidences of hemorrhagic and total strokes compared to SK.

ISIS 4

Early use of oral captopril in patients with suspected acute myocardial infarction resulted in a significant 7% reduction in 5-week mortality compared to placebo that appeared to be maintained at 1-year follow-up. Oral mononitrate and intravenous magnesium therapy offered no significant benefit in survival.

LATE

In patients with acute myocardial infarction, treatment with t-PA from 6 to 12 hours after symptom onset resulted in a significant 25% reduction in 35-day mortality compared to placebo. Treatment with t-PA from 12 to 24 hours after symptom onset revealed no significant benefit in 35-day mortality compared to placebo.

LIMIT 2

In patients with suspected acute myocardial infarction, the administration of intravenous magnesium initiated before thrombolytic agents resulted in a significant 24% reduction in 28-day mortality and a 25% reduction in the incidence of left ventricular failure compared to placebo. Follow-up at 2.7 years revealed a persistent substantial reduction in overall mortality and ischemic heart disease mortality in patients treated with magnesium.

PAMI

Immediate percutaneous transluminal coronary angioplasty in patients with acute myocardial infarction significantly reduced the combined incidence of in-hospital death or nonfatal myocardial infarction, was associated with less intracranial hemorrhage, and resulted in similar 6-month left ventricular ejection fraction compared to therapy with intravenous t-PA. However, immediate percutaneous transluminal coronary angioplasty did increase the need for surgical vascular repair and the incidence of ventricular fibrillation.

PTCA VS. SK (ZWOLLE)

In patients with acute myocardial infarction, treatment with immediate coronary angioplasty resulted in a higher long-term patency rate with less residual stenosis of the infarct-related artery, better left ventricular ejection fraction, and a lower incidence of recurrent myocardial ischemia compared to treatment with intravenous SK.

RAPID

Reteplase (r-PA) given as a double bolus of 10 + 10 million U achieved more rapid and complete thrombolysis of the infarct-related artery and resulted in a significantly higher left ventricular ejection fraction at hospital discharge compared to standard-dose t-PA. No increase in the risk of bleeding or adverse clinical events was observed with r-PA. A separate randomized trial, RAPID 2, will compare r-PA with accelerated-dose t-PA.

TAMI 1

In patients with acute myocardial infarction who achieve initial successful thrombolysis with t-PA, immediate angioplasty offered no significant benefit in mortality, reocclusion rate, or left ventricular ejection fraction compared to elective angioplasty over a 7- to 10-day follow-up.

TAMI 2

Combination therapy with t-PA and urokinase offered no significant synergistic advantage in 90-minute patency rates or reocclusion rates compared to therapy with t-PA alone in patients with acute myocardial infarction over a 7-day follow-up.

TAMI 3

The administration of t-PA and immediate high-dose intravenous heparin to patients with acute myocardial infarction did not improve 90-minute patency rates or left ventricular ejection fraction compared to t-PA and late (after 90 minutes) intravenous heparin. In addition, no significant difference in bleeding complications was found between these two groups.

TAMI 4

In patients with acute myocardial infarction, the combination of t-PA and Iloprost did not improve 90-minute vessel patency, the incidence of reocclusion, or left ventricular ejection fraction compared to t-PA alone.

TAMI 5

Combination thrombolytic therapy with t-PA and urokinase did not improve left ventricular ejection fraction or significantly improve 90-minute patency rates compared to t-PA alone or urokinase alone in patients with acute myocardial infarction. Combination therapy did significantly reduce the rate of reocclusion compared to monotherapy. The aggressive catheterization strategy did not significantly improve left ventricular ejection fraction or predischarge patency rates compared to the deferred catheterization strategy.

TAMI 6

The administration of t-PA 6 to 24 hours after the onset of acute myocardial infarction significantly improved the acute vessel patency rate only, with no significant difference observed in 6-month vessel patency, left ventricular ejection fraction, or in-hospital and 6-month mortality compared to placebo.

TAMI 7

The accelerated tissue-type plasminogen activator dosing of group C resulted in the highest infarct-related patency rate and a low reocclusion rate. The most rapid dosing schedule (60 minutes), group A, yielded a lower patency rate. Left ventricular ejection fraction and bleeding complications were not significantly different among the five dosing strategies.

TAMI 8

The use of m7E3 along with t-PA in patients with acute myocardial infarction resulted in a marked inhibition of platelet aggregation without a significant effect on bleeding complications.

TIMI 1

Treatment with t-PA produced a significantly higher reperfusion rate at 90 minutes and patency rate at 8 to 10 days compared to SK in patients with acute myocardial infarction. Neither therapy resulted in a significant overall improvement in left ventricular ejection fraction between admission and hospital discharge.

TIMI 2A

In the setting of acute myocardial infarction treated with thrombolytic therapy, no significant difference was found in cumulative mortality, discharge contrast left ventricular ejection fraction, or incidence of nonfatal reinfarction among immediate invasive, delayed invasive, and conservative strategies. Conservative therapy resulted in less morbidity and a lower use of percutaneous transluminal coronary angioplasty.

TIMI 2B

Immediate β-blocker therapy with metoprolol in the setting of acute myocardial infarction treated with thrombolytic therapy resulted in significantly less in-hospital recurrent ischemia and nonfatal reinfarction compared to delayed β-blocker therapy. However, no significant difference was observed in left ventricular ejection fraction or total mortality to 1 year.

TIMI 3A

Arteriographically apparent intraluminal thrombus was found in a low percentage (35%) of patients with unstable angina or non-Q-wave myocardial infarction. Overall, t-PA was not significantly more effective than placebo at improving coronary flow in these patients. Substantial improvement in flow, however, was more frequent with t-PA in lesions containing apparent thrombus and in patients with evolving non-Q-wave myocardial infarction. The clinical relevance of these findings was reported in the TIMI 3B study.

TIMI 3B

The administration of thrombolytic agents to patients with unstable angina or non-Q-wave myocardial infarction offered no benefit in 6-week survival and was associated with significantly greater rates of reinfarction and intracranial hemorrhage. The subgroup of patients with unstable angina treated with t-PA had a significant increase in the incidence of death or myocardial infarction compared to placebo. Early invasive strategy compared to conservative strategy did not reduce 6-week mortality but did result in significantly reduced length of hospitalization, incidence of rehospitalization, and use of antianginal medications.

TIMI 4

In the setting of acute myocardial infarction, front-loaded t-PA achieved a significantly higher 90-minute reperfusion rate compared to APSAC or combination therapy, and lower in-hospital mortality compared to

APSAC. The incidence of major hemorrhage was significantly lower with t-PA therapy. However, 1-year mortality and combined unsatisfactory end point was not significantly different between the three therapies.

TIMI 5

In this pilot study, hirudin was found to be a promising agent compared with heparin as adjunctive therapy with t-PA for acute myocardial infarction. Hirudin resulted in significantly better coronary flow at 18- to 36-hour arteriography, which was perhaps due to late reperfusion of occluded arteries. Treatment with hirudin produced a trend toward increased TIMI grade 3 flow at 90 minutes and 18 to 36 hours and reduced in-hospital mortality, although the results were not statistically significant. Reinfarction rates were also significantly lower in hirudin-treated patients.

TIMI 6

In this pilot study, hirudin appeared to be as safe as heparin when given with SK and aspirin to patients with acute myocardial infarction.

TIMI 9A

The doses of heparin and hirudin used with thrombolytic therapy and aspirin in the setting of acute myocardial infarction resulted in substantially higher hemorrhagic complications than that found in other major clinical trials. This study has been reinitiated with lower doses of heparin and hirudin and will be reported as TIMI 9B.

WARIS

Long-term treatment with warfarin in patients surviving an acute myocardial infarction who are not receiving chronic aspirin therapy significantly reduced total mortality and the incidences of recurrent myocardial infarction and cerebrovascular accidents compared to placebo during an average 37-month follow-up. The incidence of major hemorrhage was 0.6% among warfarin-treated patients.

Unstable Angina Trials (Ch. 2)

ASPIRIN–HEPARIN MONTREAL HEART INSTITUTE

In patients with acute unstable angina, the use of heparin alone significantly reduced the incidence of myocardial infarction and refractory angina, whereas aspirin alone significantly reduced the incidence of myocardial infarction only. The combination of aspirin and heparin was not superior to either medication alone and resulted in slightly more bleeding complications.

ASPIRIN VA COOPERATIVE

The use of aspirin for 12 weeks in men hospitalized with unstable angina significantly reduced the incidence of acute myocardial infarction by 55% and favored lower mortality by 51% compared to placebo at 12-week follow-up. At 1 year, mean mortality was significantly lower by 43% in the aspirin group.

CABG VA COOPERATIVE

Treatment with coronary artery bypass grafting in men with unstable angina prolonged survival only in the subgroups of patients with triple-vessel disease at 5-year follow-up and those with severe rest angina and impaired left ventricular function at 8-year follow-up compared to medical therapy. No significant difference in the incidence of myocardial infarction was observed among any subgroups.

CAPTURE: C7E3 IN UNSTABLE ANGINA

In patients undergoing angioplasty for refractory unstable angina, the use of c7E3 significantly reduced the in-hospital combined incidence of death, myocardial infarction, and recurrent ischemia requiring urgent intervention without increasing bleeding complications compared to placebo.

HEPARIN WITHDRAWAL

In patients with acute unstable angina, the abrupt discontinuation of heparin after an average of 6 days of treatment resulted in a significantly higher incidence of reactivation of disease (recurrent unstable angina, myocardial infarction, or both) compared to the other three study groups. This clinical reactivation was not observed when aspirin was administered concurrently with heparin.

Antithrombotic Trials (Ch. 3)

EPIC

The use of c7E3 bolus and infusion in patients undergoing high-risk angioplasty resulted in a significant reduction in combined end points (mortality, nonfatal reinfarction, emergency coronary artery bypass graft [CABG] or percutaneous transluminal coronary angioplasty, and requirement for stent or intra-aortic balloon pump) but at a cost of significantly more major bleeds and transfusions compared to placebo at 1 month. At 6-month follow-up, c7E3 bolus and infusion significantly reduced the combined end point (mortality, nonfatal reinfarction, or emergency CABG or percutaneous transluminal coronary angioplasty) and the need for repeat target vessel revascularization compared to placebo. The c7E3 bolus-only group was not significantly different from placebo at 1- and 6-month follow-up.

EPILOG

Among patients undergoing high- and low-risk coronary angioplasty or atherectomy, treatment with c7E3 significantly reduced the combined incidence of death, myocardial infarction, or urgent revascularization without producing an increase in bleeding complications at 30-day follow-up compared to placebo. The use of weight-adjusted low-dose heparin with c7E3 appears to provide the lowest incidence of bleeding complications.

HASI

In patients undergoing urgent angioplasty for unstable angina or postinfarction angina, no significant difference was found in the incidence of acute or 6-month ischemic complications between hirulog and heparin treatment. In the subgroup of patients with postinfarction angina treated with hirulog, a significant reduction in the incidence of myocardial infarction and combined acute ischemic complications was observed compared to heparin. Hirulog was associated with a significantly lower rate of bleeding.

IMPACT 1 (INTEGRELIN)

In this pilot study, the use of Integrelin, along with aspirin and heparin, in patients undergoing routine, elective percutaneous angioplasty or atherectomy had a favorable trend toward lowering composite end points (death, nonfatal myocardial infarction, repeat intervention, stent, or CABG for refractory ischemia) compared to placebo at 1-month follow-up without an excessive risk of major bleeding.

IMPACT 2 (INTEGRELIN)

Treatment with Integrelin significantly reduced ischemic complications compared to placebo in patients undergoing coronary angioplasty or atherectomy at 24-hr follow-up. By 30-day follow-up, however, there was no significant difference between Integrelin and placebo treatment, and at 6-month follow-up, there was no difference in the incidence of restenosis.

β-Blocker Trials (Ch. 4)

BHAT

Propranolol administered 5 to 21 days after acute myocardial infarction significantly reduced mortality by 26% compared to placebo during the 2-year follow-up.

GOTEBORG

Metoprolol treatment started immediately after admission and continued for 3 months significantly reduced total mortality by 36% and the incidence of ventricular fibrillation in patients with definite or suspected myocardial infarction at 3-month follow-up compared to placebo.

MIAMI

Early administration of metoprolol to patients with acute myocardial infarction produced a trend toward a lower 15-day mortality and reinfarction rate compared to placebo, although the results were not statistically significant. The incidences of ventricular fibrillation or ventricular tachycardia requiring cardioversion were similar between metoprolol and placebo. Metoprolol did result in less supraventricular tachycardia, need for antianginal medications, and use of digoxin and other antiarrhythmics.

NORWEGIAN PROPRANOLOL

Treatment with propranolol for 1 year after a recent myocardial infarction in selected high-risk patients significantly reduced the risk of sudden cardiac death by 52% and produced a trend toward lower total mortality compared to placebo.

NORWEGIAN TIMOLOL

Long-term treatment with timolol in patients surviving acute myocardial infarction significantly reduced total mortality by 39.4%, sudden death by 44.6%, and rate of reinfarction by 28.4% compared to placebo during a 33-month follow-up.

Calcium Channel Blocker Trials (Ch. 5)

DAVIT 1

Verapamil administered early and continued for 6 months after acute myocardial infarction had no benefit in reducing 12-month total mortality or incidence of reinfarction compared to placebo.

DAVIT 2

Late administration of verapamil in patients with acute myocardial infarction had no significant effect on total mortality but did significantly reduce the incidence of reinfarction by 17% compared to placebo over the 18-month follow-up. The subgroup of patients without heart failure treated with verapamil had significant reductions in both total mortality and reinfarction compared to placebo.

DRS

Treatment with diltiazem significantly reduced the incidence of reinfarction compared to placebo in patients with non-Q-wave myocardial infarction at 14-day follow-up. Diltiazem treatment had no significant effect on postinfarction angina or total mortality.

MDPIT

Use of diltiazem after acute myocardial infarction did not reduce total mortality or cardiac events (death and reinfarction) compared to placebo at 25-month follow-up. A retrospective subgroup analysis of patients without pulmonary congestion demonstrated lower rates of mortality and cardiac events with diltiazem compared to placebo.

NIFEDIPINE IN AORTIC REGURGITATION

In asymptomatic patients with chronic severe aortic regurgitation and normal left ventricular ejection fraction, treatment with nifedipine significantly delayed and reduced the need for aortic valve replacement compared to treatment with digoxin at 6-year follow-up. Nifedipine therapy decreased left ventricular dilatation and left ventricular mass and improved left ventricular function.

SPRINT 1

Nifedipine (30 mg daily) administered prophylactically to survivors of acute myocardial infarction had no significant effect on reducing mortality or recurrent myocardial infarction compared to placebo at 10-month follow-up.

SPRINT 2

The early administration of nifedipine (60 mg daily) to patients with suspected high-risk acute myocardial infarction resulted in no significant improvement in overall mortality, incidence of recurrent myocardial infarction, or incidence of angina during an 8-month follow-up.

Congestive Heart Failure Trials (Ch. 6)

AIRE

Ramipril, administered to patients on the third to tenth day after acute myocardial infarction with clinical evidence of heart failure, resulted in a significant 27% reduction in total mortality compared to placebo during a 15-month follow-up.

CARVEDILOL

Treatment with carvedilol significantly reduced overall mortality by 65% and reduced the risk of hospitalizations for cardiovascular causes compared to placebo in symptomatic patients with congestive heart failure who were receiving conventional therapy with digoxin, diuretics, and an ACE inhibitor during a mean follow-up of 6.5 months.

CONSENSUS 1

The addition of enalapril to conventional therapy in patients with severe congestive heart failure (New York Heart Association [NYHA] functional class IV) significantly reduced 1-year mortality by 31% and improved NYHA functional class compared to placebo.

HY-C

When added to conventional therapy, captopril significantly reduced mortality by 37% compared to hydralazine in patients with severe congestive heart failure (mean left ventricular ejection fraction, 20%) who were being evaluated for cardiac transplantation. Most of the survival benefit of captopril occurred in patients with pulmonary capillary wedge pressures greater than 16 mmHg.

MDC

The addition of metoprolol to patients with symptomatic idiopathic dilated cardiomyopathy receiving optimal heart failure therapy did not significantly decrease total mortality but did significantly reduce the need for heart transplantation and improved the left ventricular ejection fraction, hemodynamics, exercise capacity, and NYHA functional class compared to placebo at 18-month follow-up.

MTT

Immunosuppressive therapy did not have a significant effect on left ventricular ejection fraction or mortality compared to control in patients with histopathologically confirmed myocarditis and left ventricular ejection fraction less than 45% during a 1-year follow-up.

PROMISE

The use of oral milrinone in patients with severe congestive heart failure who remain symptomatic despite conventional heart failure therapy resulted in a significant 28% increase in total mortality compared to placebo with no difference in symptoms or functional capacity over a 6-month follow-up.

RADIANCE

Withdrawal of digoxin for 3 months from patients who were clinically stable while receiving optimal doses of digoxin, diuretics, and angiotensin-converting enzyme inhibitors significantly worsened the clinical severity of heart failure, NYHA functional class, patients' subjective assessment of their prognosis, and left ventricular ejection fraction and left ventricular end-diastolic dimension compared to patients continuing to receive digoxin.

SAVE

Treatment with captopril in survivors of acute myocardial infarction with asymptomatic depressed left ventricular ejection fraction (40% or less) resulted in significantly reduced total and cardiovascular mortality, reduced incidence of hospitalization for severe congestive heart failure, and reduced rate of recurrent myocardial infarction compared to placebo at 42-month follow-up.

SOLVD—PREVENTION

Enalapril significantly reduced the development of clinical heart failure and the need for hospitalization for heart failure compared to placebo among patients with asymptomatic left ventricular dysfunction (left ventricular ejection fraction 35% or less) during a 37-month follow-up period. Enalapril treatment did not significantly reduce total mortality in this group.

SOLVD—TREATMENT

Enalapril used with conventional therapy significantly reduced mortality and hospitalizations for heart failure compared to placebo at 41-month follow-up in patients with overt chronic congestive heart failure and left ventricular ejection fractions 35% or less.

VHEFT 1

The combination of hydralazine and isosorbide dinitrate significantly improved survival and left ventricular ejection fraction compared to placebo at 3-year follow-up in patients with chronic congestive heart failure. Prazosin provided no significant benefit.

VHEFT 2

Enalapril substantially reduced mortality by 28% compared to hydralazine-isosorbide dinitrate in men with chronic congestive heart failure receiving digoxin and diuretics at 2-year follow-up. At 5-year follow-up, there was a trend toward reduced mortality with enalapril, but the results were not statistically significant.

Antiarrhythmic Trials (Ch. 7)

BASIS

Prophylactic amiodarone therapy significantly reduced 12-month mortality by 62% compared to control in a high-risk group of patients with asymptomatic persistent complex ventricular arrhythmias after myocardial infarction. Individualized treatment with a variety of antiarrhythmic drugs showed no benefit in survival compared to control.

CASCADE

Amiodarone was associated with significantly better survival free of cardiac death and sustained ventricular arrhythmias compared to conventional therapy in patients surviving out-of-hospital ventricular fibrillation at 6-year follow-up. Amiodarone, however, also produced pulmonary toxicity in 10% of patients and resulted in more frequent discontinuation of therapy.

CASH

In this preliminary report at 11-month follow-up, propafenone resulted in a significantly increased incidence of sudden death and sudden death or cardiac arrest compared to patients treated with an automatic implantable cardioverter/defibrillator. The propafenone arm was therefore terminated. The study continues with metoprolol, amiodarone, and automatic implantable cardioverter/defibrillator treatments.

CAST 1

The use of encainide or flecainide in patients after myocardial infarction resulted in a significant 2.64-fold excess of death or cardiac arrest compared to placebo. The results of moricizine are reported in CAST 2.

CAST 2

The use of moricizine to reduce ventricular premature depolarizations after myocardial infarction significantly increased mortality compared to placebo during the initial 2 weeks of treatment with no benefit seen at 18-month follow-up.

ESVEM

In patients with ventricular tachyarrhythmias, no significant difference was found between invasive electrophysiologic testing and Holter monitor regarding the ability to predict the success of drug therapy in preventing recurrence of arrhythmia. In addition, patients with predictions of drug efficacy by Holter monitor or electrophysiologic study had rates of recurrence of arrhythmia similar to those of patients without predictions of drug efficacy who were treated empirically.

GESICA

Amiodarone therapy significantly reduced total mortality by 19%, reduced hospital admissions for worsening congestive heart failure, and improved New York Heart Association functional class compared to a control group in patients with severe congestive heart failure over a 13-month follow-up. This effect was independent of the presence of nonsustained ventricular tachycardia on admission Holter monitor.

IMPACT (MEXILETINE)

Use of sustained release mexiletine in patients with a recent myocardial infarction resulted in a significant reduction in the combined occurrence of frequent premature ventricular contractions, couplets, and nonsustained ventricular tachycardia at 1- and 4-month follow-up compared to placebo. However, there was a trend toward increased overall mortality at 9 months in the mexiletine group compared to placebo.

PAS

Amiodarone significantly reduced cardiac mortality and serious ventricular arrhythmias (Lown grade 4) and resulted in a trend toward less sudden death compared to placebo at 12-month follow-up in patients after acute myocardial infarction with contraindications to β-blocker therapy.

STAT CHF

The use of amiodarone in patients with congestive heart failure and asymptomatic arrhythmias had no effect on overall mortality or sudden cardiac death, despite significant suppression of ventricular arrhythmias and a substantial improvement in left ventricular ejection fraction compared to placebo over a 45-month follow-up period.

Atrial Fibrillation Trials (Ch. 8)

AFASAK

Warfarin significantly reduced the incidence of thromboembolic events by 63% in patients with chronic nonrheumatic atrial fibrillation compared to placebo. Warfarin, at the dose used in this study (international normalized ratio [INR] of 2.8 to 4.2) was also associated with higher bleeding complications. Aspirin, at a dose of 75 mg/day did not reduce the incidence of thromboembolic events compared to placebo.

BAATAF

The use of low-dose warfarin (INR 1.5 to 2.7) in patients with chronic intermittent or sustained nonrheumatic atrial fibrillation significantly reduced the incidence of ischemic stroke by 86% compared to control with no increase in the incidence of major bleeds.

CAFA

This study was terminated early as a result of available results from AFASAK and SPAF, which demonstrated the clear benefit of warfarin in preventing ischemic stroke. Warfarin reduced the annual rate of primary outcome by 37% compared to placebo at 15.2-month follow-up in this truncated study.

EAFT

In patients with nonrheumatic atrial fibrillation and a recent transient ischemic attack or minor ischemic stroke, oral anticoagulation significantly reduced the risk of recurrent stroke by 66%, whereas aspirin had no significant benefit at 2.3-year follow-up. Oral anticoagulation was also associated with a substantial excess of major and minor bleeding episodes.

SPAF 1

Warfarin and aspirin significantly reduced the rate of ischemic stroke and systemic embolism by 67% and 42%, respectively, compared to placebo in patients with sustained or intermittent nonrheumatic atrial fibrillation. No significant difference in bleeding complications was observed between the three groups.

SPAF 2

In patients of any age with sustained or intermittent nonrheumatic atrial fibrillation, only a modest benefit was found in the reduction of ischemic strokes by warfarin over aspirin; the results were not statistically significant. Patients older than 75 years of age taking warfarin (international normalized ratio [INR] 2.0 to 4.5) had significantly higher rates of major hemorrhage compared to those taking aspirin and significantly higher rates of intracranial hemorrhage compared to patients less than 75 years of age taking warfarin. In patients less than 75 years of age with no clinical risk factors for thromboembolism (history of hypertension, previous thromboembolism, or recent heart failure), the risk of ischemic stroke with aspirin was so low (0.5% per year) that use of warfarin in this population may not be advantageous.

SPINAF
Low-intensity anticoagulation with warfarin (INR 1.4 to 2.8) significantly reduced cerebral infarction by 80% compared to placebo in patients with chronic nonrheumatic atrial fibrillation without producing an excess risk of major hemorrhage.

Lipid-Lowering/Primary Prevention Trials (Ch. 9)

ACAPS
In patients with asymptomatic carotid atherosclerosis and moderately elevated low-density lipoprotein cholesterol, the use of lovastatin significantly reduced the mean intimal medial thickness in the carotid arteries and reduced the risk of cardiovascular events and mortality compared to placebo over a 3-year follow-up period. Results of low-dose warfarin therapy will be reported separately.

CARE
Treatment with pravastatin in patients surviving a recent myocardial infarction with normal or mildly elevated serum cholesterol significantly reduced a combined end point of fatal coronary heart disease or nonfatal myocardial infarction, the incidence of total myocardial infarctions, and the requirement for revascularization with percutaneous transluminal coronary angioplasty or coronary artery bypass graft compared to placebo during a 5-year follow-up.

CHAOS
Therapy with vitamin E (400–800 IU daily) to patients with angiographically proven symptomatic coronary artery disease significantly reduced the incidence of nonfatal myocardial infarction without meaningfully affecting cardiovascular mortality compared to placebo during a median follow-up of 510 days.

CLAS

Treatment with combination colestipol-niacin therapy in men with previous coronary artery bypass grafting and hypercholesterolemia resulted in significantly more nonprogression and regression of native coronary atherosclerosis and substantially fewer new lesions in native coronary arteries and bypass vein grafts compared to placebo at 4-year follow-up.

CORONARY DRUG PROJECT

Treatment with niacin in men with hypercholesterolemia and previous myocardial infarction reduced the incidence of nonfatal myocardial infarction at 5-year follow-up and total mortality at 15-year follow-up compared to placebo. Clofibrate therapy provided no beneficial effect. Estrogen and dextrothyroxine therapy produced an unfavorable trend in total mortality.

HELSINKI HEART STUDY

Among middle-aged asymptomatic men with primary dyslipidemia, defined as a non-high-density lipoprotein cholesterol 200 mg/dl or more, the use of gemfibrozil significantly reduced the incidence of combined cardiac end points (cardiac death and nonfatal myocardial infarction) by 34% and the incidence of nonfatal myocardial infarction by 37% compared to placebo over a 5-year follow-up. Total mortality was not meaningfully reduced by treatment with gemfibrozil.

LRC-CPPT

Treatment with cholestyramine in asymptomatic middle-aged men with primary hypercholesterolemia significantly reduced the incidence of coronary heart disease (death and nonfatal myocardial infarction), angina, positive exercise treadmill test, and coronary bypass surgery compared to placebo over 7.4-year follow-up. The reduction in coronary heart disease events was directly related to the degree of reduction in total and low-density lipoprotein cholesterol.

PHS—ASPIRIN

The use of aspirin in healthy male physicians for the primary prevention of cardiovascular disease resulted in a significant 44% reduction in the risk of myocardial infarction but did not reveal a substantial reduction in stroke rate or cardiovascular mortality, perhaps because of the inadequate numbers of physicians with these later two end points.

REGRESS

In men with symptomatic coronary artery disease and normal to moderately elevated serum cholesterol, use of pravastatin resulted in significantly less angiographic progression of coronary atherosclerosis and fewer new cardiovascular events compared to placebo over a 2-year follow-up.

4S

The use of simvastatin in patients with coronary artery disease and elevated total serum cholesterol significantly reduced total mortality by 29%, cardiac mortality by 42%, major coronary events by 32%, need for revascularization by 34%, and cerebrovascular events by 37% compared to placebo over a 5.4-year follow-up.

WOSCOPS

The use of pravastatin in middle-aged men with moderate hypercholesterolemia and no history of previous myocardial infarction significantly reduced the incidence of nonfatal myocardial infarction by 29%, death from all cardiovascular causes by 30%, and the need for revascularization, while producing a trend toward fewer deaths from coronary heart disease compared to placebo over a 4.9-year follow-up.

Revascularization Trials (Ch. 10)

ACME

The use of percutaneous transluminal coronary angioplasty in patients with single-vessel coronary artery disease resulted in significant improvements in total exercise duration, maximal heart rate × systolic blood pressure double product, angina-free exercise duration, incidence of clinical angina, and residual stenosis of the index lesions compared to medical therapy at 6-month follow-up.

CASS

Coronary artery bypass surgery, compared to medical therapy, did not significantly prolong survival or prevent myocardial infarction overall in patients who had mild stable angina pectoris or patients who were asymptomatic after myocardial infarction during the 10-year follow-up. Subgroup analysis according to the number of diseased vessels also revealed no significant difference in mortality or the incidence of myocardial infarction. However, the subgroup of patients with a left ventricular ejection fraction less than 50%—and particularly those with both left ventricular ejection fraction less than 50% and triple-vessel disease—had significantly higher 10-year survival and freedom from myocardial infarction with surgical treatment.

EUROPEAN CABG

A significant overall improvement in survival after CABG, compared with medical therapy, was observed in patients with stable angina pectoris and multivessel coronary artery disease with preserved left ventricular function over a 12-year follow-up. The survival advantage of CABG was especially prominent among the subgroup of patients with triple-vessel disease and patients with proximal stenosis of the left anterior descending coronary artery as a component of two-vessel disease.

VA CABG

Surgical therapy significantly improved survival compared to medical therapy only in patients with left main stenosis, high angiographic risk, and high clinical risk, but the benefits began to diminish after 5 years and lasted fewer than 11 years. No significant survival difference was observed in any group at 18-year follow-up. Patients with low clinical risk or low angiographic risk did not have a survival benefit from surgical therapy at any time over the 18-year follow-up.

Angioplasty vs. CABG Trials (Ch. 11)

CABRI

In symptomatic patients with multivessel coronary artery disease, treatment with percutaneous transluminal coronary angioplasty (PTCA) compared with coronary artery bypass graft (CABG) resulted in similar mortality and incidence of nonfatal myocardial infarction during the first year of follow-up. However, treatment with PTCA significantly increased the need for repeat revascularizations and the use of antianginal medications.

EAST

No significant difference between revascularization with PTCA or CABG was found with regard to total mortality, composite primary end point (death, Q-wave myocardial infarction, or large ischemic burden), or left ventricular ejection fraction at 3-year follow-up in patients with multivessel coronary artery disease. Patients initially treated with PTCA required significantly more subsequent revascularization with either repeat PTCA or CABG.

ERACI

In patients with multivessel coronary artery disease, treatment with PTCA or CABG resulted in similar in-hospital complication rates and similar 1-year incidence of death and acute myocardial infarction. Treatment with PTCA was associated with a significantly higher incidence of angina and the need for repeat revascularization, which was mostly due to restenosis by 6 months. The overall cost at 1 year, including all necessary repeat revascularization procedures, was significantly lower with PTCA treatment compared with CABG.

GABI

No significant difference in the freedom from angina was observed between PTCA and CABG at 1-year follow-up in patients with multivessel coronary artery disease. PTCA resulted in significantly less cumulative risk of death or myocardial infarction compared to CABG. CABG resulted in a significantly reduced need for repeat revascularization and use of antianginal medications.

RITA

At 2.5-year follow-up, no significant difference was found in total mortality or combined end points (death or nonfatal myocardial infarction) between PTCA and CABG in patients with coronary artery disease regardless of the number of diseased coronary vessels. PTCA resulted in shorter hospital stays but a substantially increased need for repeat revascularization (repeat PTCA or CABG) and antianginal medications.

New Interventional Technology Trials (Ch. 12)

BENESTENT 1

Implantation of coronary stents in patients with stable angina and a single new coronary artery lesion resulted in similar immediate success rates as balloon angioplasty but with higher in-hospital bleeding and vascular complications and longer hospital stay. At follow-up of 7 months, stent treatment resulted in substantially better clinical outcome, which was mainly due to less need for revascularization with a repeat percutaneous intervention and significantly less restenosis compared with balloon angioplasty.

BENESTENT 2

Heparin-coated stents were well tolerated, were not thrombogenic even without anticoagulation, and resulted in low bleeding complications and shortened hospital stay. Follow-up at 6 months revealed very low restenosis rates and high event-free survival.

CAVEAT 1

Directional atherectomy resulted in a significantly higher initial success rate compared to angioplasty in patients with symptomatic ischemic heart disease. However, use of atherectomy also resulted in substantially higher rates of in-hospital myocardial infarction and composite end points (death, emergency CABG, acute myocardial infarction, or abrupt vessel closure). Six-month follow-up revealed no significant difference in the restenosis rate between the two treatments; however, atherectomy resulted in significantly higher probability of death or myocardial infarction compared to angioplasty. At 1-year follow-up, atherectomy resulted in a significant excess of both death and reinfarction rate compared to angioplasty.

CAVEAT 2

In patients with a de novo saphenous vein bypass graft lesion, directional atherectomy resulted in a significantly higher initial angiographic success rate and larger luminal gain at the expense of more distal embolization and more non-Q-wave myocardial infarction compared to angioplasty. At 6-month follow-up, the two procedures were similar with respect to angiographic and clinical end points.

CCAT

Atherectomy resulted in higher initial procedural success rates in patients with lesions of the left anterior descending coronary artery compared with angioplasty with no difference in in-hospital complications. At 6-month follow-up, restenosis and clinical outcome were not significantly different between the two treatments.

STENTING ANTITHROMBOTIC REGIMEN

Antiplatelet therapy with ticlopidine and aspirin in patients after placement of intracoronary Palmaz-Schatz stents significantly reduced the incidences of myocardial infarction, repeat revascularization of the stented vessel, blood transfusions, peripheral vascular complications, and target vessel occlusion compared to anticoagulation therapy with phenprocoumon and aspirin during 30-day follow-up.

STRESS

Placement of an intracoronary stent, as compared with balloon angio-plasty, in patients with symptomatic coronary artery disease resulted in a significantly improved rate of procedural success, but with increased rates of bleeding and vascular complications and longer hospital stay. Six-month outcome revealed a significantly lower rate of restenosis and larger luminal diameter with stent placement but no substantial differ-ence in clinical outcome between the two procedures.

CHAPTER 1

Myocardial Infarction Trials

OVERVIEW

Acute myocardial infarction afflicts approximately 1.5 million people annually in the United States with an annual cost of over $50 billion. During the past 30 years, advances in the treatment of myocardial infarction have reduced the in-hospital mortality rate by approximately 80%. Initially, the widespread use of defibrillators and aggressive rhythm management in coronary care units to treat early ventricular dysrhythmias, followed by the use of β-blockers to reduce myocardial oxygen demand, and recently the use of thrombolytic agents and antiplatelet agents to treat acute coronary thrombosis, have collectively reduced the in-hospital mortality rate of acute myocardial infarction from approximately 30% to 5%. Numerous large-scale randomized clinical trials have provided valuable information regarding the benefit of various treatment modalities in patients with acute myocardial infarction.

Thrombolytic Agents

During the past two decades, the realization that unstable coronary atherosclerotic plaques lead to acute coronary thrombosis and myocardial infarction, along with the development of thrombolytic agents, provided direction for many of the initial large-scale clinical trials. The Gruppo Italiano per lo Studio della Streptochinasi nell'Infarcto Miocardico (GISSI 1) and the International Study of Infarct Survival (ISIS 2) trials, which collectively randomized approximately 30,000 patients, were the first landmark trials to clearly demonstrate a significant mortality reduction with the use of streptokinase (SK) in acute myocardial infarction. In addition, ISIS 2 showed that aspirin, given immediately, provided a reduction in mortality nearly as striking as SK and that the combination of aspirin and SK resulted in an additive benefit. These two trials also provided evidence that earlier administration of thrombolytic agents led to better clinical outcomes, presumably by reducing the duration of impaired coronary flow and reducing infarct size. In addition, a therapeutic time window was discovered beyond which the administration of thrombolytic agents provided less benefit. This later observation was confirmed in numerous trials including the Late Assessment of Thrombolytic Efficacy study (LATE) and the Thrombolysis and Angioplasty in Myocardial Infarction trial (TAMI 6), which showed reduced mortality and higher acute patency rates for the infarct-related artery, respectively, when thrombolytic agents were administered within 12 hours of symptom onset.

The emphasis on early patency of the infarct-related artery led to the development of more fibrin-specific thrombolytic agents, like tissue plasminogen activator (t-PA), which more promptly lyse fibrin-rich thrombi without inducing a systemic lytic state. The second generation of thrombolytic trials were aimed at comparing different thrombolytic interventions, such as t-PA with SK. The Thrombolysis in Myocardial Infarction (TIMI 1) trial, an angiographic study supported by the National Heart, Lung, and Blood Institute, which directly compared t-PA with SK in patients with acute myocardial infarction, found significantly higher early reperfusion and late patency with t-PA treatment. The Global Utilization of Streptokinase and Tissue Plasminogen Activator for Occluded Coronary Arteries (GUSTO 1) trial and its angiographic substudy, which randomized 41,000 patients to SK, t-PA, or a combination of the two agents, demonstrated increased 90-minute patency of the infarct-related artery and a reduced combined end point of mortality and disabling stroke with t-PA compared to SK. However, on the other side of the Atlantic, two large European trials, GISSI 2 and ISIS 3, which collectively randomized over 50,000 patients, found no significant differences in clinical end points between these two thrombolytic agents. Two criticisms of GISSI 2 and ISIS 3 have been that they did not use the "accelerated" dosing of t-PA, which was used in GUSTO, and that heparin was not given by optimal route or dose. The "accelerated" dosing was shown to provide the highest 90-minute patency rate compared to four other dosing strategies of t-PA in the TAMI 7 trial. The thrombolytic trials completed to date appear to establish a slight benefit in mortality reduction for the more fibrin-specific thrombolytic interventions, such as t-PA. However, the risk of intracranial hemorrhage may also be slightly greater with these fibrin-specific thrombolytic agents.

Heparin and Other Antithrombins

The role of heparin as an antithrombin intervention, used in conjunction with thrombolytic agents and aspirin, has been examined to clarify the role of anticoagulation in preventing reocclusion after thrombolysis and in potentially increasing the incidence of bleeding complications. ISIS 3, which randomized 41,000 patients to three different thrombolytic agents with aspirin alone or with aspirin and subcutaneous heparin, showed that the addition of subcutaneous heparin had no effect on 5-week or 6-month mortality but did increase the incidence of "major" bleeds and cerebral hemorrhage. GISSI 2 revealed that the addition of subcutaneous heparin to thrombolytics and aspirin offered no benefit in in-hospital mortality or the combined end point of mortality and extensive left ventricular damage, yet subcutaneous heparin increased the incidence of bleeding events. Furthermore, no clinical difference was observed between subcutaneous and intravenous administration of heparin in patients receiving SK and aspirin in the GUSTO 1 trial. The European Cooperative Study Group (ECSG VI) trial,[1] which randomized 650 patients with acute myocardial infarction treated with t-PA and aspirin to intravenous heparin or no heparin, demonstrated that the addition of intravenous heparin produced a small but significant increase in the 2-hour patency rate of the infarct-related artery from 75% to 83% but had no effect on mortality, incidence of recurrent ischemia, incidence of reinfarction, or bleeding events. Finally, the TAMI 3 trial revealed no significant difference in patency rates of the infarct-related artery or left ventricular function between immediate intravenous and delayed (by 90 minutes) intravenous heparin among patient with acute myocardial infarction treated with t-PA and aspirin. No large, randomized, prospective trial to date has clearly demonstrated a clinical benefit for intravenous heparin in the setting of acute myocardial infarction treated with thrombolytics and aspirin. In numerous reports of experimental animal studies, however, intravenous heparin makes t-PA a more effective thrombolytic intervention than t-PA given alone. Heparin has become standard therapy in the treatment of acute myocardial infarction, especially when t-PA is given as the thrombolytic intervention. The benefit of heparin remains controversial, however, particularly for the less fibrin-specific thrombolytic interventions. Other trials evaluating more specific thrombin inhibitors, such as hirudin, hirulog, and argatroban, are in progress, as substantial evidence in experimental animal models suggests their potential superiority over heparin. These direct thrombin inhibitors are discussed in Chapter 3, "Antithrombotic Trials."

Role of Percutaneous Transluminal Coronary Angioplasty

After percutaneous transluminal coronary angioplasty (PTCA) gained widespread acceptance as a treatment modality for coronary artery disease in the mid-1980s, trials were designed to study the role of PTCA in acute myocardial infarction. The Primary Angioplasty in Myocardial Infarction (PAMI) trial, which randomized 395 patients with acute myocardial infarction to treatment with t-PA or immediate primary angioplasty, showed that immediate angioplasty was safe and actually reduced combined in-hospital mortality and nonfatal myocardial infarction while significantly reducing the incidence of intracranial hemorrhage compared to t-PA. Zijlstra et al. compared SK to primary PTCA in the setting of acute myocardial infarction (ZWOLLE trial) and demonstrated improved long-term patency rates and better left ventricular ejection fraction with primary PTCA in 142 patients with acute myocardial infarction.

The role of early secondary PTCA following thrombolytic therapy in acute myocardial infarction was examined in the TAMI 1 and TIMI 2A trials. TAMI 1 showed that after successful thrombolysis, immediate angioplasty offered no benefit over elective angioplasty in reducing mortality or improving left ventricular function. TIMI 2A examined the benefit of immediate PTCA, delayed PTCA, and a conservative strategy after administration of t-PA in acute myocardial infarction and found no significant difference in 1-year mortality, the incidence of fatal and nonfatal reinfarctions, or left ventricular ejection fraction between the three treatment strategies.

Adjunctive Therapy

The role of adjunctive therapy like β-blockers, calcium channel blockers, angiotensin-converting enzyme (ACE) inhibitors, and nitrates in the setting of acute myocardial infarction has been examined in randomized clinical trials. The β-blocker trials are discussed in Chapter 4 and the calcium channel blocker trials in Chapter 5. The trials evaluating the role of ACE inhibitors in acute myocardial infarction include GISSI 3, ISIS 4, Survival and Ventricular Enlargement (SAVE), Acute Infarction Ramipril Efficacy (AIRE), and Cooperative New Scandinavian Enalapril Survival Study (CONSENSUS 2). GISSI 3—a randomized comparison of lisinopril, lisinopril and topical nitrates, and placebo among 19,000 patients with acute myocardial infarction—demonstrated a significant reduction in 6-week mortality with lisinopril by 11% and combination lisinopril and nitrates by 17% compared to control. The ISIS 4 trial randomized 58,000 patients with acute myocardial infarction to captopril or placebo and found that early administration of captopril provided a small but significant 7% reduction in 5-week mortality. The SAVE trial found that administration of captopril to patients with left ventricular dysfunction within 2 weeks of myocardial infarction significantly reduced total mortality, cardiovascular mortality, hospitalizations for congestive heart failure, and rate of reinfarction compared to placebo over a 42-month period. AIRE—a randomized comparison of ramipril and placebo administered between days 3 and 10 after myocardial infarction among 2,000 patients—found that ramipril reduced overall mortality by 27% and resistant congestive heart failure by 19% compared with placebo. The CONSENSUS 2 trial, however, showed no beneficial effect of enalapril among the 6,000 randomized patients with acute myocardial infarction, which was perhaps due to the short follow-up period of 6 months, the relatively small number of patients enrolled, and the low prevalence of pulmonary edema (2%) and congestive heart failure (18%) after admission. Nitrates that were evaluated in GISSI 3 (topical nitrates) and ISIS 4 (oral nitrates) were not shown to have a beneficial effect among the 60,000 collective patients with acute myocardial infarction.

Magnesium Therapy

Magnesium therapy in conjunction with thrombolytic intervention remains a controversial issue, which is due to conflicting results from large-scale clinical trials. The Leicester Intravenous Magnesium Intervention Trial (LIMIT 2), which randomized 2,000 patients with acute myocardial infarction to magnesium or placebo, demonstrated a significant 16% reduction in overall mortality at 2.7 years with magnesium treatment. Several smaller clinical trials have shown a similar benefit.[2,3] However, the ISIS 4 trial revealed no significant difference between magnesium therapy and placebo among 60,000 patients with acute myocardial infarction. Critics have argued that the timing of administration of magnesium is crucial. Animal studies have shown that magnesium must be administered before thrombolysis and reperfusion to demonstrate a beneficial effect, presumably by attenuating reperfusion injury, as was the protocol for LIMIT 2. In the ISIS 4 trial, however, no criteria for the timing of administration of magnesium were established in the protocol, and possibly as a result, many patients received magnesium after thrombolysis and reperfusion, which may explain why ISIS 4 failed to confirm a benefit for magnesium therapy.

Conclusions

Significant advances have been achieved in the treatment of myocardial infarction during the past 20 years. The administration of both thrombolytic agents and aspirin to patients with acute myocardial infarction have been clearly shown to reduce mortality. Thrombolytic interventions should be administered within the first 12 hours of symptom onset to achieve optimal results. More fibrin-specific thrombolytic agents like t-PA offer a slight reduction in mortality but with increased risk of bleeding complications compared to less fibrin-specific agents like SK. The conjunctive use of heparin with t-PA and aspirin may protect against reocclusion of the infarct-related artery after successful thrombolysis. The benefit of heparin when used with SK and aspirin is less convincing. Primary PTCA in patients with acute myocardial infarction is safe and provides better clinical outcomes with lower risk of bleeding complications compared to t-PA. However, routine use of early PTCA after successful thrombolysis with a thrombolytic agent does not appear to provide any clinical benefit. Intravenous magnesium therapy, when given before reperfusion, and early administration of ACE inhibitors substantially reduce mortality in patients with acute myocardial infarction. Early use of nitrates does not appear to offer any reduction in mortality. Clinical trials evaluating more specific thrombin inhibitors like hirudin, hirulog, and argatroban are currently in progress.

CONSENSUS 2

Cooperative New Scandinavian Enalapril Survival Study

PURPOSE
Determine the effect of early administration of enalapril on mortality in patients with acute myocardial infarction (MI).

STUDY DESIGN

General

- 6,090 patients enrolled in this prospective, randomized, double-blinded, placebo controlled, multicenter trial.
- Eligible patients were randomized to one of two treatment groups:
  1. Enalapril: enalapril at 1 mg intravenous (IV) infusion over 2 hr, then after 6 hr 2.5 mg PO bid titrated up to 20 mg PO qd by day 5 as tolerated until completion of the study
  2. Placebo
- Treatment was started within 24 hr of the acute myocardial infarction (MI).
- All patients received standard therapy including analgesics, nitrates, β-blockers, calcium channel blockers, thrombolytic agents, aspirin, diuretics, and anticoagulation as indicated.
- Treatment with thrombolytic agents and/or β-blockers was completed before administration of the study drugs.

Inclusion. Patients included presented within 24 hr of onset of chest pain that was due to myocardial infarction associated with ST-segment elevation in two or more contiguous electrocardiogram leads, new pathologic Q waves, or elevated cardiac enzymes.

Exclusion. The criteria for exclusion were supine blood pressure < 105/65, need for vasopressor agents, hemodynamically severe valvular stenosis, untreated third-degree atrioventricular block, use of angiotensin-converting enzyme (ACE) inhibitors within 1 week before the MI, history of transient ischemic attack that was due to hypotension within 6 months, a clear indication for or contraindication to ACE inhibitors, or other serious illness.

End Points. The criterion for end point was 6-month mortality.

RESULTS

No significant difference in 6-month mortality was observed between enalapril and placebo treatment (11.0% enalapril vs. 10.2% placebo, P = 0.26). Significantly more patients receiving placebo required a change in treatment because of worsening heart failure (27% enalapril vs. 30%

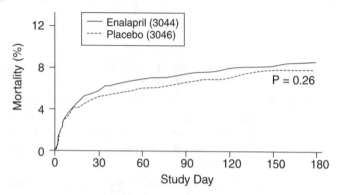

Figure 1-1. Kaplan-Meier Life-Table Mortality curves for the placebo and enalapril groups. (From Swedberg et al.,[4] with permission.)

placebo, P < 0.006). Subgroup analysis revealed a trend toward increased mortality with enalapril in elderly patients ≥ 70 years of age (17% enalapril vs. 15% placebo, P = 0.07). In addition, no significant difference in mortality between enalapril and placebo was found among patients with previous myocardial infarction, Q-wave infarction, anterior infarction, or patients with pulmonary edema or heart failure complicating the acute MI (Fig. 1-1).

CONCLUSIONS
In patients receiving standard therapy for acute MI, the administration of enalapril within 24 hr of onset of chest pain did not improve 6-month survival compared to placebo.

(Data from Swedberg et al.[4]) ∎

GISSI 1

Gruppo Italiano per lo Studio della Streptochinasi nell'Infarcto Miocardico

PURPOSE
Determine the effect of intravenous (IV) streptokinase (SK) on reducing mortality in patients with acute myocardial infarction.

STUDY DESIGN

General

- 11,806 patients enrolled in this prospective, randomized, controlled, unblinded multicenter trial.
- Eligible patients were randomized to one of two treatment groups:
  1. Streptokinase: 1.5 million U IV over 60 min
  2. No thrombolytic therapy
- Subgroup analysis of time elapsed from symptom onset to randomization.
- Use of other medications, including heparin, was left to the discretion of each coronary care unit.

Inclusion. Patients included presented with chest pain accompanied by ST-segment elevation or depression of 1 mm or more in any electrocardiogram limb lead and/or of 2 mm or more in any precordial lead and were admitted within 12 hr of symptom onset.

Exclusion. Patients excluded had a contraindication to thrombolytics.

End Points. Criteria for end points were in-hospital (14–21 days) morbidity and mortality.

RESULTS

Treatment with SK produced a statistically significant 18% reduction in overall in-hospital mortality at 21 days compared to the control group (10.7% SK vs. 13.0% control, P = 0.0002). Infusion of SK within 1, 3, and 3–6 hr of symptom onset resulted in a significant 47%, 23%, and 17% respective reduction in 21-day mortality. Streptokinase administered after 6 hr of symptom onset did not significantly reduce mortality. At 12-month follow-up, a significant reduction in mortality with SK was observed for the whole group (17.2% SK vs. 19.0% control, P = 0.008) and for the subsets of patients treated within 0–1 hr (12.9% SK vs. 21.2% control, P = 0.00001), treated within 0–3 hr (15.1% SK vs. 17.3% control, P = 0.02), and treated within 3–6 hr (18.3% SK vs. 21.2% control, P = 0.02). No significant difference in mortality at 12 months was apparent among patients treated with SK after 6 hr. The incidence of ischemic and hemorrhagic strokes with SK was very low (<1%) and comparable to the control group (Fig. 1-2).

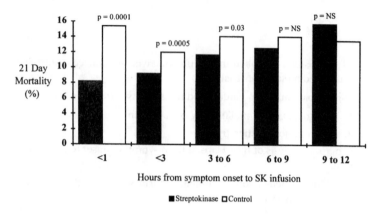

Figure 1-2. Twenty-one-day mortality rates according to the time from symptom onset to SK infusion.

CONCLUSIONS
Intravenous infusion of 1.5 million U of SK over 60 min produced a significant 18% reduction in overall in-hospital mortality compared to no thrombolytic therapy in patients with acute myocardial infarction. The reduction in mortality was persistent up to 12-month follow-up and was limited to patients who received SK within 6 hr of onset of symptoms.

(Data from Gruppo Italiano per lo Studio della Streptochinasi nell'Infarto Micardico [GISSI].[5]) ■

GISSI 2

Gruppo Italiano per lo Studio della Streptochinasi nell'Infarcto Miocardico

PURPOSE
Compare the effect of streptokinase (SK) with tissue plasminogen activator (t-PA), both with and without subcutaneous (SQ) heparin, on mortality and left ventricular function in patients with acute myocardial infarction.

STUDY DESIGN

General

- 12,490 patients enrolled in this prospective, randomized, multicenter trial.
- Eligible patients were randomized to one of four treatment groups:
  1. Streptokinase alone
  2. Streptokinase and heparin SQ
  3. Tissue plasminogen activator alone
  4. Tissue plasminogen activator and heparin SQ
- Streptokinase: 1.5 million U intravenously (IV) over 30–60 min.
- Tissue plasminogen activator: 100-mg total dose administered as a 10-mg IV bolus, then 50 mg over 1 hr, then 20 mg/hr over 2 hr.
- Heparin: 12,500 U SQ q 12 hr started 12 hr after thrombolytic infusion and continued until hospital discharge.
- All patients were treated with aspirin 325 mg/day and atenolol (5–10 mg slow IV injection according to ISIS 1 protocol) if not contraindicated.

Inclusion. Patients included had chest pain accompanied by ST-segment elevation of 1 mm or more in any limb lead and/or 2 mm or more in any precordial lead of the electrocardiogram and were admitted within 6 hr of symptom onset.

Exclusion. Patients excluded had a contraindication to thrombolytic therapy or heparin or had previous treatment with SK within the past 6 months.

End Points. Criteria for end points were combined end point of in-hospital mortality and late (after 4 days) clinical congestive heart failure or extensive left ventricular damage (left ventricular ejection fraction < 35%).

RESULTS

No significant difference between t-PA and SK was observed with respect to in-hospital mortality (9.0% t-PA vs. 8.6% SK, P = not significant [NS]) or combined end points (23.1% t-PA vs. 22.5% SK, P = NS). The

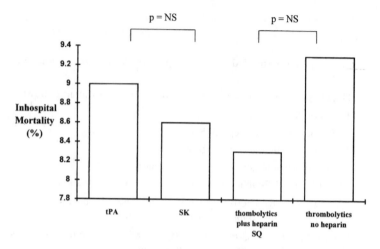

Figure 1-3. In-hospital mortality rates for the two treatment comparisons. No significant differences were observed.

addition of SQ heparin to thrombolytic therapy did not significantly reduce in-hospital mortality (8.3% heparin vs. 9.3% no heparin, P = NS) or combined end points (22.7% heparin vs. 22.9% no heparin, P = NS). The rate of major bleeds (requiring ≥ 2 U of blood transfusions) was increased with SK compared to t-PA (1.0% SK vs. 0.5% t-PA) and also with heparin compared to no heparin (1.0% heparin vs. 0.6% no heparin). No significant difference in the incidence of hemorrhagic stroke was observed between t-PA and SK (Fig. 1-3).

CONCLUSIONS
Streptokinase and t-PA are equally effective in reducing in-hospital mortality and preserving left ventricular function when administered with aspirin and atenolol in the setting of acute myocardial infarction. The addition of SQ heparin started 12 hr after thrombolytic therapy offered no significant benefit.

(Data from Gruppo Italiano per lo Studio della Streptochinasi nell'Infarto Micardico [GISSI].[6]) ∎

GISSI 3

Gruppo Italiano per lo Studio della Streptochinasi nell'Infarcto Miocardico

PURPOSE

Determine the effects of lisinopril, transdermal glyceryl trinitrate (GTN), and their combination on improving survival and left ventricular function in patients with acute myocardial infarction.

STUDY DESIGN

General

- 19,394 patients enrolled in this prospective, controlled, randomized multicenter trial.

- Eligible patients were randomized to one of four treatment groups:

  1. Lisinopril: 5 mg PO at randomization, 5 mg after 24 hr, 10 mg after 48 hr, then 10 mg/day for 6 weeks.

  2. Transdermal GTN: intravenous (IV) infusion during the first 24 hr starting at 5 µg/min, and increased by 5–20 µg/min every 5 min for the first 30 min until systolic blood pressure fell by at least 10%. After 24 hr, dosage changed to transdermal GTN 10 mg/day applied in the morning and removed at bedtime, continued for 6 weeks. If the patch was not tolerated, a single dose of 50 mg isosorbide mononitrate was used.

  3. Combination lisinopril and transdermal GTN.

  4. Control.

- Individualized treatment with thrombolytics (72%), β-blockade (31%), and aspirin (84%) was used.

- Left ventricular ejection fraction (LVEF) was measured by echocardiography at baseline and 6 weeks.

Inclusion. Patients included had chest pain accompanied by ST-segment elevation or depression of at least 1 mm in one or more electrocardiogram limb leads or of at least 2 mm in one or more precordial leads and were admitted within 24 hr of symptom onset.

Exclusion. Patients excluded had contraindications to lisinopril or nitrates, severe heart failure requiring any of the study treatments, Killip class IV, systolic blood pressure < 100 mmHg, creatinine > 177 µmol/L, proteinuria > 500 mg/day, bilateral renal artery stenosis, or other life-threatening disorders.

End Points. The criterion for primary end point was total 6-week mortality. The combined end point was defined as total mortality and late (after 4 days) clinical congestive heart failure or extensive left ventricular damage (LVEF < 35%).

RESULTS

Lisinopril significantly reduced 6-week mortality by 11% (6.3% lisinopril vs. 7.1% control, P = 0.03) and combined end point events by 8.2% (15.6% lisinopril vs. 17.0% control, P = 0.009) compared to control. Transdermal GTN did not significantly improve 6-week mortality or combined end point events. The combination of lisinopril and transdermal GTN produced the greatest benefit, reducing 6-week mortality by 17% (6.0% combination vs. 7.2% control, P = 0.021) and combined end point events by 13% (14.8% combination vs. 17.0% control, P = 0.003) compared to control. There were no significant differences in the rates of reinfarction, postinfarction angina, or revascularization procedures among all four groups (Fig. 1-4).

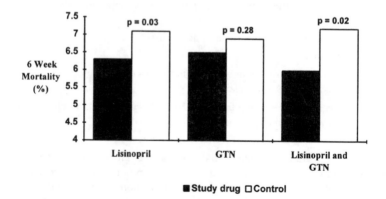

Figure 1-4. Six-week mortality rates for the three treatment comparisons.

CONCLUSIONS

In the setting of acute myocardial infarction, lisinopril alone and in combination with transdermal GTN significantly reduced 6-week mortality by 11% and 17%, respectively, and also significantly reduced 6-week combined end point events (deaths, congestive heart failure, and LVEF < 35%) by 8% and 13%, respectively, compared to control. Transdermal GTN alone provided no significant benefit.

(Data from Gruppo Italiano per lo Studio della Streptochinasi nell'Infarto Miocardico.[7]) ■

GUSTO 1

Global Utilization of Streptokinase and Tissue Plasminogen Activator for Occluded Coronary Arteries

PURPOSE

Compare the effects of tissue plasminogen activator (t-PA), streptokinase (SK), or both on reducing mortality in patients with acute myocardial infarction.

STUDY DESIGN

General

- 41,021 patients enrolled in this prospective, randomized, blinded, multicenter trial.
- Eligible patients were randomized to one of four treatment groups:
  1. Streptokinase and subcutaneous (SQ) heparin: SK 1.5 million U intravenously (IV) over 60 min, and heparin SQ 12,500 U bid × 7 days beginning 4 hr after start of thrombolytics.
  2. Streptokinase and heparin IV: SK 1.5 million U IV over 60 min and heparin IV given immediately as a 5,000-U bolus, then 1,000 U/hr (or 1,200 U/hr if weight > 80kg) with dose adjusted to keep partial thromboplastin time between 60 and 85 sec continued for at least 48 hr.
  3. Accelerated t-PA and heparin IV: t-PA 15-mg IV bolus, then 0.75 mg/kg (up to 50 mg) over 30 min, then 0.5 mg/kg (up to 35 mg) over 60 min and heparin IV as described above.

4. Combination t-PA, streptokinase, and heparin IV: t-PA 1 mg/kg (up to 90 mg) over 60 min with 10% given as bolus, SK 1.5 million U IV over 60 min, and heparin IV as described above.

- All patients were given aspirin ≥ 160 mg PO immediately, then 160–325 mg/day PO and atenolol 5 mg IV given in two divided doses followed by 50–100 mg/day PO if not contraindicated.

- The use of other medications was left to the discretion of the physician.

Inclusion. Patients included had chest pain lasting ≥ 20 min presenting within 6 hr of symptom onset associated with ≥ 0.1 mV ST-segment elevation in two or more limb leads or ≥ 0.2 mV in two or more contiguous precordial electrocardiogram leads.

Exclusion. Patients excluded had a contraindication to thrombolytic therapy.

End Points. The criterion for end point was total 30-day mortality. The combined end point was death and hemorrhagic or nonhemorrhagic stroke.

RESULTS

Thirty-day mortality rates were as follows: SK and heparin SQ, 7.2%; SK and heparin IV, 7.4%; accelerated t-PA and heparin IV, 6.3%; and combination t-PA, SK, and heparin IV, 7.0%. Accelerated t-PA provided a 14% reduction in mortality when compared to the two SK-only strategies (P = 0.001) (Fig. 1-5). Combination therapy offered no significant advantage over SK alone or t-PA alone. Among patients treated with SK, there was no significant difference in total mortality or the incidence of hemorrhagic stroke between heparin administered by IV or SQ route. Hemorrhagic stroke rates in the four treatment groups were 0.49%, 0.54%, 0.72%, and 0.94%, respectively, which represents a significant excess of hemorrhagic stroke for accelerated t-PA (P = 0.03) and combination therapy (P < 0.001) when compared to SK-only strategies (Fig. 1-6). However, the combined end point of death or disabling stroke was significantly lower for the accelerated t-PA group compared to both SK groups (6.9% vs. 7.8%, P = 0.006).

CONCLUSIONS

In the setting of acute myocardial infarction, accelerated dose t-PA and heparin IV resulted in a significant 14% reduction in total 30-day mortality compared with SK and intravenous or subcutaneous heparin. Accelerated

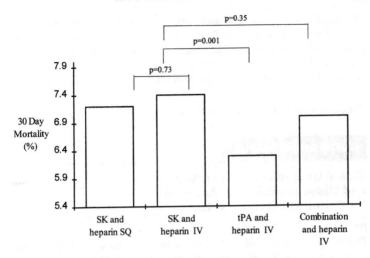

Figure 1-5. Thirty-day mortality rates demonstrating a significant reduction in mortality with accelerated t-PA compared to both SK groups.

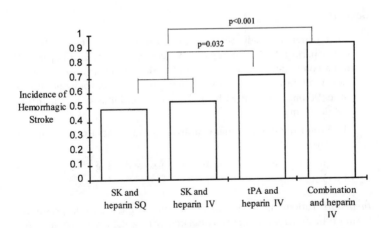

Figure 1-6. The incidence of hemorrhagic strokes showing a significant increase with accelerated t-PA and combination therapy compared to both SK groups.

t-PA was associated with a significantly higher incidence of hemorrhagic stroke compared to SK. Overall benefit, as assessed by the combined end point of total mortality and disabling stroke, was significantly better with accelerated t-PA. Accelerated t-PA led to an actual survival benefit of 10 additional lives saved per 1,000 patients treated when compared with SK.

(Data from The GUSTO Investigators.[8])   ■

GUSTO ANGIOGRAPHIC

Global Utilization of Streptokinase and Tissue Plasminogen Activator for Occluded Coronary Arteries

PURPOSE
Determine the effects of accelerated tissue plasminogen activator (t-PA), streptokinase (SK), and a combination of both thrombolytics on coronary artery patency and ventricular function in the setting of acute myocardial infarction

STUDY DESIGN

General

- 2,431 patients already randomized to the four arms of GUSTO (SK and heparin SQ, SK and heparin IV, accelerated t-PA and heparin IV, and a combination of accelerated t-PA, SK, and heparin IV) were further randomly assigned to angiography and ventriculography at either 90 min, 180 min, 24 hr, or 5–7 days after initiation of the thrombolytic agent.

- The group undergoing angiography at 90 min had a repeat study at 5–7 days.

- Flow in the infarct-related artery was assessed using TIMI grade flow of 0–3.

Inclusion. Patients included had chest pain lasting ≥ 20 min presenting within 6 hr of symptom onset associated with ≥ 0.1-mV ST-segment elevation in two or more electrocardiogram limb leads or ≥ 0.2 mV in two or more contiguous precordial leads.

Exclusion. Patients excluded had a contraindication to thrombolytic therapy.

Table 1-1. Patency and Reocclusion of the Infarct-Related Artery, According to Treatment Group

VARIABLE	STREPTOKINASE SQ HEPARIN (%)	STREPTOKINASE IV HEPARIN (%)	ACCELERATED t-PA (%)	t-PA+STREP-TOKINASE (%)
Patency				
Open vessels, TIMI grades 2 and 3 combined				
At 90 min	54	60	$81^{a,b}$	73^b
At 180 min	73	74	76	85
At 24 hr	77	80	86	94^c
At 5–7 days	72	84	84^d	80
Complete reperfusion, TIMI grade 3				
At 90 min	29	32	$54^{b,e}$	38
At 180 min	35	41	43	53
At 24 hr	51	41	45	60
At 5–7 days	51	58	58	55
Reocclusion				
Overall reocclusion	6.4	5.5	5.9	4.9

[a]P = 0.032 for the comparison of this group with the group given t-PA with streptokinase.

[b]P < 0.001 for the comparison of this group with the groups given streptokinase with subcutaneous or intravenous heparin.

[c]P < 0.001 for the comparison of this group with the group given streptokinase with subcutaneous heparin.

[d]P = 0.032 for the comparison of this group with the group given streptokinase with subcutaneous heparin.

[e]P < 0.001 for the comparison of this group with the group given t-PA with streptokinase.

(Adapted from The GUSTO Angiographic Investigators,[9] with permission.)

End Points. Criteria for end points were patency and reocclusion rates of the infarct-related artery and contrast left ventricular ejection fraction.

RESULTS

The patency rate (TIMI grade 2 and 3 flow) of the infarct-related artery at 90 min was significantly higher with accelerated t-PA (81%) compared to SK and heparin SQ (54%, P < 0.001), SK and heparin IV (60%, P < 0.001), and combination therapy (73%, P = 0.032). TIMI grade 3 flow at 90 min was higher with accelerated t-PA (54%) than with the two SK groups (31%, P < 0.001). By 180 min, 24 hr, and 5–7 days, patency rates were similar in the four treatment groups (72–84%). Reocclusion rates were similar among all groups (4.9–6.4%). No significant difference in contrast left ventricular ejection fraction was seen at 90 min or 5–7 days, although other indicators of left ventricular function (end-systolic volume index, regional wall motion in the infarct zone, abnormal chords) were significantly better in the accelerated t-PA group (Table 1-1).

CONCLUSIONS

Accelerated t-PA provided more rapid and complete flow in the infarct-related artery at 90 min compared to SK in patients with acute myocardial infarction. Patency rates by 180 min and later were not significantly different among the four treatment groups. No significant difference in left ventricular ejection fraction was found at 90 min or 5–7 days among the four treatment groups, although other indicators of ventricular function were better in the accelerated t-PA group.

(Data from The GUSTO Angiographic Investigators.[9]) ■

GUSTO 2A

Global Utilization of Streptokinase and Tissue Plasminogen Activator for Occluded Coronary Arteries

PURPOSE

Compare the effect of intravenous (IV) heparin with IV hirudin on mortality and incidence of myocardial infarction in acute coronary syndromes.

STUDY DESIGN

General

- 2,564 patients enrolled in this prospective, double-blinded, randomized multicenter trial.

- Eligible patients were randomized to heparin or hirudin infusions for 72–120 hr as follows:

  1. Heparin: 5,000-U IV bolus, then 1,000 U/hr if weight < 80 kg, or 1,300 U/hr if weight > 80 kg titrated to maintain partial thromboplastin time between 60 and 90

  2. Hirudin: 0.6-mg/kg IV bolus, then 0.2 mg/kg/hr; only titrated if partial thromboplastin time > 150

- Patients with ST-segment elevation were eligible to receive thrombolytics.

Inclusion. Patients included had chest pain associated with either ST-segment elevation or depression of > 0.05 mV or T-wave inversion ≥ 0.1 mV in two or more contiguous electrocardiogam leads presenting within 12 hr of symptom onset.

Exclusion. Criteria for exclusion were active bleeding, serum creatinine > 2.5 mg/dl, prior stroke within 1 year, or contraindications to heparin.

End Points. Criteria for end points were death or myocardial infarction within 30 days.

RESULTS
The study was terminated early because of a significant excess of intracranial hemorrhage in the heparin (0.7%) and hirudin (1.3%) groups when compared to the results of GUSTO 1. Intracranial hemorrhage was highest in those patients receiving thrombolytics and heparin (1.5%) or hirudin (2.2%).

CONCLUSIONS
The use of heparin and hirudin in acute coronary syndromes in the doses used in this study resulted in a significantly higher rate of intracranial hemorrhage compared to the results of GUSTO 1. The trial has been reinitiated, as GUSTO 2B, at lower doses of heparin and hirudin.

(Data from The Global Use of Strategies to Open Occluded Coronary Arteries [GUSTO] IIa Investigators.[10]) ∎

ISIS 1

International Study of Infarct Survival

PURPOSE
Determine the effects of atenolol, administered immediately and continued for 1 week, on vascular mortality in the setting of acute myocardial infarction.

STUDY DESIGN

General

- 16,027 patients enrolled in this prospective, controlled, randomized multicenter trial.
- Eligible patients were randomized to one of two treatment groups:
    1. Atenolol: 5-mg intravenous (IV) bolus given immediately over 5 min ± an additional 5 mg after 10 min if tolerated, then atenolol 50 mg PO given followed by 50 mg additional after 12 hr, then atenolol 100 mg PO qd for 6 days or until discharge with the option to continue as an outpatient.
    2. Control.
- After hospital discharge, all patients had the option to take atenolol.
- The control arm avoided β-blockers unless clearly indicated.
- Other medical therapy was left to the discretion of each physician.

Inclusion. Patients included had suspected myocardial infarction presenting within 12 hr of symptom onset.

Exclusion. Patients excluded had a contraindication to or clear indication for β-blockade or were currently taking β-blockers or verapamil at the time of admission.

End Points. Criteria for end points were vascular mortality (cardiac, cerebral, other vascular, and unknown etiologies of death) during the treatment period (1 week) and at 20-month follow-up.

RESULTS

During the treatment period of 1 week, the vascular mortality rate was 15% lower in the atenolol group compared to control (3.89% atenolol vs. 4.57% control, $P < 0.04$). All of the benefit occurred during days 0–1, which resulted in a 30% reduction in vascular mortality; during days 2–7, there was no significant difference in vascular mortality. Rates of nonfatal reinfarction (2.5% atenolol vs. 2.8% control) and sudden cardiac death (2.4% atenolol vs. 2.5% control) were not significantly different. There was no significant reduction in vascular mortality between the atenolol and control groups at an average of 20-month follow-up (12.5% atenolol vs. 13.4% control, $P = 0.07$). The use of atenolol was associated with a significantly higher need

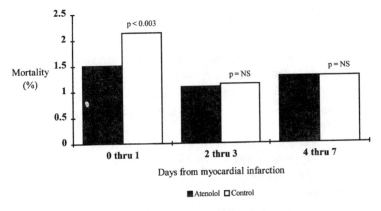

Figure 1-7. Mortality rates according to the number of days from acute myocardial infarction demonstrating a significant reduction in mortality with atenolol therapy only during days 0 through 1.

for inotropic agents (dobutamine, dopamine, or isoprenaline) than control (5.0% atenolol vs. 3.4% control, $P < 0.0001$) (Fig. 1-7).

CONCLUSIONS
The use of atenolol, administered immediately and continued for 1 week, in the setting of acute myocardial infarction reduced 1-week vascular mortality by 15% compared to placebo with most of the benefit occurring during days 0–1. There was no significant difference in vascular mortality at 20-month follow-up.

(Data from ISIS-1 [First International Study of Infarct Survival].[11]) ■

ISIS 2

International Study of Infarct Survival

PURPOSE
Determine the effect of intravenous (IV) streptokinase (SK), aspirin, or a combination of both on mortality during the first 5 weeks and a median of 15-month follow-up in patients with acute myocardial infarction.

STUDY DESIGN

General

- 17,187 patients enrolled in this prospective, randomized, placebo-controlled, blinded, multicenter trial.
- Eligible patients were randomized to one of four treatment groups:
  1. Streptokinase alone: 1.5 million U IV over 60 min started immediately
  2. Aspirin alone: 162.5 mg chewed immediately, then 162.5 mg/day enteric coated continued for 1 month
  3. Both SK and aspirin
  4. Control
- Other therapy (i.e., β-blockers, anticoagulants) was left to the discretion of the physician.

Inclusion. Patients included had suspected myocardial infarction presenting within 24 hr of symptom onset. Electrocardiogram changes at entry were not a requirement.

Exclusion. Patients excluded had a contraindication to or clear indication for aspirin or thrombolytic agents.

End Points. Criteria for end points were vascular (cardiac, cerebral, other vascular, and unknown causes of death) mortality at 5 weeks and at a median of 15 months. A subgroup analysis of 5-week vascular mortality was performed among patients randomized to SK 0–4, 5–12, and 13–24 hr after symptom onset.

RESULTS

Streptokinase Alone. Intravenous SK resulted in a 23% reduction in 5-week vascular mortality compared to control (9.2% SK vs. 12.0% control, $P < 0.00001$), which remained statistically significant at 15-month follow-up. Streptokinase resulted in a statistically significant 0.1% excess of cerebral hemorrhage ($P < 0.01$), all occurring on day 0–2. The overall incidence of in-hospital strokes, however, was not significantly different from control, which was due to a slight protective effect of SK against strokes after day 2. Among patients randomized to

SK 0-4, 5-12, and 13-24 hr after symptom onset, the reductions in the odds of 5-week vascular mortality were 35% (P < 0.00001), 16% (P = 0.01), and 21% (P = 0.04), respectively.

Aspirin Alone. Aspirin resulted in a 21% reduction in 5-week vascular mortality compared to control (9.4% aspirin vs. 11.8% control, P < 0.00001), which remained statistically significant at 15-month follow-up. Aspirin also significantly reduced the incidence of nonfatal reinfarctions (1.0% aspirin vs. 2.0% control) and nonfatal strokes (0.3% aspirin vs. 0.6% control). No significant bleeding complications occurred from aspirin alone.

Streptokinase Plus Aspirin Combination. Streptokinase and aspirin used in combination resulted in a 40% reduction in 5-week vascular

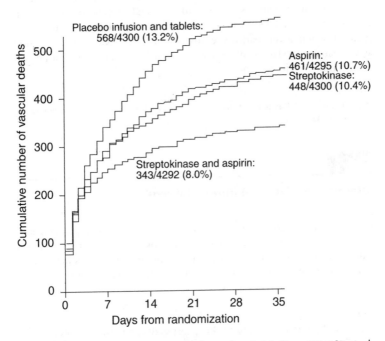

Figure 1-8. Cumulative vascular mortality in days 0–35. (From ISIS-2 [Second International Study of Infarct Survival] Collaborative Group,[12] with permission.)

mortality compared to control (8.0% combination vs. 13.2% control, P < 0.00001), which remained statistically significant at 15-month follow-up. The combination was significantly better than SK or aspirin treatment alone. Among patients randomized to SK and aspirin 0–4, 5–12, and 13–24 hr after symptom onset, the reductions in the odds of 5-week vascular mortality were 53% (P < 0.00001), 32% (P < 0.0001), and 38% (P < 0.01), respectively. The combination of SK and aspirin resulted in a 0.3% excess of major bleeds and a 0.1% excess of cerebral hemorrhage (Fig. 1-8).

CONCLUSIONS

In the setting of acute myocardial infarction, SK alone, aspirin alone, and the combination of SK/aspirin significantly reduced 5-week vascular mortality by 23%, 21%, and 40%, respectively, over control. This survival benefit remained statistically significant during the 15-month follow-up period. Treatment with SK significantly reduced vascular mortality even for patients treated 13–24 hr after symptom onset, but the benefit was greatest when given early. Streptokinase therapy was also associated with a small but significant excess of major bleeds and cerebral hemorrhage compared to control.

(Data from ISIS-2 [Second International Study of Infarct Survival] Collaborative Group.[12]) ∎

ISIS 3

International Study of Infarct Survival

PURPOSE

Compare the effects of streptokinase (SK), tissue plasminogen activator (t-PA), and acylated plasminogen streptokinase activator complex (APSAC), combined with either aspirin alone or aspirin plus heparin, on mortality in patients with acute myocardial infarction.

STUDY DESIGN

General

- 41,299 patients enrolled in this prospective, randomized multicenter trial.

- Eligible patients were randomized to one of six treatment groups:

1. Streptokinase and aspirin plus heparin
2. Streptokinase and aspirin alone
3. Tissue plasminogen activator and aspirin plus heparin
4. Tissue plasminogen activator and aspirin alone
5. APSAC and aspirin plus heparin
6. APSAC and aspirin alone

- Streptokinase: 1.5 million U intravenously (IV) over 60 min.
- Tissue plasminogen activator: 0.04 million U/kg IV bolus, then 0.36 million U/kg over 1 hr, then 0.067 million U/kg/hr over 3 hr.
- APSAC: 30 U IV over 30 min.
- Aspirin: 162 mg chewed immediately, then 162 mg/day enteric coated continued for 1 month.
- Heparin: 12,500 U subcutaneously (SQ) q 12 hr started 4 hr after thrombolytics and continued for 7 days.
- The use of oral anticoagulants and heparin beyond 1 week was to be avoided unless clearly indicated.
- The use of other medications was left to the discretion of the physician.
- Statistical comparisons were made between thrombolytic/aspirin plus heparin vs. thrombolytic/aspirin alone, SK vs. APSAC, and SK vs. t-PA.

Inclusion. Patients included presented within 24 hr of symptom onset for suspected or definite myocardial infarction. There were no specific electrocardiographic criteria.

Exclusion. Patients excluded had contraindications to thrombolytic therapy.

End Points. Criteria for end points were total mortality at 5 weeks and at 6-month follow-up and the incidence of hemorrhagic stroke and total stroke.

RESULTS

Thrombolytic/Aspirin Plus Heparin vs. Thrombolytic/Aspirin Alone. No significant difference in 5-week or 6-month mortality was observed between thrombolytic/aspirin plus heparin and thrombolytic/aspirin

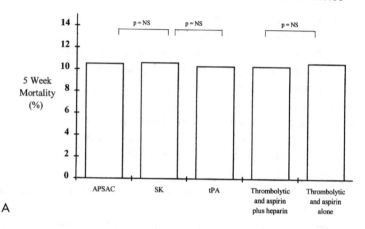

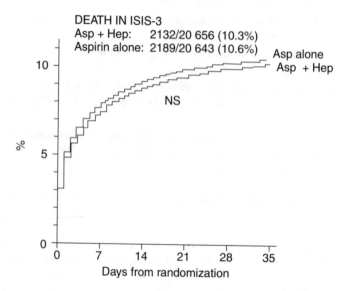

Figure 1-9. *(A)* Five-week mortality rates for the three treatment comparisons. No significant differences observed. *(B)* Cumulative mortality in days 0–35 for aspirin plus heparin vs. aspirin alone. (Fig. B from ISIS-3 [Third International Study of Infarct Survival] Collaborative Group,[13] with permission.)

alone (5-week mortality: 10.3% thrombolytic/aspirin plus heparin vs. 10.6% thrombolytic/aspirin alone, P = not significant [NS]). A small but significant increase in major bleeds (1.0% thrombolytic/aspirin plus heparin vs. 0.8% thrombolytic/aspirin alone, P < 0.01) and cerebral hemorrhage (0.56% thrombolytic/aspirin plus heparin vs. 0.40% thrombolytic/aspirin alone, P < 0.05) was observed in the thrombolytic/aspirin plus heparin group. However, there was no significant difference in overall risk of stroke between the two groups.

Streptokinase vs. APSAC. No significant difference in 5-week or 6-month mortality was observed between APSAC and SK (5-week mortality: 10.5% APSAC vs. 10.6% SK, P = NS). No significant difference in the incidence of major bleeds was observed. APSAC produced a significant increase in hemorrhagic stroke (0.55% APSAC vs. 0.24% SK, P < 0.001) and total stroke (1.26% APSAC vs. 1.04% SK, P = 0.04) compared to SK. This increase in hemorrhagic strokes was observed in patients given APSAC plus aspirin and heparin and also in patients given APSAC with aspirin alone.

Streptokinase vs. t-PA. No significant difference in 5-week or 6-month mortality was observed between t-PA and SK (5-week mortality: 10.3% t-PA vs. 10.6% SK, P = NS). Tissue plasminogen activator produced a significant excess of hemorrhagic stroke (0.66% t-PA vs. 0.24% SK, P < 0.00001) and total strokes (1.39% t-PA vs. 1.04% SK, P < 0.01) compared to SK. This increase in hemorrhagic strokes was observed in patients given t-PA plus aspirin and heparin and also in patients given t-PA with aspirin alone (Fig.1-9).

CONCLUSIONS

In patients with acute myocardial infarction, no significant difference in 5-week or 6-month mortality was observed between treatment with SK, t-PA, or acylated plasminogen streptokinase activator complex (APSAC). The addition of SQ heparin to thrombolytic/aspirin therapy resulted in no significant difference in 5-week or 6-month mortality but did result in a significant increase in major bleeds and hemorrhagic strokes compared to thrombolytic/aspirin alone. Tissue plasminogen activator and APSAC, both with aspirin alone or with aspirin and heparin, were associated with significantly higher incidences of hemorrhagic and total strokes compared to SK.

(Data from ISIS-3 [Third International Study of Infarct Survival] Collaborative Group.[13]) ∎

ISIS 4

International Study of Infarct Survival

PURPOSE

Determine the benefit of early oral captopril, oral mononitrate, and intravenous (IV) magnesium on total mortality in patients with suspected acute myocardial infarction.

STUDY DESIGN

General

- 58,050 patients were enrolled in this randomized, prospective, double-blinded, placebo-controlled trial.
- Eligible patients were randomized to one of four treatment groups:
  1. Captopril: 6.25-mg initial oral dose, 12.5 mg PO 2 hr later, 25 mg PO 10–12 hr later, then 50 mg PO bid for 28 days
  2. Mononitrate: Imdur 30-mg PO initial dose, 30 mg PO 10–12 hr later, then 60 mg PO every morning for 28 days
  3. Magnesium: Magnesium sulfate 8-mmol IV bolus over 15 min followed by 72 mmol infused over 24 hr
  4. Placebo
- In general, all study treatments were to be started immediately (within 1 hr) of any fibrinolytic therapy.
- Antiplatelet therapy was used in 94%, and fibrinolytic therapy was used in 70% of patients.
- Additional therapy was left to the discretion of each physician.

Inclusion. Patients included had suspected acute myocardial infarction presenting within 24 hr of symptom onset with no clear indication or contraindication to any of the study regimens. Patients given IV or other nonstudy nitrates for a few days could still be enrolled.

Exclusion. Contraindications were suggested, not absolute, and included cardiogenic shock, severe hypotension especially with right ventricular infarction, severe fluid depletion, and low risk of cardiac death or other life-threatening illness. The decision to enroll patients remained with the local physician.

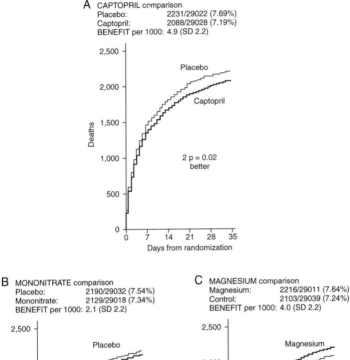

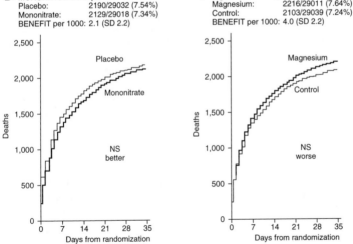

Figure 1-10. *(A–C)* Cumulative mortality rates in days 0–35. (From ISIS-4 [Fourth International Study of Infarct Survival] Collaborative Group,[14] with permission.)

End Points. The criterion for end points was total mortality at 5 weeks.

RESULTS

Definite myocardial infarction was confirmed in 92% of patients.

Oral Captopril vs. Placebo. Oral captopril resulted in a significant 7% reduction in 5-week mortality (7.19% captopril vs. 7.69% placebo, P = 0.02), which corresponds to 4.9 fewer deaths per 1,000 patients treated. At 1 year the survival advantage appeared to be maintained (5.4 fewer deaths per 1,000 patients treated). Captopril was also associated with a small but significant excess of second- or third-degree heart block, cardiogenic shock, and hypotension requiring termination of captopril, especially in patients with presenting systolic blood pressure < 100 mmHg.

Oral Mononitrate vs. Placebo. No significant difference was observed in total mortality at 5 weeks or at 1 year between oral mononitrate and placebo (5-week mortality: 7.34% mononitrate vs. 7.54% placebo, P = 0.3). Correcting for patients receiving IV or nonstudy nitrates did not change this result. In addition there was no significant reduction in postinfarction angina with mononitrate use.

Intravenous Magnesium vs. Open Control. No significant difference was observed in total mortality at 5 weeks or at 1 year between IV magnesium and control (5-week mortality: 7.64% magnesium vs. 7.24% control, P = 0.07). Patients given magnesium had significantly less ventricular fibrillation but slightly more other forms of cardiac arrest, so that there was no significant difference in the overall incidence of cardiac arrest. Magnesium treatment resulted in a small but significant increase in heart failure, cardiogenic shock, and bradycardia (Fig. 1-10).

CONCLUSIONS

Early use of oral captopril in patients with suspected acute myocardial infarction resulted in a significant 7% reduction in 5-week mortality compared to placebo, which appeared to be maintained at 1-year follow-up. Oral mononitrate and IV magnesium therapy offered no significant benefit in survival.

(Data from ISIS-4 [Fourth International Study of Infarct Survival] Collaborative Group.[14]) ∎

Late Assessment of Thrombolytic Efficacy

PURPOSE

Determine the benefit of late administration of tissue plasminogen activator (t-PA), 6–24 hr after the onset of symptoms, in patients with acute myocardial infarction.

STUDY DESIGN

General

- 5,711 patients enrolled in this prospective, randomized, double-blinded, placebo-controlled, multicenter trial.
- Eligible patients were randomized to one of two treatment groups:
  1. Tissue plasminogen activator: 10-mg intravenous (IV) bolus, then 50 mg over the first hour, then 20 mg/hr over the next 2 hr
  2. Placebo
- All patients received chewable aspirin immediately, then 75–360 mg/day, heparin IV 5,000-U initial bolus followed by a second 5,000-U bolus after completion of study medication infusion, then 1,000 U/hr.
- Prophylactic β-blockers were recommended.
- All other medications and interventions were left to the discretion of each physician.

Inclusion. Patients included were 18–75 years old with chest pain for ≥ 30 min presenting within 6–24 hr after onset of symptoms with associated electrocardiogram findings of transmural or non-Q-wave myocardial infarction.

Exclusion. Patients excluded had contraindications to thrombolytics, cardiogenic shock, or other serious illness.

End Points. The criterion for end point was mortality.

RESULTS

Myocardial infarction was confirmed in 93% of patients. Q-wave and non-Q-wave infarctions occurred in 60% and 23% of patients, respectively, while 10 % of patients were diagnosed with possible infarction. Mortality at 35 days for all patients was 8.9% for t-PA and 10.3% for placebo (P = 0.07). The subgroup of patients treated 6–12 hr after onset of myocardial infarction had a significant 25% reduction in 35-day mortality compared to placebo (8.9% t-PA vs. 12.0% placebo, P = 0.02), whereas the subgroup treated 12–24 hr after myocardial infarction showed no significant difference in 35-day mortality (8.7% t-PA vs. 9.2% placebo, P = 0.65). Although treatment with t-PA resulted in an excess of hemorrhagic strokes (1.74% t-PA vs. 0.38% placebo), by 6 months the number of disabled survivors was the same in both treatment groups (Fig. 1-11).

CONCLUSIONS

In patients with acute myocardial infarction, treatment with t-PA from 6–12 hr after symptom onset resulted in a significant 25% reduction in

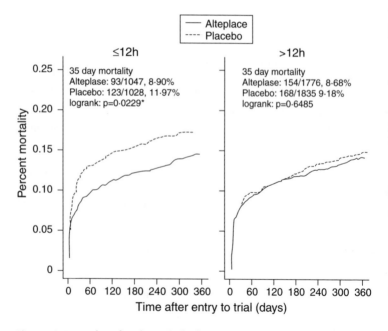

Figure 1-11. Thirty-five-day mortality by time to randomization from onset of symptoms. (From LATE Study Group,[15] with permission.)

35-day mortality compared to placebo. Treatment with t-PA from 12–24 hr after symptom onset revealed no significant benefit in 35-day mortality compared to placebo.

_____

(Data from LATE Study Group.[15])   ■

LIMIT 2

Leicester Intravenous Magnesium Intervention Trial

PURPOSE
Determine the effect of early intravenous (IV) magnesium administration on mortality in patients with suspected acute myocardial infarction.

STUDY DESIGN

General

- 2,316 patients enrolled in this prospective, randomized, double-blinded, placebo-controlled trial.
- Eligible patients were randomized to one of two treatment groups:
  1. Magnesium: 8-mmol IV immediate bolus over 5–10 min followed by a continuous infusion of 65 mmol over 24 hr
  2. Placebo
- Routine use of aspirin and thrombolytics was introduced when the results of ISIS 2 became available.
- The bolus injection of the study drug was given immediately before initiation of thrombolytic therapy.
- Other medical therapy was left to the discretion of each physician.

Inclusion. Patients included were judged likely to have an acute myocardial infarction with onset of symptoms within 24 hr. No electrocardiographic criteria were specified.

Exclusion. Patients excluded had complete heart block, a clear indication for magnesium therapy, or serum creatinine > 300 μmol/L.

End Points. The criterion for end point was 28-day mortality.

RESULTS

A diagnosis of acute myocardial infarction was confirmed in 65% of randomized patients (55% Q-wave, 10% non-Q-wave) and angina without myocardial infarction in 26%. Overall, 36% of patients received thrombolytics and 65% received aspirin. Administration of magnesium significantly reduced 28-day mortality by 24% compared to placebo (7.8% magnesium vs. 10.3% placebo, 2P = 0.04). This survival benefit of magnesium was observed in both thrombolysed and nonthrombolysed patients. Subgroup analysis by age, delay time of magnesium administration, use of thrombolytics or aspirin, and prior use of β-blockers, diuretics, calcium antagonists, or nitrates did not reveal any effect on mortality. The incidence of clinical left ventricular failure was significantly reduced by 25% with magnesium therapy (11.2% magnesium vs. 14.9% placebo, 2P = 0.009). Long-term follow-up at a mean of 2.7 years revealed a persistently significant reduction in total mortality by 16% (22.7% magnesium vs. 26.3% placebo, P = 0.03) and ischemic heart disease mortality by 21% (16.2% magnesium vs. 20.2% placebo, P = 0.01) with magnesium therapy compared to placebo (Figs. 1-11 to 1-13).

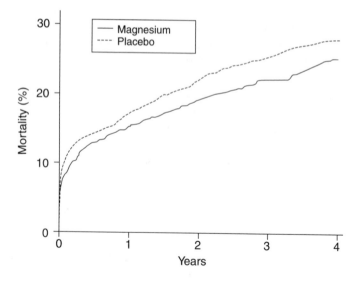

Figure 1-12.   All-cause mortality. (From Woods et al.,[17] with permission.)

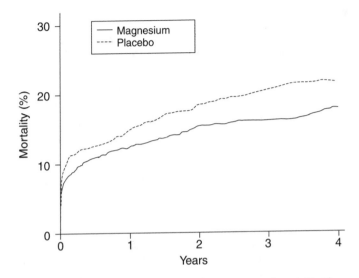

Figure 1-13. Ischemic heart disease mortality. (From Woods et al.,[17] with permission.)

CONCLUSIONS

In patients with suspected acute myocardial infarction, the administration of IV magnesium initiated before thrombolytic agents resulted in a significant 24% reduction in 28-day mortality and a 25% reduction in the incidence of left ventricular failure compared to placebo. Follow-up at 2.7 years revealed a persistent substantial reduction in overall mortality and ischemic heart disease mortality in patients treated with magnesium.

(28-day follow-up data from Woods et al.[16]; long-term follow-up data from Woods et al.[17]) ■

Primary Angioplasty in Myocardial Infarction

PURPOSE

Compare the effect of immediate percutaneous transluminal coronary angioplasty (PTCA) with intravenous (IV) thrombolytic therapy on clinical outcomes in patients with acute myocardial infarction.

STUDY DESIGN

General

- 395 patients enrolled in this prospective, randomized, multicenter trial.

- Patients initially received oxygen, IV nitroglycerin, aspirin 325 mg chewed immediately, and IV heparin 10,000-U bolus and were then randomized to one of two treatment groups:

  1. Intravenous tissue plasminogen activator (t-PA): 100 mg IV (or 1.25 mg/kg for patients < 65 kg) infused over 3 hr followed by conservative therapy according to the TIMI 2B protocol

  2. Immediate PTCA: Immediate coronary angiography, and if coronary anatomy suitable, standard PTCA performed after additional heparin IV 5,000–10,000 U bolus with the goal to reduce residual stenosis to < 50%

- Both treatment groups received heparin IV for 3–5 days with the dose titrated to maintain partial thromboplastin time 1.5–2.0 × control, nitroglycerin IV followed by oral nitrates, aspirin 325 mg/day, and diltiazem 30–60 mg PO qid. The use of β-blockers and lidocaine IV was left to the discretion of each physician.

- Resting radionuclide ventriculography was performed within 24 hr of admission, exercise thallium before hospital discharge, and stress/rest radionuclide ventriculogram (RVG) at 6 weeks.

Inclusion. Patients included were of any age presenting within 12 hr of symptom onset of ischemic chest pain with ST-segment elevation of ≥ 1 mm in two or more contiguous electrocardiogram leads.

Exclusion. Patients excluded presented with dementia, complete left bundle branch block, cardiogenic shock, high risk of bleeding, left main

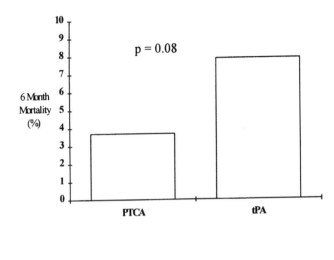

A

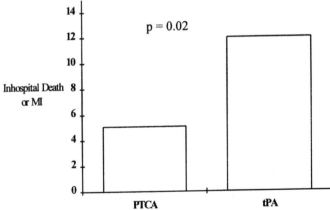

B

Figure 1-14. *(A)* Six-month mortality demonstrating a trend toward reduced mortality with primary angioplasty. *(B)* Incidence of in-hospital death or myocardial infarction demonstrating a significant reduction with primary angioplasty.

stenosis > 70%, patent infarct-related artery, triple-vessel disease or high-risk lesion for PTCA, small coronary vessels, stenosis < 70% in the infarct-related artery, or unidentifiable infarct-related artery.

End Points. The criteria for end points were mortality, ventricular function, bleeding complications, and recurrent ischemia.

RESULTS

Patients undergoing immediate PTCA had a 97.1% success rate with no requirement for emergency coronary artery bypass graft. The in-hospital mortality rate was 2.6% for the PTCA group compared to 6.5% for the t-PA group (P = 0.06); reinfarction rates were coincidentally the same (2.6% PTCA vs. 6.5% t-PA, P = 0.06). The combined end point of in-hospital death or nonfatal reinfarction was significantly lower in the PTCA group (5.1% PTCA vs. 12.0% t-PA, P = 0.02). Hemorrhagic strokes occurred more often in patients treated with t-PA (0% PTCA vs. 2.0% t-PA, P = 0.05), whereas treatment with PTCA resulted in more ventricular fibrillation (6.7% PTCA vs. 2.0% t-PA, P = 0.02) and the need for surgical vascular repair (2.1% PTCA vs. 0% t-PA, P = 0.05). Predischarge exercise testing was clinically positive more often in the t-PA group (2.9% PTCA vs. 8.6% t-PA, P = 0.04). Left ventricular ejection fraction at 6 months was similar between the two groups, both at rest (average 53%) and during exercise (average 56%). Death at 6 months had occurred in 3.7% of the PTCA group compared to 7.9% in the t-PA group (P = 0.08) (Fig. 1-14).

CONCLUSIONS

Immediate PTCA in patients with acute myocardial infarction significantly reduced the combined incidence of in-hospital death or nonfatal myocardial infarction, was associated with less intracranial hemorrhage, and resulted in similar 6-month left ventricular ejection fraction compared to IV t-PA therapy. Immediate PTCA, however, did increase the need for surgical vascular repair and the incidence of ventricular fibrillation.

———————

(Data from Grines et al.[18])   ■

Immediate PTCA vs. Intravenous Streptokinase in Acute Myocardial Infarction

PURPOSE

Compare the effects of immediate angioplasty with intravenous (IV) streptokinase (SK) on clinical events and vessel patency in patients with acute myocardial infarction.

STUDY DESIGN

General

- 142 patients enrolled in this prospective, randomized, trial.
- Eligible patients were randomized to one of two treatment groups:
  1. Intravenous SK: 1.5 million U IV infused over 60 min
  2. Immediate angioplasty
- All patients received aspirin 300 mg immediately and then daily, IV nitroglycerin to maintain systolic blood pressure at 110 mmHg, and IV heparin to maintain partial thromboplastin time 2.0–3.0 × control for at least 2 days.
- Use of calcium channel blockers, lidocaine, and β-blockers was left to the discretion of each physician.
- Radionuclide ventriculography was performed before hospital discharge.
- Coronary arteriography was performed at 3 weeks in the SK group and at 3 months in the percutaneous transluminal coronary angioplasty (PTCA) group.

Inclusion. Patients included were < 76 years old with symptoms of acute myocardial infarction persisting for > 30 min and presenting within 6 hr of symptom onset with associated ST-segment elevation > 1 mm in two or more contiguous electrocardiogram leads.

Exclusion. Patients excluded had contraindications to thrombolytic therapy.

End Points. The criteria for end points were recurrent ischemia before hospital discharge, left ventricular ejection fraction, and vessel patency.

RESULTS

Immediate PTCA of the infarct-related artery had a success rate of 98%; one patient underwent emergency coronary artery bypass surgery because the culprit artery could not be reopened. Significantly fewer patients in the angioplasty group had recurrent ischemia compared to the SK group (9% PTCA vs. 38% SK, P < 0.001). Radionuclide left ventricular ejection fraction at hospital discharge was significantly better with immediate PTCA, both at rest (51% PTCA vs. 45% SK, P = 0.004) and with exercise (52% PTCA vs. 46% SK, P = 0.02). Ischemic ST-segment depression on predischarge treadmill testing occurred less often with PTCA treatment (21% PTCA vs. 41% SK, P = 0.01). In patients treated with primary angioplasty, follow-up angiography revealed a substantially higher patency rate (91% PTCA vs. 68% SK, P = 0.001) and less average residual stenosis (residual stenosis of 36% with PTCA vs. residual stenosis of 76% with SK, P < 0.001) (Fig. 1-15).

CONCLUSIONS

In patients with acute myocardial infarction, treatment with immediate coronary angioplasty resulted in a higher long-term patency rate with less residual stenosis of the infarct-related artery, better left ventricular

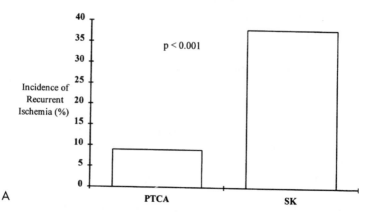

Figure 1-15. Bar graphs demonstrating a significant reduction in *(A)* the incidence of recurrent ischemia. *(Figure continues.)*

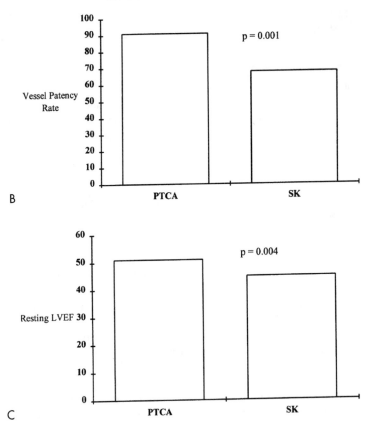

Figure 1-15 *(Continued). (B)* Improved vessel patency rate. *(C)* Bar graph demonstrating improved resting left ventricular ejection fraction with primary angioplasty.

ejection fraction, and a lower incidence of recurrent myocardial ischemia compared to treatment with IV SK.

(Data from Zijlstra et al.[19]) ∎

RAPID

Reteplase Angiographic Patency International Dose-Ranging Trial

PURPOSE

Compare the effects of r-PA, a nonglycosylated deletion mutant of tissue plasminogen activator (t-PA), with standard-dose t-PA on coronary patency and perfusion rates in patients with acute myocardial infarction.

STUDY DESIGN

General

- 606 patients enrolled in this prospective, randomized, dose-ranging, multicenter trial.

- Eligible patients were randomized to one of four treatment groups:

  1. r-PA: 15 million U IV bolus only

  2. r-PA: 10 million U initial IV bolus followed by 5 million U IV bolus after 30 min

  3. r-PA: 10 million U initial IV bolus followed by 10 million U IV bolus after 30 min

  4. Tissue plasminogen activator (standard dose): 60 mg IV over the first hour with 6–10 mg given as a bolus followed by 20 mg/hr for 2 hr (total dose 100 mg)

- All patients received aspirin 200–325 mg PO immediately and then daily and heparin 5,000-U IV bolus immediately followed by 1,000 U/hr titrated to maintain partial thromboplastin time 1.5–2.0 × control.

- Coronary arteriography and left ventriculography were performed at 30, 60, and 90 min after initiation of thrombolytic therapy and again after 5 days of hospitalization.

- Mechanical intervention was performed only when there was clear evidence of ongoing ischemia.

Inclusion. Patients included were 18–75 years old with ≥ 30 min of ischemic chest pain not relieved by nitroglycerin presenting within 6 hr of symptom onset with associated ST-segment elevation of ≥ 0.1 mV in the limb leads or ≥ 0.2 mV in the precordial leads.

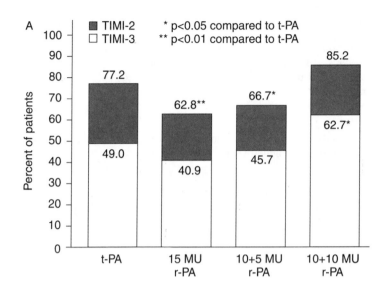

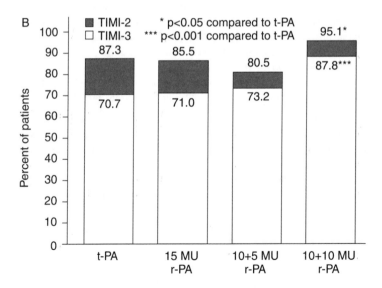

Figure 1-16. Patency rates at *(A)* 90 min and *(B)* hospital discharge in the four treatment groups. (From Smalling et al.,[20] with permission.)

Exclusion. Patients excluded presented with left bundle branch block, previous coronary artery bypass graft, previous Q-wave myocardial infarction in the same distribution as the current event, percutaneous transluminal coronary angioplasty within 2 weeks, or contraindications to thrombolytic therapy.

End Points. The criteria for end points were TIMI grade 2 or 3 flow, reocclusion rate, and left ventricular ejection fraction (LVEF).

RESULTS

The r-PA 10 + 10 million U dose resulted in a trend toward higher patency rates (TIMI grade 2 or 3 flow) at both 60 min (78% r-PA 10 + 10 vs. 66% t-PA, P = 0.079) and at 90 min (85% r-PA 10 + 10 vs. 78% t-PA, P = 0.084) compared to t-PA. At hospital discharge, r-PA 10 + 10 produced a significantly better patency rate compared to t-PA (95% r-PA 10 + 10 vs. 88% t-PA, P = 0.04). TIMI 3 flow was significantly higher with r-PA 10 + 10 at all angiographic study times compared to t-PA (60 min: 51% r-PA 10 + 10 vs. 33% t-PA, P = 0.009; 90 min: 63% r-PA 10 + 10 vs. 49% t-PA, P = 0.019; hospital discharge: 88% r-PA 10 + 10 vs. 71% t-PA, P < 0.001). r-PA 10 + 10 also resulted in a substantial improvement in LVEF compared to t-PA at hospital discharge (53% LVEF r-PA 10 + 10 vs. 49% LVEF t-PA, P = 0.034). Patency rates and LVEF were not significantly different between the r-PA 15 million U, 10 + 5 million U, and t-PA groups. The need for transfusions, the incidence of intracranial hemorrhage, and the mortality and reinfarction rates were similar among the four groups (Fig. 1-16).

CONCLUSIONS

Reteplase (r-PA) given as a double bolus of 10 + 10 million U achieved more rapid and complete thrombolysis of the infarct-related artery and resulted in a significantly higher LVEF at hospital discharge compared to standard-dose t-PA. No increase in the risk of bleeding or adverse clinical events were observed with r-PA. A separate randomized trial, RAPID 2, will compare r-PA with accelerated-dose t-PA.

(Data from Smalling et al.[20]) ∎

TAMI 1

Thrombolysis and Angioplasty in Myocardial Infarction

PURPOSE

Determine the clinical benefit of immediate vs. late coronary angioplasty in patients with acute myocardial infarction who have a patent infarct-related artery after treatment with tissue plasminogen activator (t-PA).

STUDY DESIGN

General

- 197 patients enrolled in this prospective, randomized, multicenter trial.
- Eligible patients underwent coronary angiography within 90 min of receiving t-PA. Patients with TIMI grade 2 or 3 flow in the infarct-related artery with a residual stenosis of $\geq$ 50% and suitable coronary anatomy were randomized to one of two treatment groups:
  1. Immediate angioplasty
  2. Elective angioplasty
- Angioplasty was performed by day 7 if persistent residual stenosis of $\geq$ 50% without total occlusion, or a positive exercise stress test was found.
- All patients received t-PA 150 mg infused over 6–8 hr, heparin 500–1,000 U/hr titrated to maintain partial thromboplastin time 1.5–2.0 × control for $\geq$ 24 hr, aspirin 325 mg/day, dipyridamole 75 mg PO tid, diltiazem 30–60 mg PO qid, and lidocaine IV for 24 hr.
- β-Blockers were avoided if possible.
- Repeat coronary angiography was performed 7–10 days after randomization.

Inclusion. Patients included were $\leq$ 75 years old presenting within 4–6 hr of onset of acute myocardial infarction with associated ST-segment elevation of $\geq$ 1 mm in two or more contiguous electrocardiom leads.

Exclusion. Patients excluded had a contraindication to thrombolytics, previous coronary artery bypass graft (CABG), previous Q-wave myocardial infarction in the same distribution of the infarct-related artery, cardiogenic shock, left main or equivalent stenosis of ≥ 50%, severe diffuse multivessel disease, residual stenosis of < 50%, or an unidentifiable infarct-related artery.

End Points. The criteria for end points were mortality, recurrent ischemia, reocclusion rate, and left ventricular ejection fraction (LVEF).

RESULTS

Seventy-five percent of patients treated with t-PA had a patent infarct-related artery at 90 min. The 25% of patients with an occluded infarct-related artery at 90 min after initiation of t-PA therapy were excluded from the study and suffered a high, 10.4%, mortality rate. Among patients with a patent infarct-related artery, no significant difference was observed between immediate and elective percutaneous transluminal coronary angioplasty (PTCA) with respect to overall mortality (4.0% immediate vs. 1.0% elective, P = 0.37), incidence of reocclusion (11% immediate vs. 13% elective, P = 0.67), or requirement for emergency CABG (7% immediate vs. 2% elective, P = 0.17). Immediate angioplasty resulted in a significant reduction in the need for emergency PTCA (5% immediate vs. 16% elective, P = 0.01). No significant difference in LVEF was observed between the two strategies at 7 days (Fig. 1-17).

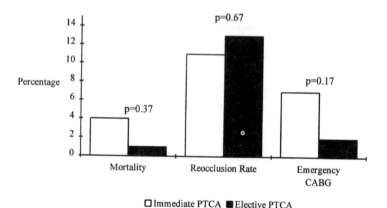

Figure 1-17. Major clinical end points demonstrating no significant difference between the immediate and elective PTCA.

CONCLUSIONS

In patients with acute myocardial infarction who achieved initial successful thrombolysis with t-PA, immediate angioplasty offered no significant benefit in mortality, reocclusion rate, or LVEF compared to elective angioplasty over a 7–10 day follow-up period.

(Data from Topol et al.[21]) ■

TAMI 2

Thrombolysis and Angioplasty in Myocardial Infarction

PURPOSE

Determine the clinical benefit of combination therapy with tissue plasminogen activator (t-PA) and urokinase (UK) in patients with acute myocardial infarction.

STUDY DESIGN

General

- 146 patients enrolled in this prospective, randomized, multicenter trial.

- Eligible patients were randomized to one of five treatment groups:

  1. Tissue plasminogen activator 25 mg intravenously (IV) and UK 0.5 million U IV

  2. Tissue plasminogen activator 25 mg IV and UK 1.0 million U IV

  3. Tissue plasminogen activator 1.0 mg/kg IV (maximum of 90 mg) and UK 0.5 million U IV

  4. Tissue plasminogen activator 1.0 mg/kg IV (maximum of 90 mg) and UK 1.0 million U IV

  5. Tissue plasminogen activator 1.0 mg/kg IV (maximum of 90 mg) and UK 2.0 million U IV

- Tissue plasminogen activator and UK were infused simultaneously over 60 min.

- All patients received heparin 500–800 U/hr titrated to maintain partial thromboplastin time 2.0–2.5 × control for ≥ 3 days, aspirin 325

mg/day, diltiazem 30–60 mg PO qid, and lidocaine IV and nitroglycerin IV for 24 hr.
- β-Blockers were avoided if possible.
- Coronary angiography was performed at 90 min and at 7 days after
  initiation of thrombolytic therapy with angioplasty performed at the
  discretion of the physician.

Inclusion. Patients included were ≤ 75 years old presenting within 4–6
hr of onset of acute myocardial infarction with associated ST-segment
elevation of ≥ 1 mm in two or more contiguous electrocardiogram leads.

Exclusion. Patients excluded had a contraindication to thrombolytics,
previous Q-wave myocardial infarction in the same distribution of the
infarct-related artery, or cardiogenic shock.

End Points. The criteria for end points were patency and reocclusion
rates. Study groups in TAMI 2 were compared to the results from TAMI 1
(t-PA 150 mg/6–8 hr in a similar patient population).

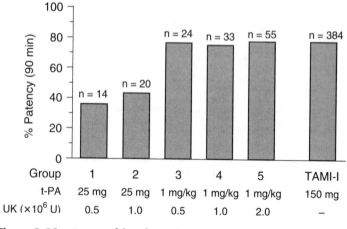

Figure 1-18. Patency of the infarct-related artery at 90 min for the five treatment groups compared to the t-PA alone in the TAMI 1 trial. (From Topol et al.,[22]
with permission.)

RESULTS

Patency rates of the infarct-related artery at 90 min were as follows: group 1, 36%; group 2, 42%; groups 3–5, average 72%; TAMI 1, 75%. These data reveal a significantly worse outcome for groups 1 and 2 compared to TAMI 1 (these two groups were subsequently terminated from the study) and no difference for groups 3–5 compared to TAMI 1 ($P = 0.66$). The reocclusion rates at day 7 were as follows: group 3, 11%; group 4, 6%; group 5, 11%; and TAMI 1, 15%. These data also reveal no significant difference (group 3–5 vs. TAMI 1, $P = 0.11$) (Fig. 1-18).

CONCLUSIONS

Combination therapy with t-PA and UK offered no significant synergistic advantage in 90-min patency rates or reocclusion rates compared to therapy with t-PA alone in patients with acute myocardial infarction over a 7-day follow-up period.

(Data from Topol et al.[22]) ■

TAMI 3

Thrombolysis and Angioplasty in Myocardial Infarction

PURPOSE

Determine the thrombolytic efficacy of treatment with tissue plasminogen activator (t-PA) and immediate high-dose intravenous (IV) heparin compared to t-PA and delayed IV heparin in patients with acute myocardial infarction.

STUDY DESIGN

General

- 134 patients enrolled in this prospective, randomized, multicenter trial.
- Eligible patients were randomized to one of two treatment groups:
  1. Tissue plasminogen activator 1.5 mg/kg IV over 4 hr and immediate heparin IV 10,000-U bolus
  2. Tissue plasminogen activator 1.5 mg/kg IV over 4 hr and delayed heparin IV 5,000-U bolus given 90 min after t-PA

- Patients underwent coronary arteriography within 90 min of treatment.
- All patients then received heparin 500–1,000 U/hr titrated to maintain partial thromboplastin time 1.5–2.0 × control for ≥ 24 hr, aspirin 325 mg/day, and diltiazem 30–60 mg PO qid.
- β-Blockers were avoided if possible.
- Repeat coronary angiography was performed 7–10 days after randomization.

Inclusion. Patients included were ≤ 75 years old presenting within 4–6 hr of onset of acute myocardial infarction with associated ST segment elevation of ≥ 1 mm in two or more contiguous electrocardiogram leads.

Exclusion. Patients excluded had a contraindication to thrombolytics, previous Q-wave myocardial infarction in the same distribution of the infarct-related artery, or cardiogenic shock.

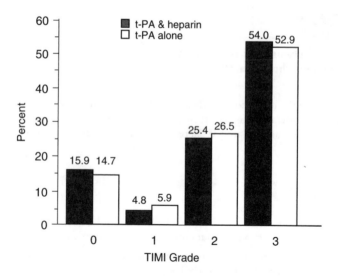

Figure 1-19. Recanalization of the infarct-related artery at 90 min by TIMI grade for the t-PA and heparin vs. t-PA alone. (From Topol et al.,[23] with permission.)

End Points. Criteria for end points were patency rate, reocclusion rate, and LVEF.

RESULTS

Patency rates of the infarct-related artery at 90 min were 79% for both the t-PA plus immediate heparin group and the t-PA plus delayed heparin group. The success rate of immediate rescue angioplasty was not significantly different between the two groups (92% t-PA plus immediate heparin vs. 77% t-PA plus delayed heparin, P = not significant). Bleeding complications, requirement for transfusions, and intracranial hemorrhage were also not significantly different between the two groups. There was no improvement in left ventricular ejection fraction (LVEF) at 7 days in both groups (49.0% t-PA plus immediate heparin vs. 50.2% t-PA plus delayed heparin). The predischarge patency rates of the infarct-related artery were 62% for t-PA plus immediate heparin compared to 54% for t-PA plus delayed heparin (Figs. 1-19 and 1-20).

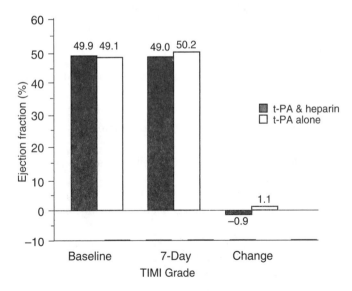

Figure 1-20. Global left ventricular ejection fraction. No significant difference observed between t-PA and heparin vs. t-PA alone. (From Topol et al.,[23] with permission.)

CONCLUSIONS

The administration of t-PA and immediate high-dose IV heparin to patients with acute myocardial infarction did not improve 90-min patency rates or LVEF compared to t-PA and late (after 90 min) IV heparin. In addition, no significant difference in bleeding complications was found between these two groups.

———————

(Data from Topol et al.[23]) ∎

Thrombolysis and Angioplasty in Myocardial Infarction

PURPOSE

Determine the effect of Iloprost, an analogue of prostacyclin PGI_2, on clinical outcome in patients with acute myocardial infarction.

STUDY DESIGN

General

- 50 patients enrolled in this prospective, randomized, multicenter trial.
- Eligible patients were randomized to one of two treatment groups:
  1. Tissue plasminogen activator (t-PA) and Iloprost
  2. Tissue plasminogen activator alone
- Tissue plasminogen activator: 100 mg intravenously (IV) over 3 hr (1 mg/kg (maximum of 80 mg) over the first hour with 10% as bolus, with the remainder infused over the next 2 hr.
- Iloprost: initial dose of 0.5 ng/kg/min titrated up to 2 ng/kg/min and continued for 48 hr.
- All patients received heparin IV 1,000 U/hr titrated to maintain partial thromboplastin time 2.0–2.5 × control for ≥ 72 hr, aspirin 325 mg/day, and lidocaine IV for 24 hr.
- β-Blockers were avoided unless clearly indicated.
- Coronary angiography was performed at 90 min and 7 days.

Inclusion. Patients included were ≤ 75 years old with chest discomfort of ≥ 20-min but < 6-hr duration with associated ST-segment elevation of ≥ 1 mV in two or more contiguous leads.

Exclusion. Patients excluded had contraindications to thrombolytics or had a previous myocardial infarction in the same territory of the current event.

End Points. Criteria for end points were patency rates of the infarct-related artery, reocclusion rates, and left ventricular ejection fraction (LVEF).

RESULTS

Patency rates of the infarct-related artery at 90 min were 44% for patients receiving t-PA and Iloprost compared to 60% for patients receiving t-PA alone (P = 0.26). Reocclusion at day 7 was not significantly different between the two groups (14% t-PA and Iloprost vs. 26% t-PA alone, P = 0.46). A significant improvement in LVEF was observed with treatment with t-PA alone (+3.1%) compared to t-PA and Iloprost (-2.3, P = 0.05) (Fig. 1-21).

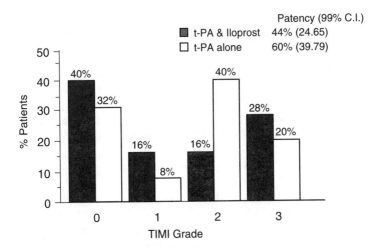

Figure 1-21. Recanalization of the infarct-related artery at 90 min by the TIMI grade for t-PA and Iloprost vs. t-PA alone. (From Topol et al.,[24] with permission.)

CONCLUSIONS

In patients with acute myocardial infarction, the combination of t-PA and Iloprost did not improve 90-min vessel patency, the incidence of reocclusion, or LVEF compared to t-PA alone.

(Data from Topol et al.[24]) ■

TAMI 5

Thrombolysis and Angioplasty in Myocardial Infarction

PURPOSE

Determine the benefit of combination therapy with tissue plasminogen activator (t-PA) and urokinase (UK) vs. monotherapy and the role for aggressive vs. deferred cardiac catheterization in patients with acute myocardial infarction.

STUDY DESIGN

General

- 575 patients enrolled in this prospective, randomized, multicenter trial.
- Eligible patients were randomized to one of three thrombolytic treatment groups and then randomized a second time to aggressive or deferred cardiac catheterization:
  1. Tissue plasminogen activator alone: 100-mg total dose given as 60 mg intravenously (IV) over the first hour with a 6-mg bolus, then 20 mg/hr for next 2 hr
  2. UK alone: 1.5 million U IV bolus, followed by 1.5 million U IV infusion over 90 min
  3. Combination t-PA and UK: t-PA 1 mg/kg (maximum of 90 mg) over 60 min and UK 1.5 million U IV over 60 min given simultaneously
- Aggressive catheterization: coronary angiography at 90 min with rescue angioplasty attempted if thrombolysis failed and anatomy was suitable.
- Deferred catheterization: coronary angiography at 5–7 days.

- All patients received heparin initiated at the end of the thrombolytic infusion as 1,000 U/hr IV titrated to maintain partial thromboplastin time 1.5-2.0 × control for ≥ 48 hr, aspirin 325 mg/day, diltiazem 30-60 mg PO tid, and lidocaine IV for 24 hr.
- β-Blockers were avoided unless clearly indicated.
- Repeat cardiac catheterization was attempted on all patients before discharge.

Inclusion. Patients included were ≤ 75 years old with chest discomfort of < 6-hr duration with associated ST-segment elevation of ≥ 1 mV in two or more contiguous leads.

Exclusion. Patients excluded had contraindications to thrombolytics, previous coronary artery bypass surgery, cardiogenic shock, or a previous myocardial infarction in the same territory of the current event.

End Points. Criteria for end points were patency rates of the infarct-related artery, reocclusion rates, and left ventricular ejection fraction (LVEF).

RESULTS

Predischarge LVEF was almost identical (54%) among all three thrombolytic groups and both catheterization strategies (P = 0.98). There was a trend toward higher patency rates at 90 min with combination thrombolytic therapy compared to monotherapy. Combination thrombolytic therapy was associated with a lower reocclusion rate (2%) compared to UK alone (7%) and t-PA alone (12%) (P = 0.04). Aggressive catheterization led to an initial patency rate of 96%. Predischarge patency rate with aggressive catheterization was 94% compared to 90% with the deferred strategy (P = 0.065). No significant difference in bleeding complications was observed with any thrombolytic regimen or catheterization strategy.

CONCLUSIONS

Combination thrombolytic therapy with t-PA and UK did not improve LVEF or significantly improve 90-min patency rates compared to t-PA alone or UK alone in patients with acute myocardial infarction. Combination therapy did significantly reduce the rate of reocclusion compared to monotherapy. The aggressive catheterization strategy did not significantly improve LVEF or predischarge patency rates compared to the deferred catheterization strategy.

(Data from Califf et al.[25]) ■

TAMI 6

Thrombolysis and Angioplasty in Myocardial Infarction

PURPOSE

Determine the benefit of late administration of tissue plasminogen activator (t-PA), 6–24 hr after symptom onset, in patients with acute myocardial infarction.

STUDY DESIGN

General

- 197 patients enrolled in this prospective, randomized, double-blind, placebo-controlled, multicenter trial.
- Eligible patients were randomized to one of two treatment groups:
  1. Tissue plasminogen activator: 1.0 mg/kg (maximum of 80 mg) intravenously (IV) over the first hour with 10% given as a bolus, then 20 mg infused over the next hour (total maximum dose of 100 mg)
  2. Placebo
- All patients received heparin 5,000-U IV bolus given 120 min after initiation of study drug infusion and then a continuous infusion of 1,000 U/hr IV titrated to maintain partial thromboplastin time 1.5–2.0 × control, and aspirin 325 mg/day.
- β-Blockers, lidocaine, nitrates, and angiotensin-converting enzyme inhibitors were avoided unless clearly indicated.
- Coronary angiography was performed 6–24 hr after the study drug was given and again at 4–6 months.

Inclusion. Patients included were ≤ 75 years old presenting with acute myocardial infarction within 6–24 hr of onset of symptoms with associated ST-segment elevation of ≥ 1 mV in two or more contiguous leads.

Exclusion. Patients excluded had chest pain relieved by nitroglycerin, contraindications to thrombolytics, or a previous myocardial infarction in the same territory of the current event.

End Points. Criteria for end points were patency rates of the infarct-related artery, mortality, and left ventricular ejection fraction (LVEF).

RESULTS

At an average of 16 hr after the study medication was administered, patients treated with t-PA had significantly higher vessel patency rates compared to placebo (65% patency t-PA vs. 27% patency placebo, P < 0.0001). This effect remained significant among the subgroup of patients treated 6–12 hr and 12–24 hr after symptom onset. At 6-month follow-up, vessel patency was identical in the t-PA and placebo groups (59%). There was no significant difference between the two groups with respect to in-hospital mortality (9.4% t-PA vs. 8.9% placebo, P = not significant [NS]) or 6-month mortality (12.5% t-PA vs. 9.9% placebo, P = 0.56). At 6 months, there were no significant differences in rein-farction rates (3.2% t-PA vs. 5.0% placebo, P = 0.42), rates of coronary angioplasty (32% t-PA vs. 38% placebo, P = 0.40), or LVEF (52.5% t-PA

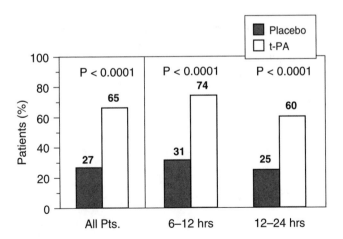

Figure 1-22. Patency of the infarct-related vessel at 16 hr for all patients and according to the duration of time from symptom onset to study medication. (From Topol et al.,[26] with permission.)

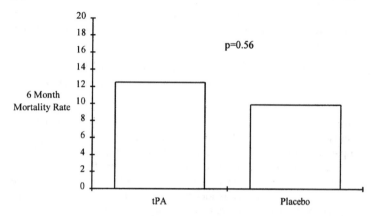

Figure 1-23. Six-month mortality. No significant difference was observed.

vs. 51.4% placebo, P = NS). No differences in bleeding complications, intracranial hemorrhage, or transfusion rates were observed between the two treatment groups (Figs. 1-22 and 1-23).

CONCLUSIONS
The administration of t-PA 6–24 hr after the onset of acute myocardial infarction significantly improved the acute vessel patency rate only, with no significant difference observed in 6-month vessel patency, LVEF, or in-hospital and 6-month mortality compared to placebo.

(Data from Topol et al.[26]) ∎

TAMI 7

Thrombolysis and Angioplasty in Myocardial Infarction

PURPOSE

Determine the benefit of various accelerated dosing regimens of tissue plasminogen activator (t-PA) in patients with acute myocardial infarction.

STUDY DESIGN

General

- 232 patients enrolled in this prospective, randomized, multicenter trial.
- Eligible patients were randomized to one of five t-PA dosing regimens:
  - A. Tissue plasminogen activator 1.0 mg/kg over 30 min (10% given as bolus), then 0.25 mg/kg over 30 min (maximum of 120 mg)
  - B. Tissue plasminogen activator 1.25 mg/kg over 90 min (20 mg given as bolus) (maximum of 120 mg)
  - C. Tissue plasminogen activator 0.75 mg/kg over 30 min (10% given as bolus), then 0.50 mg/kg over 60 min (maximum of 120 mg)
  - D. Tissue plasminogen activator 20-mg bolus, wait 30 min, then 80 mg over 120 min (maximum of 100 mg)
  - E. Tissue plasminogen activator 1.0 mg/kg over 30 min and urokinase 1.5 million U over 60 min
- All patients received heparin intravenously (IV) 1,000 U/hr titrated to maintain partial thromboplastin time 2.0 × control continued until the second angiography, aspirin 325 mg/day, and metoprolol 15 mg IV over three divided doses.
- Coronary angiography was performed within 90 min and at 5–7 days.

Inclusion. Patients included were 18–75 years old with chest discomfort of ≥ 30-min but < 6-hr duration with associated ST-segment elevation of ≥ 1 mV in two or more contiguous leads.

Exclusion. Patients excluded had contraindications to thrombolytics, had > 10 min of cardiopulmonary resuscitation within the previous 2

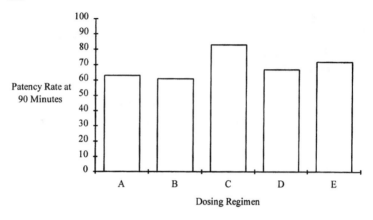

Figure 1-24. Patency rate of the infarct-related artery at 90 min according to the five accelerated dosing strategies of t-PA.

weeks, were women of childbearing potential, had previous coronary artery bypass surgery, had a previous myocardial infarction in the same territory as the current event, or had another serious illness.

End Points. Criteria for end points were patency rates of the infarct-related artery and left ventricular ejection fraction (LVEF).

RESULTS

Vessel patency of the infarct-related artery at 90 min angiography was as follows: (A) 63%, (B) 61%, (C) 83%, (D) 67%, and (E) 72%. Reocclusion rates at 5–7 days were as follows: (A) 11%, (B) 3%, (C) 4%, (D) 14%, and (E) 13%. No significant differences in predischarge LVEF or severe bleeding complications were observed for any of the five treatment groups (Fig. 1-24).

CONCLUSIONS

The accelerated t-PA dosing of group C resulted in the highest infarct-related patency rate and a low reocclusion rate. The most rapid dosing schedule (60 min), group A, yielded a lower patency rate. LVEF and bleeding complications were not significantly different among the five dosing strategies.

(Data from Wall et al.[27]) ■

TAMI 8

Thrombolysis and Angioplasty in Myocardial Infarction

PURPOSE
Determine the effect of m7E3, a monoclonal Fab antibody against the platelet glycoprotein (GP) IIb/IIIa integrelin, on platelet function and safety in patients with acute myocardial infarction treated with tissue plasminogen activator (t-PA).

STUDY DESIGN

General

- 60 patients enrolled in this prospective, nonrandomized, multicenter trial.

- Eligible patients were treated with m7E3 from 3-15 hr after initiation of t-PA with bolus-only doses of m7E3 ranging from 0.10 to 0.25 mg/kg intravenously (IV).

- All patients received t-PA 100 mg (60 mg IV on the first hour with 6 mg given as a bolus, then 20 mg/hr for 2 hr), aspirin 160-325 mg/day, heparin 2,500-5,000 U IV bolus followed by 800-1,000 U/hr infusion titrated to maintain partial thromboplastin time between 65 and 80 sec, and metoprolol 15 mg IV in three divided doses.

- Platelet aggregation and GP IIb/IIIa receptor studies were performed at certain centers.

Inclusion. Patients included were 18-76 years old with chest pain within 6 hr of symptom onset with associated ST-segment elevation of ≥ 0.1 mV in two or more contiguous electrocardiograph leads.

Exclusion. Patients excluded had contraindications to thrombolytics or m7E3, were women of childbearing potential, and had a previous splenectomy, a history of vasculitis, acute angioplasty, or another serious illness.

End Points. Criteria for end points were the results of platelet aggregation studies and bleeding events.

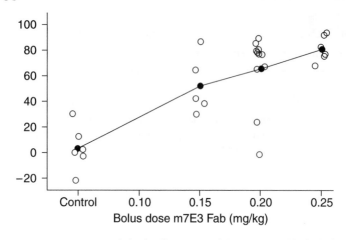

Figure 1-25. Percent of platelet glycoprotein IIb/IIIa receptors blocked after bolus doses of m7E3. (From Kleiman et al.,[28] with permission.)

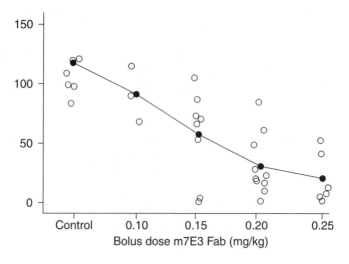

Figure 1-26. Inhibition of in vitro platelet aggregation to 20 μmol/l adenosine diphosphate after bolus doses of m7E3. (From Kleiman et al.,[28] with permission.)

RESULTS

There was a dose–response effect of m7E3 on blocking GP IIb/IIIa receptors and inhibiting platelet aggregation, with the 0.25-mg/kg bolus having the greatest effect. Major hemorrhages and requirement for transfusion, respectively, occurred in 25% and 20% of patients treated with m7E3 compared to 50% and 40% of control patients. There were no intracranial hemorrhages. Serum human anti-murine antibodies of the immunoglobulin G isotype were detected in 52% of patients after treatment with m7E3 (Figs. 1-25 and 1-26).

CONCLUSIONS

The use of m7E3 along with t-PA in patients with acute myocardial infarction resulted in a marked inhibition of platelet aggregation without a significant effect on bleeding complications.

——————

(Data from Kleiman et al.[28]) ■

TIMI 1

Thrombolysis in Myocardial Infarction

PURPOSE

Compare the effects of intravenous (IV) streptokinase (SK) with IV tissue plasminogen activator (t-PA) on the rate of reperfusion and left ventricular function in patients with acute myocardial infarction.

STUDY DESIGN

General

- 290 patients enrolled in this prospective, blinded, randomized trial.

- Eligible patients had immediate cardiac catheterization after heparin 5,000-U IV bolus was administered.

- Patients with ≥ 50% stenosis in the infarct-related artery were randomized to one of two thrombolytic therapies:

  1. Streptokinase: 1.5 million U IV infusion over 1 hr

  2. Tissue plasminogen activator: 40 mg IV over the first hour, then 20 mg/hr IV for 2 hr (total dose 80 mg)

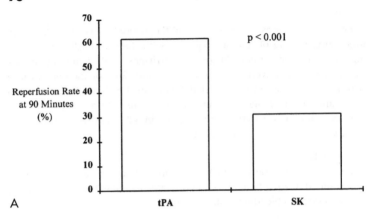

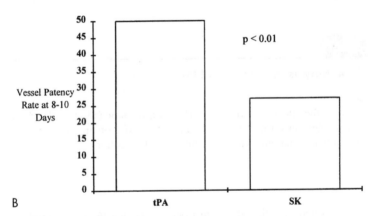

Figure 1-27. *(A & B)* Angiographic outcome for t-PA vs. streptokinase.

- Angiograms were performed at 10, 20, 30, 45, 60, 75, and 90 min after initiating thrombolytic therapy.

- Patients then received routine coronary care including heparin 1,000 U/hr starting 3 hr after the initial bolus and adjusted to keep partial thromboplastin time 1.5–2.0 × control.

- Repeat cardiac catheterization after 8–10 days was performed.

Inclusion. Patients included had > 30 min of ischemic chest pain presenting within 7 hr of symptom onset associated with ≥ 0.1-mV ST-segment elevation in at least two contiguous electrocardiogram leads.

Exclusion. Patients excluded were > 75 years old, had previous coronary artery bypass surgery, left bundle branch block, prosthetic heart valve, dilated cardiomyopathy, stroke, shock unresponsive to volume expansion or vasopressors, other serious illness, or contraindications to thrombolytic therapy.

End Points. Criteria for end points were left ventricular ejection fraction measured by contrast ventriculography and angiographically confirmed reperfusion of the infarct-related artery and patency rate at 8–10 days, both defined as TIMI grade 2 or 3 flow.

RESULTS

Treatment with t-PA resulted in a significantly higher reperfusion rate after 90 min of treatment (62% t-PA vs. 31% SK, $P < 0.001$) and also a significantly higher patency rate after 8–10 days (50% t-PA vs. 27% SK, $P < 0.01$) compared to SK. Left ventricular ejection fraction (LVEF) did not change significantly in either group between admission and hospital discharge (t-PA: 49.1% LVEF baseline vs. 49.9% LVEF predischarge, $P = 0.35$; SK: 48.1% LVEF baseline vs. 49.1% LVEF predischarge, $P = 0.32$). LVEF did improve in the subgroup of patients who achieved reperfusion earlier than 4 hr after symptom onset and in patients with collaterals to the infarct region (Fig. 1-27).

Table 1-2. Definitions of Perfusion in the TIMI Trial

Grade 0 (no perfusion): There is no antegrade flow beyond the point of occlusion.

Grade 1 (penetration with minimal perfusion): The contrast material passes beyond the area of obstruction, but "hangs up" and fails to opacify the entire coronary bed distal to the obstruction for duration of the cine run.

Grade 2 (partial perfusion): The contrast material passes across the obstruction and opacifies the coronary bed distal to the obstruction. However, the rate of entry of contrast material into the vessel distal to the obstruction or its rate of clearance from the distal bed (or both) are perceptibly slower than its entry into or clearance from comparable areas not perfused by the previously occluded vessel, e.g., the opposite coronary artery or the coronary bed proximal to the obstruction.

Grade 3 (complete perfusion): Antegrade flow into the bed distal to the obstruction occurs as promptly as antegrade flow into the bed proximal to the obstruction, and clearance of contrast material from the involved bed is as rapid as clearance from an uninvolved bed in the same vessel or the opposite artery.

(From Sheehan et al.,[29] with permission.)

CONCLUSIONS

Treatment with t-PA produced a significantly higher reperfusion rate at 90 min and patency rate at 8–10 days compared to SK in patients with acute myocardial infarction. Neither therapy resulted in a significant overall improvement in LVEF between admission and hospital discharge.

———————

(Data from Sheehan et al.[29])   ■

TIMI 2A

Thrombolysis in Myocardial Infarction

PURPOSE

Compare the benefit of immediate invasive, delayed invasive, and conservative strategies after tissue plasminogen activator (t-PA) therapy in the setting of acute myocardial infarction.

STUDY DESIGN

General

- 586 patients enrolled in this prospective, randomized trial.

- Three treatment groups as follows:

  1. Immediate invasive: immediate coronary arteriography (within 2 hr) followed by percutaneous transluminal angioplasty (PTCA) of the infarct-related artery if appropriate

  2. Delayed invasive: deferred arteriography and PTCA for 18–48 hr

  3. Conservative strategy: PTCA used only if ischemia occurred spontaneously or at the time of predischarge exercise testing

- Tissue plasminogen activator was administered initially as 150 mg/6 hr (195 patients) but subsequently reduced to 100 mg/6 hr because of excessive bleeding. The dosing schedule was 6-mg intravenous (IV) bolus, 54 mg over the first hour, 20 mg over the second hour, then 5 mg over each next hour × 4 hr. Tissue plasminogen activator was administered within 4 hr of symptom onset.

- Immediate heparin 5,000-U IV bolus, then 1,000 U/hr × 5 days titrated to keep partial thromboplastin time 1.5–2.0 × control. On day 6, heparin changed to 10,000 U subcutaneously (SQ) q 12 hr until discharge.

- Aspirin 81 mg PO qd × 5 days (initiated on day 1–2), then 325 mg qd starting on day 6.
- All patients also received sublingual nitroglycerin, prophylactic lidocaine, morphine, nifedipine 10–20 mg PO tid given for 96 hr, and metoprolol, started after predischarge contrast and radionuclide studies, at 50 mg PO bid for 1 day, then 100 mg PO bid for 1 year unless contraindicated.

Inclusion. Patients included were < 76 years old with ischemic chest pain ≥ 30-min duration associated with ST-segment elevation of ≥ 1.0 mV in at least two contiguous electrocardiogram leads.

Exclusion. Patients excluded had a contraindication to thrombolytic therapy.

End Points. Criteria for end points were patency rates of the infarct-related artery, left ventricular ejection fraction, and clinical outcomes.

RESULTS

Predischarge contrast left ventricular ejection fraction was not significantly different among all three treatment groups, averaging 49.3%. Patency rates of the infarct-related artery at the time of discharge angiography were equal among the three groups (mean 83.7%); however, patients in the conservative strategy had significantly greater stenosis of the infarct-related artery. Immediate invasive strategy led to a higher rate of coronary artery bypass graft (CABG) after PTCA (7.7%) and bleeding requiring transfusion (13.8%) than delayed invasive strategy (2.1% CABG after PTCA, P < 0.01, 3.1% bleeding, P < 0.01) or conservative strategy (2.5% CABG after PTCA, P < 0.001, 2.0% bleeding, P < 0.001). Severe or prolonged recurrent ischemia in the conservative strategy resulted in early (before hospital discharge) coronary angiography in 17.8%, PTCA in 7.1%, and CABG in 3.0% of patients. At 1-year follow-up, the three treatment groups had similar cumulative rates of death (average, 8.7%), fatal and nonfatal reinfarctions (8.5%), combined death and reinfarction (14.5%), and CABG (17.2%). The cumulative use of PTCA remained significantly higher in both invasive groups (immediate invasive 75.8%, delayed invasive 64.3% vs. conservative strategy 23.9%, P < 0.001) (Fig. 1-28).

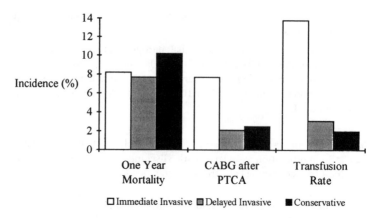

Figure 1-28. Bar graphs of clinical outcomes demonstrating similar 1-year mortality rates. Immediate invasive strategy resulted in increased CABG after PTCA and need for transfusions.

CONCLUSIONS
In the setting of acute myocardial infarction treated with thrombolytic therapy, there was no significant difference in cumulative mortality, discharge contrast left ventricular ejection fraction, or incidence of nonfatal reinfarction among immediate invasive, delayed invasive, and conservative strategies. Conservative therapy resulted in less morbidity and a lower use of PTCA.

(Data from Rogers et al.[30]) ■

TIMI 2B

Thrombolysis in Myocardial Infarction

PURPOSE
Compare the effects of immediate vs. delayed β-blockade therapy on mortality and the incidence of reinfarction in patients with acute myocardial infarction treated with intravenous (IV) tissue plasminogen (t-PA) therapy.

STUDY DESIGN

General

- 1,434 patients enrolled in this prospective, randomized, double-blinded, multicenter trial.
- Eligible patients were randomized to one of two treatments groups:
  1. Immediate therapy: within 2 hr of initiating t-PA, metoprolol was given as 5 mg IV q 2 min × 3 for a total of 15 mg followed by 50 mg PO q 12 hr × 24 hr, then 100 mg PO q 12 hr thereafter
  2. Delayed therapy: metoprolol 50 mg PO q 12 hr × 2 doses starting on day 6, then 100 mg PO q 12 hr thereafter
- All patients received the following:

  Tissue plasminogen activator: Initially, 150 mg IV over 6 hr, later the dose was reduced to 100 mg IV over 6 hr (6-mg IV bolus, 54 mg infused in the first hour, 20 mg infused in the second hour, then 5 mg/hr infused for 4 hr). Treatment with t-PA was started within 4 hr of onset of chest pain.

  Heparin: Initiated at the same time as t-PA as a 5,000-U IV bolus, followed by 1,000 U/hr titrated to keep partial thromboplastin time 1.5–2.0 × control for 6 days. Then the heparin dose was changed to 10,000 U subcutaneously (SQ) bid until hospital discharge.

  Aspirin: 80 mg/day initiated on day 1–2 for 6 days, then 325 mg/day thereafter.

  Lidocaine: 1–1.5 mg/kg IV bolus, then 2–4 mg/min infusion for maximum of 24 hr.

Inclusion. Patients included were < 75 years old with chest pain suggestive of myocardial infarction lasting ≥ 30 min associated with ST-segment elevation of ≥ 0.1 mV in two contiguous electrocardiogram leads.

Exclusion. Criteria for exclusion were as follows: percutaneous transluminal coronary angioplasty within 6 months; previous coronary artery bypass surgery; prosthetic heart valves; left bundle branch block; dilated cardiomyopathy; implanted pacemaker; resting heart rate < 55 bpm; systolic blood pressure consistently < 100 mmHg; rales or pulmonary edema on chest x-ray; greater than first-degree atrioventricular block; asthma/chronic obstructive pulmonary disease; pre-existing ther-

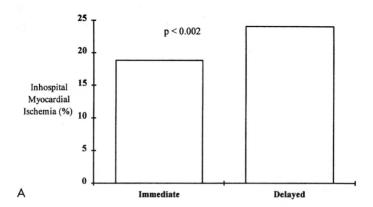

A

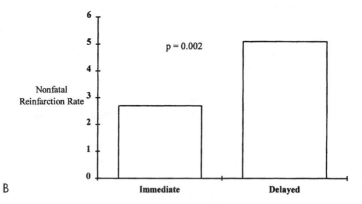

B

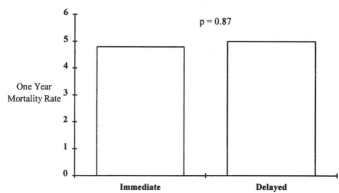

C

apy with β-blockers, verapamil, or diltiazem on admission; or contraindications to thrombolytic therapy.

End Points. Criteria for end points were global left ventricular function measured by radionuclide ventriculography before hospital discharge; in-hospital recurrent ischemia and reinfarction; and total mortality at 6 days, 6 weeks, and 1 year.

RESULTS

Immediate β-blockade therapy resulted in significantly decreased rates of in-hospital myocardial ischemia (18.8% immediate vs. 24.1% deferred, P < 0.002) and nonfatal reinfarction (2.7% immediate vs. 5.1% deferred, P = 0.002) compared to delayed β-blockade therapy. Global resting left ventricular ejection fraction averaged 50.5% and was identical in both groups at discharge and 6-week follow-up. Total mortality was not significantly different in the two groups at hospital discharge (2.4%), 6-week follow-up (3.5%), and 1-year follow-up (5.0%) (Fig. 1-29).

CONCLUSIONS

Immediate β-blocker therapy with metoprolol in the setting of acute myocardial infarction treated with thrombolytic therapy resulted in significantly less in-hospital recurrent ischemia and nonfatal reinfarction compared to delayed β-blocker therapy. However, no significant difference was observed in left ventricular ejection fraction or total mortality to 1 year.

(Data from Roberts et al.[31]) ■

Figure 1-29. *(A–C)* Bar graphs of clinical outcomes demonstrating reduced in-hospital recurrent ischemia and reinfarction rates with immediate metoprolol therapy compared to delayed therapy. Mortality rates at 1 year were not significantly different.

TIMI 3A

Thrombolysis in Myocardial Infarction

PURPOSE

Determine the early effects of tissue plasminogen activator (t-PA) on quantitative arteriography of the culprit coronary artery in patients with unstable angina or non-Q-wave myocardial infarction.

STUDY DESIGN

General

- 306 patients enrolled in this prospective, randomized, double-blind, placebo-controlled, multicenter trial.

- Eligible patients were randomized to one of two treatment groups:

    1. Tissue plasminogen activator: 0.8 mg/kg (up to maximum of 80 mg) given as 1/3 total dose up to 20 mg as initial bolus, the remainder infused over 90 min

    2. Placebo

- All patients received heparin 5,000-U intravenous (IV) bolus, then a continuous infusion to keep partial thromboplastin time 1.5–2.0 × control, and antianginal drug combinations including PO or IV nitrates, calcium channel antagonists, and/or β-blocking drugs.

- Aspirin was withheld until 4 hr before anticipated percutaneous transluminal coronary angioplasty (PTCA) or after heparin was stopped.

- Quantitative coronary arteriography and left ventriculography were performed within 12 hr of enrollment and again at 18–48 hr.

Inclusion. Patients included were 21–75 years old with ischemic chest discomfort at rest lasting $\geq$ 5 min but $\leq$ 6 hr and occurring within 24 hr of enrollment with objective evidence of ischemic heart disease consisting of the following:

1. $\geq$ 0.1-mV ST-segment elevation lasting < 30 min, or $\geq$ 0.1-mV ST-segment depression or T-wave inversion in at least two contiguous leads OR
2. Documented coronary artery disease: history of previous myocardial infarction, > 70% luminal diameter stenosis on previous coronary angiograms, or positive exercise thallium scan

Exclusion. Criteria for exclusion were as follows: treatable cause of unstable angina, myocardial infarction within the preceding 3 weeks, coronary arteriography within 30 days, PTCA within 6 months, coronary artery bypass graft in the past, pulmonary edema or shock, left bundle branch block, coexisting severe illness, woman of childbearing potential, pre-existing therapy with oral anticoagulants, or contraindications to t-PA or heparin.

End Points. Criteria for end points were measurable improvement in the culprit artery lesion caliber of ≥ 10% reduction of diameter stenosis or improvement in flow by at least two TIMI flow grades between baseline and 18–48 hr studies.

RESULTS

Arteriographically apparent thrombus was present at the baseline angiographic study in only 35% of patients. No significant difference was found in the primary study end point of improved coronary flow among t-PA- and placebo-treated patients (25% t-PA vs. 19% placebo achieved improved flow, $P = 0.25$). Angiographic improvement was significantly more frequent with t-PA treatment among lesions containing apparent thrombus (36% t-PA vs. 15% placebo, $P < 0.01$) and in patients evolving a non-Q-wave myocardial infarction (33% t-PA vs. 8% placebo, $P < 0.005$).

CONCLUSIONS

Arteriographically apparent intraluminal thrombus was found in a low percentage (35%) of patients with unstable angina or non-Q-wave mycardial infarction. Overall, t-PA is not significantly more effective than placebo at improving coronary flow in these patients. Substantial improvement in flow, however, was more frequent with t-PA in lesions containing apparent thrombus and in patients with evolving non-Q-wave MI. Clinical relevance of these findings was reported in the TIMI 3B study.

(Data from The TIMI IIIA Investigators.[32]) ■

Thrombolysis in Myocardial Infarction

PURPOSE

Compare the effects of tissue plasminogen activator (t-PA) with placebo and early invasive with conservative strategies in unstable angina and non-Q-wave myocardial infarction.

STUDY DESIGN

General

- 1,473 patients enrolled in this prospective, randomized, placebo controlled, multicenter trial.

- Patients were first randomized to t-PA or placebo treatment, and then randomized a second time to early invasive strategy or conservative strategy as follows:

  Tissue plasminogen activator: 0.8 mg/kg (up to maximum of 80 mg) given as ⅓ total dose up to 20 mg as initial bolus, the remainder infused over 90 min.

  Early invasive: coronary arteriography and left ventriculography in all patients 18–48 hr after randomization with immediate percutaneous transluminal coronary angioplasty (PTCA) of suitable culprit vessels. Coronary artery bypass graft (CABG) within 6 weeks if > 50% left main, triple-vessel disease with left ventricular ejection fraction < 40%, or recurrent ischemia despite maximal medical therapy in patients not suitable for PTCA or in whom PTCA was already performed.

  Conservative: cardiac catheterization only after failure of initial medical therapy.

- All patients received heparin 5,000-U IV bolus, then a continuous infusion to keep partial thromboplastin time 1.5–2.0 × control, aspirin 325 mg/day starting on day 2 and continued for 1 year, β-blockade (metoprolol 50 mg PO q 12 hr), calcium channel antagonist (diltiazem 30 mg PO q 6 hr), and long-acting nitrates (isosorbide dinitrate 10 mg PO q 8 hr).

Inclusion. Patients included were 21–75 years old with ischemic chest discomfort at rest lasting ≥ 5 min but ≤ 6 hr occurring within 24 hr of enrollment with objective evidence of ischemic heart disease consisting of the following:

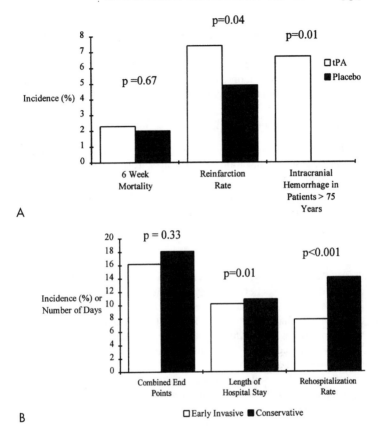

Figure 1-30. (A) Bar graph of clinical outcomes demonstrating increased reinfarction rate and intercranial hemorrhage with t-PA therapy compared to placebo. (B) Bar graph of clinical outcomes demonstrating reduced length of hospital stay and rehospitalization rate with early invasive strategy compared to conservative strategy.

1. ≥ 0.1-mV ST-segment elevation lasting < 30 min, or ≥ 0.1-mV ST-segment depression or T-wave inversion in at least two contiguous leads OR
2. Documented coronary artery disease: history of previous myocardial infarction, > 70% luminal diameter stenosis on previous coronary angiograms or positive exercise thallium scan

Exclusion. Criteria for exclusion were as follows: treatable cause of unstable angina, myocardial infarction within preceding 3 weeks, coronary arteriography within 30 days, PTCA within 6 months, CABG in the past, pulmonary edema or shock, left bundle branch block, coexisting severe illness, woman of childbearing potential, pre-existing therapy with oral anticoagulants, or contraindications to t-PA or heparin.

End Points. Criteria for end points were as follows:

- Tissue plasminogen activator vs. placebo: combined end point of death, postrandomization nonfatal myocardial infarction, or failure of initial therapy at 6-week follow-up
- Early invasive vs. conservative strategy: combined end point of death, postrandomization myocardial infarction, or unsatisfactory exercise treadmill test at 6-week follow-up

RESULTS

Tissue Plasminogen Activator vs. Placebo. No significant difference was observed at 6 weeks between t-PA and placebo treatment in total mortality (2.3% t-PA vs. 2.0% placebo, P = 0.67) or combined end points (54.2% t-PA vs. 55.5% placebo, P = 0.61). Tissue plasminogen activator treatment was associated with significantly greater reinfarction by 6 weeks (7.4% t-PA vs. 4.9% placebo, P = 0.04) and intracranial hemorrhage in patients over 75 years of age (6.7% t-PA vs. 0.0% placebo, P = 0.01). The subgroup of patients with unstable angina treated with t-PA had a significant 84% increase in the incidence of death or myocardial infarction compared to placebo at 6 weeks.

Early Invasive vs. Conservative Strategy. No significant difference in combined end points was observed at 6 weeks between early invasive and conservative strategy (16.2% early invasive vs. 18.1% conservative, P = 0.33). Early invasive treatment did result in a significantly reduced length of initial hospitalization, incidence and length of rehospitalization at 6 weeks, and use of antianginal medications (Fig. 1-30).

CONCLUSIONS

The administration of thrombolytic agents to patients with unstable angina or non-Q-wave myocardial infarction offered no benefit in 6-week survival and was associated with significantly greater rates of reinfarction and intracranial hemorrhage. The subgroup of patients with unstable angina treated with t-PA had a significant increase in the incidence of death or myocardial infarction compared to placebo. Early invasive strategy compared with conservative strategy did not reduce 6-week mortality but did result in a significantly reduced length of hospitalization, incidence of rehospitalization, and use of antianginal medications.

(Data from The TIMI IIIB Investigators.[33]) ■

TIMI 4

Thrombolysis in Myocardial Infarction

PURPOSE

Compare the effects of front-loaded tissue plasminogen activator (t-PA), APSAC, and the combination of both on mortality and morbidity in patients with acute myocardial infarction.

STUDY DESIGN

General

- 382 patients enrolled in this randomized, prospective, double-blinded trial.

- Eligible patients were randomized to one of three treatment groups:

  1. Tissue plasminogen activator: 15-mg intravenous (IV) bolus, then 0.75 mg/kg (up to 50 mg) infused over 30 min followed by 0.50 mg/kg (up to 35 mg) infused over 60 min
  2. APSAC: 30-U IV bolus over 2–5 min
  3. Combination: t-PA—15-mg IV bolus, then 0.75 mg/kg (up to 50 mg) over 30 min, and APSAC—20-U IV bolus over 2–5 min

- All patients received heparin 5,000-U IV bolus immediately, then 1,000 U/hr titrated to keep partial thromboplastin time 1.5–2.0 × control, and aspirin 325 mg chewed immediately and then 325 mg PO qd. Metoprolol was also used if not contraindicated.

- All other medications were left to the discretion of the physician.

- Coronary arteriography was performed 90 min after thrombolytic therapy was initiated and again after 18–36 hr to determine patency of the infarct-related artery.

- Sestamibi scanning immediately after the 18–36 hr catheterization and before hospital discharge was performed as well as radionuclide ventriculograms before hospital discharge.

Inclusion. Patients included had ischemic chest pain for $\geq$ 30-min duration presenting within 6 hr of symptom onset associated with ST-segment elevation of $\geq$ 0.1 mV in at least two contiguous leads or with new left bundle branch block (LBBB).

Exclusion. The criteria for exclusion were as follows: age $\geq$ 80 years, treatment with t-PA within previous 2 weeks or APSAC or streptokinase at any time, oral anticoagulation, women of childbearing age, previous LBBB, other serious illness, or contraindications to thrombolytic therapy.

End Points. The criteria for end points were as follows: primary study end point of "unsatisfactory outcome" was defined as any of the following: death, severe congestive heart failure, left ventricular ejection fraction < 40%, reinfarction, TIMI grade flow < 2 during either catheterization, reocclusion assessed by sestamibi imaging, major spontaneous hemorrhage, or severe anaphylaxis.

RESULTS

TIMI grade 2 or 3 flow at 60 and 90 min was achieved significantly more often in patients treated with t-PA than APSAC (84.2% t-PA vs. 72.9% APSAC at 90 min, P = 0.02) or the combination (84.2% t-PA vs. 67.7% combination at 90 min, P < 0.01). In addition TIMI grade 3 flow at 90 min was achieved with a significantly higher proportion with t-PA than APSAC (60.2% t-PA vs. 42.9% APSAC, P < 0.01) or the combination (60.2% t-PA vs. 44.8% combination, P = 0.02). At 18–36 hr, TIMI grade 2 or 3 flow was not significantly different among the three groups (72.6% t-PA vs. 64.8% APSAC vs. 71.0% combination, P = NS). Tissue plasminogen activator achieved significantly lower in-hospital mortality when compared to APSAC (2.2% t-PA vs. 8.8% APSAC, P = 0.02); however, mortality at 1 year was not significantly different among the three groups (5.3% t-PA vs. 11% APSAC, P = 0.07, and vs. 10.5% combination, P = 0.13). No significant difference in combined unsatisfactory outcome was found. The incidence of intracranial hemorrhage was similar among the three groups (0% t-PA, 0.7% APSAC, 1.0% combination, P = NS); however, t-PA resulted in significantly less major hemorrhage (10.9% t-PA vs. 21.8% APSAC, P = 0.01, and vs. 21.6% combination, P = 0.02).

CONCLUSIONS

In the setting of acute myocardial infarction, front-loaded t-PA achieved a significantly, higher 90-min reperfusion rate compared to APSAC or combination therapy and lower in-hospital mortality compared to APSAC. The incidence of major hemorrhage was significantly lower with t-PA therapy. However, 1-year mortality and combined unsatisfactory end point were not significantly different between the three therapies.

(Data from Cannon et al.[34]) ■

TIMI 5

Thrombolysis in Myocardial Infarction

PURPOSE

Compare the effect of hirudin and heparin on mortality and reperfusion rates in patients with acute myocardial infarction treated with front-loaded tissue plasminogen activator (t-PA) and aspirin.

STUDY DESIGN

General

- 246 patients enrolled in this prospective, randomized, dose-ranging, pilot trial.

- Eligible patients were randomized to one of five treatment groups:

  1. Heparin: 5,000-U intravenous (IV) bolus, then 1,000 U/hr titrated to keep partial thromboplastin time 65–90 sec
  2. Hirudin: in one of four ascending doses
     A. 0.15-mg/kg IV bolus (B), then 0.05 mg/kg/hr infusion (I)
     B. 0.1 mg/kg B, then 0.1 mg/kg/hr I
     C. 0.3 mg/kg B, then 0.1 mg/kg/hr I
     D. 0.6 mg/kg B, then 0.2 mg/kg/hr I

- Heparin and hirudin infusions were continued for 5 days.

- All patients received IV t-PA (15-mg IV bolus, 0.75 mg/kg (up to 50 mg) over 30 min, then 0.50 mg/kg (up to 35 mg) over 60 min, aspirin 160 mg chewed immediately and then 160 mg/day, and IV followed by oral metoprolol.

- The use of other medications was left to the discretion of the physician.
- Coronary arteriography was performed 90 min after initiation of thrombolytic therapy and again at 18– 36 hr.

Inclusion. Patients included had ischemic chest pain lasting at least 30 min with associated ST-segment elevation ≥ 0.1 mV in at least two contiguous electrocardiogram leads or new left bundle branch block (LBBB).

Exclusion. Criteria for exclusion were as follows: pulmonary edema, cardiogenic shock, coronary artery bypass graft or prosthetic valve, cardiac catheterization or angioplasty within the previous 2 weeks, anticoagulation, previous LBBB, women of childbearing age, probable pericarditits, renal dysfunction, other serious illness, and contraindications to thrombolytic therapy.

End Points. The primary end point was achievement of TIMI grade 3 flow at both 90 min and 18–36 hr arteriography without death or reinfarction.

RESULTS

A trend toward increased TIMI grade 3 flow was observed with hirudin therapy at both 90 min (64.8% hirudin vs. 57.1% heparin, P = NS) and

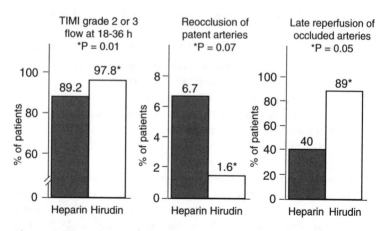

Figure 1-31. Angiographic results at 18 to 36 hr after the start of thrombolytic antithrombotic therapy. (From Cannon et al.,[35] with permission.)

18–36 hr arteriography (84.1% hirudin vs. 73.8% heparin, P = 0.09) compared to heparin therapy. There was no difference in TIMI 3 flow among the four dose groups of hirudin. Hirudin resulted in significantly better TIMI grade 2 or 3 flow at 18–36 hr, better late reperfusion of occluded arteries, and a favorable trend toward less reocclusion of patent arteries (Fig. 1-31). Reinfarction rates were significantly lower in hirudin-treated patients (4.3% hirudin vs. 11.9% heparin, P = 0.03). There was a trend toward less in-hospital mortality in hirudin-treated patients (2.5% hirudin vs. 6.0% heparin, P = 0.17). No significant difference in safety end points (major hemorrhage, intracranial hemorrhage, and hemorrhage at instrumented sites) was observed.

CONCLUSIONS

In this pilot study, hirudin was found to be a promising agent compared with heparin as adjunctive therapy with t-PA for acute myocardial infarction. Hirudin resulted in significantly better coronary flow at 18–36 hr arteriography, which perhaps was due to late reperfusion of occluded arteries. Treatment with hirudin produced a trend toward increased TIMI grade 3 flow at 90 min and 18–36 hr and reduced in-hospital mortality, although the results were not statistically significant. Reinfarction rates were also significantly lower in hirudin-treated patients.

(Data from Cannon et al.[35]) ∎

TIMI 6

Thrombolysis in Myocardial Infarction

PURPOSE

Compare the safety of intravenous (IV) hirudin with IV heparin when administered with streptokinase (SK) and aspirin in patients with acute myocardial infarction.

STUDY DESIGN

General

- 193 patients enrolled in this prospective, randomized, dose-ranging trial.

- Eligible patients were randomized to one of two treatment groups:

1. IV heparin: 5,000-U IV bolus, followed by a continuous infusion of 1,000 U/hr titrated to maintain partial thromboplastin time 65–90 sec
2. IV hirudin: one of three dosing schedules
   A. 0.15-mg/kg IV bolus, then 0.05-mg/kg/hr continuous infusion
   B. 0.30-mg/kg IV bolus, then 0.10-mg/kg/hr continuous infusion
   C. 0.60-mg/kg IV bolus, then 0.20-mg/kg/hr continuous infusion

- Both heparin and hirudin were infused for 5 days.
- All patients received SK (1.5 million U IV infused over 60 min) and aspirin 325 mg/day administered immediately after enrollment.
- Metoprolol, IV followed by oral, was given to all patients unless contraindicated.
- The use of other medications was left to the discretion of each physician.

Inclusion. Patients included were 21–75 years old with ischemic chest pain at rest of > 30-min duration and within 6 hr of symptom onset associated with ST-segment elevation of > 0.1 mV in more than two contiguous electrocardiogram leads, or new left bundle branch block.

Exclusion. Criteria for exclusion were as follows: acute pulmonary edema, serum creatinine > 1.5 mg/dl, clear indication for anticoagulation, previous coronary artery bypass graft or valve replacement, cardiac catheterization or angioplasty within 2 weeks, thrombolytic therapy within 2 weeks, women of childbearing age, contraindication to thrombolytic therapy, or other serious illness.

End Points. The criteria for end points follow:

- Safety: incidence of major hemorrhage (overt bleeding with decrease in hematocrit $\geq$ 15% or decrease in hemoglobin of $\geq$ 5 g/dl, intracranial hemorrhage, or pericardial hemorrhage or tamponade)
- Efficacy: composite unsatisfactory outcome of death, nonfatal reinfarction, new-onset congestive heart failure, cardiogenic shock, or reduced left ventricular ejection fraction of < 40%

RESULTS

The incidence of major hemorrhage was similar between heparin and each of the hirudin dose groups (5.6% heparin, 5.5% hirudin A, 6.5%

hirudin B, 5.6% hirudin C, P = not significant). No intracranial or pericardial hemorrhages occurred in the trial. The composite end point of unsatisfactory outcome was not different between any of the treatment groups (32.3% heparin, 37.3% hirudin A, 32.2% hirudin B, 34.3% hirudin C). There was a trend toward less death, reinfarction, severe congestive heart failure, or cardiogenic shock in the two highest hirudin doses (B and C) compared to the lowest hirudin dose (A).

CONCLUSIONS

In this pilot study, hirudin appeared to be as safe as heparin when given with SK and aspirin to patients with acute myocardial infarction.

(Data from Lee.[36]) ■

TIMI 9A

Thrombolysis in Myocardial Infarction

PURPOSE

Compare the efficacy and safety of intravenous (IV) hirudin and heparin as adjunctive therapy to thrombolytic agents and aspirin in patients with acute myocardial infarction.

STUDY DESIGN

General

- 757 patients enrolled in this prospective, randomized, double-blinded, multicenter trial.

- Two treatment groups as follows:

  1. Heparin: 5,000-U IV bolus, then 1,000 U/hr if weight < 80 kg, or 1,300 U/hr if weight > 80 kg titrated to keep partial thromboplastin time 2.0–3.0 × control (partial thromboplastin time 60–90 sec.)

  2. Hirudin: 0.6-mg/kg IV bolus followed by 0.2-mg/kg/hr infusion for 96 hr with no titration to partial thromboplastin time

- All patients received either front-loaded tissue plasminogen activator (t-PA) (maximum of 100 mg) IV over 90 min or 1.5 million U SK IV over 60 min and aspirin 150 mg to 325 mg immediately chewed and then daily.

Inclusion. Patients included had acute myocardial infarction exhibiting ≥ 0.1-mV ST-segment elevation in at least two contiguous electrocardiogram leads presenting within 12 hr of onset of ischemic discomfort.

Exclusion. Patients excluded had a contraindication to thrombolytic therapy.

End Points. Criteria for end points follow:

- Primary efficacy end point: death, recurrent myocardial infarction, development of congestive heart failure or cardiogenic shock, or left ventricular ejection fraction < 40% at 1 month
- Primary safety end point: major hemorrhage defined as either an intracranial hemorrhage or overt hemorrhage in association with an absolute reduction in hematocrit of 15% or anaphylaxis

RESULTS

The study was suspended early on recommendation of the Data Safety Monitoring Board because of a substantially higher rate of major hemorrhage for heparin (10.1%) and hirudin (13.9%) compared to that in TIMI 5, TIMI 6, and GUSTO 1. No significant difference in intracranial hemorrhage or major hemorrhage was apparent between heparin and hirudin.

CONCLUSIONS

The doses of heparin and hirudin used with thrombolytic therapy and aspirin in the setting of acute myocardial infarction resulted in substantially higher hemorrhagic complications than that found in other major clinical trials. This study has been reinitiated with lower doses of heparin and hirudin and will be reported as TIMI 9B.

(Data from Antman.[37])   ∎

WARIS

Warfarin Reinfarction Study

PURPOSE

Determine the effects of long-term warfarin therapy on mortality and cardiovascular events in patients with acute myocardial infarction.

STUDY DESIGN

General

- 1,214 patients enrolled in this prospective, randomized, double-blinded, placebo-controlled, multicenter trial.
- Eligible patients were randomized to one of two treatment groups:
  1. Warfarin: dose titrated to maintain an INR of 2.8–4.8 (corresponding to a typical prothombin time of 1.5–2.0 × control)
  2. Placebo
- All patients received standard medical therapy during the hospitalization including β-blockers.
- Patients were advised not to take aspirin or other antiplatelet drugs during the study to minimize the risk of bleeding.

Inclusion. Patients included were ≤ 75 years old, discharged from the hospital for an acute myocardial infarction according to the World Health Organization (WHO) criteria.

Exclusion. Patients excluded had malignant disease, life expectancy of < 2 years, high risk of bleeding, concurrent or clear indication for anticoagulants, or anticipated poor compliance.

End Points. Criteria for end points were total mortality, incidence of reinfarction, and incidence of cerebrovascular accident.

RESULTS

Baseline characteristics included a mean age of 61 years, with 48% of patients receiving β-blockers, 70% having Q-wave myocardial infarctions, and 11% in New York Heart Association class III or IV. During an average follow-up of 37 months, treatment with warfarin significantly reduced total mortality by 24% (15% warfarin vs. 20% placebo, P = 0.027) and the incidence of recurrent myocardial infarction by 34% (13.5% warfarin vs. 20.6% placebo, P = 0.0007) compared to placebo. This beneficial effect of warfarin was present regardless of the use of concomitant β-blockers. Chronic warfarin therapy also substantially reduced the incidence of cerebrovascular accidents by 55% (3.3% warfarin vs. 7.2% placebo, P = 0.0015). Major bleeding (requiring blood transfusions or an operation) occurred in 0.6% of patients taking warfarin compared to no patients

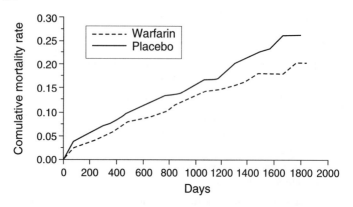

Figure 1-32. Cumulative rates of death from all causes. (From Smith et al.,[38] with permission.)

taking placebo. Five patients in the warfarin group had intracranial hemorrhages (four were fatal) (Figs. 1-32 and 1-33).

CONCLUSIONS

Long-term treatment with warfarin in patients surviving an acute myocardial infarction who are not receiving chronic aspirin therapy sig-

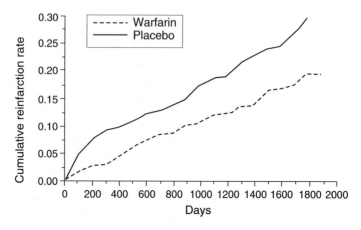

Figure 1-33. Cumulative rates of reinfarction. (From Smith et al.,[38] with permission.)

nificantly reduced total mortality and the incidences of recurrent myocardial infarction and cerebrovascular accidents compared to placebo during an average 37-month follow-up. The incidence of major hemorrhage was 0.6% among warfarin-treated patients.

(Data from Smith et al.[30]) ■

References

1. deBono DP, Simoons ML, Tijssen J et al: Effects of early intravenous heparin on coronary patency, infarct size, and bleeding complications after alteplase thrombolysis: results of a randomized double-blind European Cooperative Study Group trial. Br Heart J 67:122, 1992

2. Smith LF, Heagerty AM, Bing RF et al: Intravenous infusion of magnesium sulphate after acute myocardial infarction: effects on arrhythmias and mortality. Int J Cardiol 12:175, 1986

3. Rasmussen HS, Gronbach M, Cintin C et al: One-year death rate in 270 patients with suspected acute myocardial infarction, initially treated with intravenous magnesium or placebo. Clin Cardiol 11:377, 1988

4. Swedberg K, Held P, Kjekshus J et al: Effects of the early administration of enalapril on mortality in patients with acute myocardial infarction: results of the Cooperative New Scandinavian Enalapril Survival Study II (CONSENSUS II). N Engl J Med 327:678-84, 1992

5. Gruppo Italiano per lo Studio della Streptochinasi nell'Infarto Miocardico (GISSI): Effectiveness of intravenous thrombolytic treatment in acute myocardial infarction. Lancet I:397-402, 1986

6. Gruppo Italiano per lo Studio della Streptochinasi nell'Infarto Miocardico (GISSI): GISSI-2: a factorial randomised trial of alteplase versus streptokinase and heparin versus no heparin among 12,490 pateints with acute myocardial infarction. Lancet 336:65-71, 1990

7. Gruppo Italiano per lo Studio della Sopravvivenza nell'Infarto Miocardico: GISSI-3: effects of Lisinopril and transdermal glyceryl trinitrate singly and together on 6-week mortality and ventricular function after acute myocardial infarction. Lancet 343:1115-22, 1994

8. The GUSTO Investigators: An international randomized trial comparing four thrombolytic strategies for acute myocardial infarction. N Engl J Med 329:673-82, 1993

9. The GUSTO Angiographic Investigators: The effects of tissue plasminogen activator, streptokinase, or both on coronary-artery patency, ventricular function, and survival after acute myocardial infarction. N Engl J Med 329:1615-22, 1993

10. The Global Use of Strategies to Open Occluded Coronary Arteries (GUSTO) IIa Investigators: Randomized trial of intravenous heparin versus recombinant hirudin for acute coronary syndromes. Circulation 90:1631-7, 1994

11. ISIS-1 (First International Study of Infarct Survival) Collaborative Group: Randomised trial of intravenous atenolol among 16,027 cases of suspected acute myocardial infarction: ISIS-1. Lancet II:57-66, 1986

12. ISIS-2 (Second International Study of Infarct Survival) Collaborative Group: Randomised trial of intravenous streptokinase, oral aspirin, both, or neither among 17,187 cases of suspected acute myocardial infarction: ISIS-2. Lancet II:349-60, 1988

13. ISIS-3 (Third International Study of Infarct Survival) Collaborative Group: ISIS-3: a randomised comparison of streptokinase vs. tissue plasminogen activator vs. anistreplase and of aspirin plus heparin vs. aspirin alone among 41,299 cases of suspected acute myocardial infarction. Lancet 339:753-70, 1992

14. ISIS-4 (Fourth International Study of Infarct Survival) Collaborative Group: ISIS-4: a randomised factorial trial assessing early oral captopril, oral mononitrate, and intravenous magnesium suphate in 58,050 patients with suspected acute myocardial infarction. Lancet 345:669-82, 1995

15. LATE Study Group: Late Assessment of Thrombolytic Efficacy (LATE) study with alteplase 6-24 hours after onset of acute myocardial infarction. Lancet 342:759-66, 1993

16. Woods KL, Fletcher S, Roffe C et al: Intravenous magnesium sulphate in suspected acute myocardial infarction: results of the second Leicester Intravenous Magnesium Intervention Trial (LIMIT-2). Lancet 339:1553-8, 1992

17. Woods KL, Fletcher S: Long-term outcome after intravenous magnesium sulphate in suspected acute myocardial infarction: the second Leicester Intravenous Magnesium Intervention Trial (LIMIT-2). Lancet 343:816-9, 1994

18. Grines CL, Browne KF, Marco J et al: A comparison of immediate angioplasty with thrombolytic therapy for acute myocardial infarction. N Engl J Med 328:673-9, 1993

19. Zijlstra F, de Boer MJ, Hoorntje JCA et al: A comparison of immediate coronary angioplasty with intravenous streptokinase in acute myocardial infarction. N Engl J Med 328:680-4, 1993

20. Smalling RW, Bode C, Kalbfleisch J et al: More rapid, complete, and stable coronary thromblysis with bolus administration of reteplase compared with alteplase infusion in acute myocardial infarction. Circulation 91:2725-32, 1995

21. Topol EJ, Califf RM, George BS et al: A randomized trial of immediate versus delayed elective angioplasty after intravenous tissue plasminogen activator in acute myocardial infarction. N Engl J Med 317:581-8, 1987

22. Topol EJ, Califf RM, George BS et al: Coronary arterial thrombolysis with combined infusion of recombinant tissue-type plasminogen activator and urokinase in patients with acute myocardial infarction. Circulation 77:1100-7, 1988

23. Topol EJ, George BS, Kereiakes DJ et al: A randomized controlled trial of intravenous tissue plasminogen activator and early intravenous heparin in acute myocardial infarction. Circulation 79:281-6, 1989

24. Topol EJ, Ellis SG, Califf RM et al: Combined tissue-type plasminogen activator and prostacyclin therapy for acute myocardial infarction. J Am Coll Cardiol 14:877-84, 1989

25. Califf RM, Topol EJ, Stack RS et al: Evaluation of combination thrombolytic therapy and timing of cardiac catheterization in acute myocardial infarction: results of thrombolysis and angioiplasty in myocardial infarction—phase 5 randomized trial. Circulation 83:1543-56, 1991

26. Topol EJ, Califf RM, Candormael M et al: A randomized trial of late reperfusion therapy for acute myocardial infarction. Circulation 85:2090–99, 1992

27. Wall TC, Califf RM, George BS et al: Accelerated plasminogen activator dose regimens for coronary thrombolysis. J Am Coll Cardiol 19:482–9, 1992

28. Kleiman NS, Ohman EM, Califf RM et al: Profound inhibition of platelet aggregation with monoclonal antibody 7E3 fab after thrombolytic therapy: results of the Thrombolysis and Angioplasty in Myocardial Infarction (TAMI) 8 pilot study. J Am Coll Cardiol 22:381–9, 1993

29. Sheehan FH, Braunwald E, Canner P et al: The effect of intravenous thrombolytic therapy on left ventricular function: a report on tissue-type plasminogen activator and streptokinase from the Thrombolysis in Myocardial Infarction (TIMI Phase I) trial. Circulation 75:817–29, 1987

30. Rogers WJ, Baim DS, Gore JM et al: Comparison of immediate invasive, delayed invasive, and conservative strategies after tissue-type plasminogen activator: results of the Thrombolysis in Myocardial Infarction (TIMI) Phase II-A trial. Circulation 81:1457–76, 1990

31. Roberts R, Rogers WJ, Mueller HS et al: Immediate versus deferred β-blockade following thrombolytic therapy in patients with acute myocardial infarction: results of the Thrombolysis in Myocardial Infarction (TIMI) II-B study. Circulation 83:422–37, 1991

32. The TIMI IIIA Investigators: Early effects of tissue-type plasminogen activator added to conventional therapy on the culprit coronary lesion in patients presenting with ischemic cardiac pain at rest: results of the Thrombolysis in Myocardial Ischemia (TIMI IIIA) trial. Circulation 87:38–52, 1993

33. The TIMI IIIB Investigators: Effects of tissue-type plasminogen activator and a comparison of early invasive and conservative strategies in unstable angina and non-Q-wave myocardial infarction: results of the TIMI IIIB trial. Circulation 89:1145–56, 1994

34. Cannon CP, McCabe CH, Diver DJ et al: Comparison of front-loaded recombinant tissue-type plasminogen activator, anistreplase and combination thrombolytic therapy for acute myocardial infarction: results of the Thrombolysis in Myocardial Infarction (TIMI) 4 trial. J Am Coll Cardiol 24:1602–10, 1994

35. Cannon CP, McCabe CH, Henry TD et al: A pilot trial of recombinant desulfatohiruden compared with heparin in conjunction with tissue-type plasminogen activator and aspirin for acute myocardial infarction: results of the Thrombolysis in Myocardial Infarction (TIMI) 5 trial. J Am Coll Cardiol 23:993–1003, 1994

36. Lee LV: Initial experience with hirudin and streptokinase in acute myocardial infarction: results of the Thrombolysis in Myocardial Infarction (TIMI) 6 trial. Am J Cardiol 75:7–13, 1995

37. Antman EM: Hirudin in acute myocardial infarction: safety report from the Thrombolysis and Thrombin Inhibition in Myocardial Infarction (TIMI) 9a trial. Circulation 90:1624–30, 1994

38. Smith P, Arnesen H, Holme I: The effect of warfarin on mortality and reinfarction after myocardial infarction. N Engl J Med 323:147–52, 1990

CHAPTER 2

Unstable Angina Trials

OVERVIEW

For the past 200 years, physicians have recognized a syndrome of cardiac chest pain occurring at rest. Heberden in 1772 mentioned nonexertional angina during his classic dissertation of angina pectoris. Only limited progress was made in further understanding rest angina until the 1930s. Nonexertional angina became descriptively termed "impending or threatening myocardial infarction," "preinfarction angina," and "prethrombotic syndrome" as it was realized that this clinical pattern heralded acute myocardial infarction. More recently, this premonitory syndrome has been called *unstable angina* and defined as anginal pain of new onset within 2 months, occurring in an accelerated pattern, and/or occurring at rest. The development of unstable angina confers a 10% to 20% incidence of death and a 20% to 30% incidence of nonfatal myocardial infarction at 1 year. The pathophysiologic mechanism underlying unstable angina appears to be intermittent coronary thrombosis and coronary spasm.

During the early phase of unstable angina, atherosclerotic plaques rupture or fissure, exposing thrombogenic substances, including collagen, fibronectin, and von Willebrand factor, to circulating blood elements. Platelet adhesion and aggregation occur, forming a platelet–fibrin thrombus. When this thrombus repetitively forms and lyses, a syndrome of intermittent coronary ischemia develops, clinically defined as *unstable angina*. Furthermore, the local accumulation of vasoactive substances, such as thromboxane A_2, serotonin, thrombin, and platelet-activating factor, promotes platelet aggregation and thrombus propagation and also contributes to vasoconstriction further contributing to myocardial ischemia. Treatment is aimed at preventing intermittent coronary thrombus formation with antiplatelet agents and anticoagulants, reducing coronary vasoconstriction with nitrates and selected calcium channel blockers, and where appropriate, stabilizing the active plaque with revascularization techniques and lipid-lowering therapy.

Aspirin and Heparin

Theroux et al. examined the effect of aspirin, heparin, or both on the incidence of ischemic complications in 479 patients with unstable angina. Treatment with heparin alone significantly reduced the incidence of myocardial infarction and refractory angina compared to placebo. Treatment with aspirin alone reduced the incidence of myocardial infarction compared to placebo. The combination of aspirin and heparin was not superior to either medication alone. The use of heparin, either alone or in combination with aspirin, significantly increased the risk of bleeding complications.

The effect of aspirin therapy was examined in the Veterans Affairs Cooperative study of 1,266 men with unstable angina. Treatment with aspirin for 12 weeks significantly reduced the incidence of myocardial infarction by 55% and total mortality by 51% compared to placebo. Despite termination of the study drugs at 12 weeks, the mean mortality at 1 year remained significantly lower by 43% in the aspirin-treated group. Similar results were obtained in a Canadian Multicenter trial[1] evaluating the effects of aspirin (1,300 mg/day), sulfinpyrazone, or both in 555 patients with unstable angina. Treatment with aspirin significantly reduced the combined incidence of cardiac death and nonfatal myocardial infarction by 51% and overall mortality by 43% during an 18-month follow-up. Sulfinpyrazone provided no apparent benefit.

Medical treatment for unstable angina therefore should consist initially of aspirin along with other antianginal agents as tolerated (nitrates and either β-blockers or selected calcium channel blockers) to reduce the incidence of nonfatal myocardial infarction. Heparin is added to treat recurrent rest angina, bearing in mind the concomitant increased risk of bleeding associated with heparin therapy alone and with combined heparin and aspirin. Aspirin should be continued long term, hoping to reduce the incidence of myocardial infarction and total mortality.

Newer Antithrombotic Agents

The recent development of new antithrombotic agents like the platelet glycoprotein IIb/IIIa receptor antagonists (c7E3, Integrelin, and MK-383) and direct thrombin inhibitors (hirudin, hirulog, argatroban) has generated considerable interest in studying the effects of these agents in patients with unstable angina. The Chimeric 7E3 Antiplatelet Therapy in Unstable Angina Refractory to Standard Treatment (CAPTURE) trial randomized 1,266 patients with refractory unstable angina scheduled to undergo treatment with percutaneous transluminal coronary angioplasty (PTCA) to treatment with c7E3 bolus plus sustained infusion or placebo administered 18 to 24 hours before PTCA and continuing for 1 hour after PTCA. This trial was terminated early because of a significant 34% reduction in the combined end point of death, myocardial infarction, or need for urgent intervention with c7E3 treatment compared to placebo at 30-day follow-up. The final results of CAPTURE should be published in 1996.

The Hirudin in a European Trial vs. Heparin in the Prevention of Restenosis after PTCA (HELVETICA) trial[2] compared the effect of hirudin with heparin on the prevention of restenosis among 1,141 patients with unstable angina who were scheduled for angioplasty. The administration of hirudin was associated with a significant reduction in early cardiac events compared to heparin. Event-free survival at 7 months and mean minimal luminal diameter at 6-month angiography were not meaningfully different between the treatment groups. Bleeding events were similar among heparin- and hirudin-treated groups. Thus, hirudin reduced early cardiac events although no substantial reduction in restenosis was observed.

The Hirulog Angioplasty Study Investigation (HASI) trial examined the role of hirulog to prevent ischemic complications in 4,098 patients undergoing coronary angioplasty for unstable or postinfarction angina. No significant difference was observed in the incidence of acute or 6-month ischemic complications between hirulog and heparin. In the subgroup of patients with postinfarction angina, however, a meaningful reduction in the incidence of myocardial infarction and combined ischemic complications was observed with hirulog treatment. In addition, treatment with hirulog resulted in significantly fewer transfusions and "major" hemorrhages compared to heparin.

Heparin (and Other Antithrombins) Rebound

The abrupt discontinuation of heparin in patients with unstable angina has been shown to reactivate myocardial ischemia by Théroux et al. This phenomenon, known as *heparin rebound,* occurred in 13% of patients with unstable angina treated with heparin alone compared to 4.6% of patients treated with combination heparin and aspirin when heparin was abruptly withdrawn from patients with unstable angina. The reactivation of myocardial ischemia occurred earlier and was more likely to be clinically severe in patients treated with heparin alone compared to combination heparin and aspirin therapy. Reactivation of angina was also observed after abrupt discontinuation of argatroban,[3] a direct thrombin inhibitor, in patients with unstable angina. Postulated mechanisms for this phenomenon include generation and accumulation of thrombin during the infusion of the antithrombins and possible upregulation of thrombin receptors on platelets. Current recommendations are to taper heparin therapy over approximately 4 to 6 hours instead of abruptly discontinuing the infusion and to have the patient treated with aspirin concomitantly. Empirically, this approach has appeared to reduce the incidence of the heparin rebound phenomenon.

Thrombolytic Agents in Unstable Angina

Since intermittent coronary thrombosis and associated vasoconstriction are postulated to result in the syndrome of unstable angina, the use of thrombolytic agents has been considered in the treatment of these patients. Several small clinical trials[4,5] produced conflicting results regarding the benefit of tissue plasminogen activator (t-PA) in patients with unstable angina. A meta-analysis of these trials suggested an increase in the incidence of myocardial infarction associated with thrombolytic therapy. The Thrombolysis in Myocardial Infarction (TIMI 3A) trial was designed to more clearly define the benefit of t-PA in 1,473 patients with unstable angina or non-Q-wave myocardial infarction. The subgroup of patients with unstable angina who were treated with t-PA had a significant 84% increase in the incidence of death or myocardial infarction compared to placebo at 6 weeks. Furthermore, treatment with t-PA was associated with a substantially greater incidence of reinfarction among all patients and increased intracranial hemorrhage among patients older than 75 years. Thus, t-PA did not provide any benefit and, in fact, appeared to be harmful in patients with unstable angina.

Revascularization in Unstable Angina

The benefit of routine early revascularization with PTCA or coronary artery bypass graft (CABG) compared with an initial strategy of medical treatment has been examined in randomized clinical trials of patients with unstable angina. The TIMI 3B trial evaluated the effects of an early invasive strategy using routine angioplasty compared with a conservative strategy using angioplasty only for failure of medical treatment in 1,473 patients with unstable angina or non-Q-wave myocardial infarction. At 1-year follow-up, the subgroup of patients with unstable angina had no significant difference in the incidence of death or myocardial infarction between early invasive and conservative strategies. The early invasive strategy resulted in significantly more angioplasty procedures, whereas the conservative strategy resulted in longer initial hospitalization and significantly more subsequent readmissions for angina.

The Veterans Affairs Cooperative Study examined the benefit of early CABG compared with medical therapy in 468 patients with unstable angina. Patients were subgrouped according to the severity of unstable angina as follows: type I, those with progressive effort angina or recent angina at rest; type II, those with severe rest angina associated with ST-segment abnormalities on the electrocardiogram. Among patients presenting with type II unstable angina, the prevalence of single-, double-, and triple-vessel coronary artery disease was 21%, 38%, and 41%, respectively. After 5-year follow-up, a subgroup of patients with triple-vessel disease demonstrated significantly improved survival with surgical therapy. After 8 years of follow-up, an additional subgroup of patients with both type II unstable angina and abnormal left ventricular function (left ventricular ejection fraction < 50% or a pulmonary capillary wedge pressure ≥ 16 mmHg) had significantly better survival with CABG therapy. Patients with type II unstable angina and normal left ventricular function and all patients with type I unstable angina had no reduction in mortality or the incidence of nonfatal myocardial infarction with surgical therapy compared with medical therapy.

Conclusions

Unstable angina is a clinical syndrome caused by intermittent coronary thrombosis and vasoconstriction. The development of unstable angina confers a 10% to 20% incidence of death and a 20% to 30% incidence of myocardial infarction over 1 year, with most events occurring within the first 3 months. Acute treatment with aspirin reduces the risk of nonfatal myocardial infarction. Administration of heparin reduces the risk of nonfatal myocardial infarction and recurrent ischemia. The combination of aspirin and heparin provides no additive benefit but does increase the risk of bleeding. Therefore, aspirin and other antianginal medications, such as nitrates, β-blockers, or selected calcium channel blockers, should be used as first-line therapy, with heparin added for the patient with recurrent ischemia at rest. Heparin infusions should be tapered over 4 to 6 hours to prevent the reactivation of ischemia observed with abrupt termination of heparin (the previously mentioned heparin rebound phenomenon), and these patients should receive an antiplatelet agent as well, such as aspirin. Chronic administration of aspirin to patients with unstable angina significantly reduces the long-term incidence of myocardial infarction and total mortality. Thrombolytic agents should probably not be administered to patients with unstable angina because of the increased incidence of death or myocardial infarction and increased hemorrhagic risk associated with this therapy. Early routine use of angioplasty reduces hospital stay and readmissions for angina but results in more angioplasty procedures compared to medical therapy and provides no benefit in mortality or the incidence of myocardial infarction. CABG appears to prolong survival in the subgroup of patients with significant triple-vessel disease and those with more severe angina and impaired left ventricular function. The use of newer antithrombotic agents, like the platelet glycoprotein IIb/IIIa receptor antagonists and direct thrombin inhibitors, are being investigated in clinical trials; developing evidence indicates that they improve clinical outcomes compared to aspirin and heparin therapy.

ASPIRIN, HEPARIN, OR BOTH TO TREAT ACUTE UNSTABLE ANGINA

Montreal Heart Institute

PURPOSE

Determine the effect of aspirin, heparin, or both on the incidence of death, myocardial infarction, and refractory angina in patients during the acute phase of unstable angina.

STUDY DESIGN

General

- 479 patients enrolled in this prospective, randomized, double-blinded, placebo-controlled trial.

- Eligible patients were randomized to one of four treatment groups:

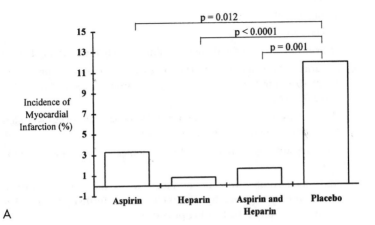

A

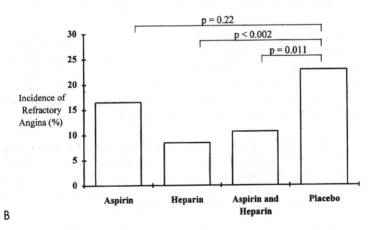

B

Figure 2-1. *(A)* Bar graph demonstrating significant reductions in the incidence of myocardial infarction with aspirin, heparin, and both compared to placebo. *(B)* Bar graph demonstrating significant reductions in the incidence of refractory angina in both heparin groups only compared to placebo. (From Théroux et al.,[6] with permission.)

1. Aspirin/heparin
2. Aspirin alone
3. Heparin alone
4. Placebo

- Aspirin: initial dose of 650 mg given immediately, then 325 mg PO bid
- Heparin: 5,000-U intravenous (IV) bolus, then continuous infusion of 1,000 U/hr titrated to maintain partial thromboplastin time (PTT) 1.5–2.0 × control.
- Medications other than antiplatelet and anticoagulant drugs were left to the discretion of the treating physician.
- Coronary arteriography was performed a mean of 6 days after enrollment.
- Study medications were discontinued when the patient returned from coronary angiography with the option of further treatment left to the discretion of the treating physician.
- All study medications were stopped abruptly, without tapering.

Inclusion. Patients included were < 75 years old presenting within 24 hr of symptom onset with a history of an accelerating pattern of chest pain occurring at rest or with minimal exertion or with chest pain lasting ≥ 20 min. Serum creatine kinase levels were less than twice the upper limit of normal on admission. Electrocardiogram changes compatible with myocardial ischemia were required.

Exclusion. The criteria for exclusion were as follows: the pre-existing use of aspirin, other active platelet drugs or warfarin, percutaneous transluminal coronary angioplasty within the previous 6 months, coronary artery bypass surgery within the past year, identifiable precipitating cause of angina, or contraindications to aspirin or heparin.

End Points. The criteria for end points were death, nonfatal myocardial infarction, and refractory recurrent angina.

RESULTS

The in-hospital incidence of myocardial infarction was significantly lower in all three treatment groups compared to placebo: 3.3% aspirin alone (P = 0.012), 0.8% heparin alone (P < 0.0001), 1.6% aspirin/heparin combination (P = 0.001), and 11.9% placebo. The in-hospital incidence of refractory angina was significantly reduced with the heparin alone and aspirin/heparin combination but not with aspirin alone compared to placebo: 16.5% aspirin alone (P = 0.22), 8.5% heparin alone (P = 0.002), 10.7% aspirin/heparin combination (P = 0.011), and 22.9% placebo. No deaths occurred in any of the treatment groups, compared with two in the placebo group. There were no statistically significant differences between the three treatment groups with respect to the study end points. Bleeding complications were more common in patients receiving heparin (20 patients receiving heparin vs. 10 patients receiving no heparin) (Fig. 2-1).

CONCLUSIONS

In patients with acute unstable angina, the use of heparin alone significantly reduced the incidence of myocardial infarction and refractory angina, whereas aspirin alone significantly reduced the incidence of myocardial infarction only. The combination of aspirin and heparin was not superior to either medication alone and resulted in slightly more bleeding complications.

(Data from Théroux et al.[6]) ■

PROTECTIVE EFFECTS OF ASPIRIN IN UNSTABLE ANGINA

VA Cooperative Study

PURPOSE

Determine the effect of aspirin on mortality and the incidence of acute myocardial infarction in men with unstable angina.

STUDY DESIGN

General

- 1,266 men enrolled in this prospective, randomized, double-blinded, placebo controlled, multicenter trial.

- Eligible men with chest pain suggestive of unstable angina were screened within 48 hr of hospital admission and randomized to one of two treatment groups:

  1. Aspirin: 324 mg in an effervescent powder taken immediately and then once a day for 12 weeks
  2. Placebo

- Other medical therapy was left to the discretion of the treating physician.

- After 12 weeks, study drugs were discontinued.

Inclusion. Patients included were men with unstable angina beginning within the previous month and still present within the previous week. They had evidence of coronary artery disease and the absence of baseline evidence of acute myocardial infarction by electrocardiogram or measurement of cardiac enzymes.

Exclusion. Patients excluded had acute myocardial infarction on admission, New York Heart Association functional class IV congestive heart failure, tachyarrhythmia, anemia, hypoxemia, a contraindication to aspirin, a

Figure 2-2. Bar graphs demonstrating significant reductions in *(A)* the incidence of myocardial infarction, with *(B)* 12-week and *(C)* 1-year mortality with aspirin therapy compared to placebo. (From Lewis et al.,[7] with permission.)

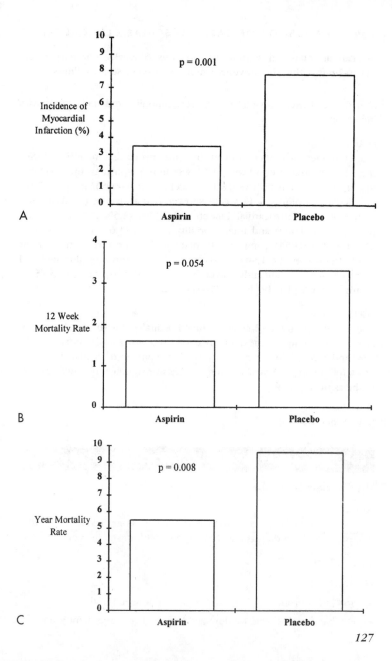

A

B

C

myocardial infarction within the previous 6 weeks, coronary artery bypass graft within the previous 3 months, or other serious illness.

End Points. Criteria for end points were mortality and acute myocardial infarction.

RESULTS

The combined incidence of death or acute myocardial infarction during the 12-week study period was 51% lower in the aspirin group compared to placebo (5.0% aspirin vs. 10.1% placebo, P = 0.0005). Analysis of the individual end points at 12 weeks showed that aspirin reduced the incidence of acute myocardial infarction by 55% (3.5% aspirin vs. 7.8% placebo, P = 0.001) and total mortality by 51% (1.6% aspirin vs. 3.3% placebo, P = 0.054) compared to placebo. Despite termination of the study drugs after the 12-week trial period, the mean mortality rate at 1 year remained significantly lower by 43% in the aspirin group (5.5% aspirin vs. 9.6% placebo, P = 0.008) (Fig. 2-2).

CONCLUSIONS

The use of aspirin for 12 weeks in men hospitalized with unstable angina significantly reduced the incidence of acute myocardial infarction by 55% and favored lower mortality by 51% compared to placebo at 12-week follow-up. At 1 year, mean mortality was significantly lower by 43% in the aspirin group.

(Data from Lewis et al.[7]) ■

CORONARY ARTERY BYPASS SURGERY IN UNSTABLE ANGINA

VA Cooperative Study

PURPOSE

Determine the benefit of coronary artery bypass graft surgery (CABG) compared with medical therapy in patients with unstable angina.

STUDY DESIGN

General

- 468 men enrolled in this prospective, randomized trial.

- Eligible patients were randomized to one of two treatment groups:

1. CABG
2. Medical therapy
- Subgroups were predefined according to the severity of unstable angina:

    Type I. Patients with stable exertional angina who had an increase in the frequency or severity of angina, new onset angina, or rest angina

    Type II. Resistant prolonged rest angina associated with 1-mm ST-segment elevation or depression or T-wave inversion on electrocardiogram (ECG)

- Myocardial infarction was excluded in all patients by serial ECGs and cardiac enzymes.
- Abnormal left ventricular function was defined as a left ventricular ejection fraction (LVEF) < 50% or a pulmonary capillary wedge pressure ≥ 16 mmHg.

Inclusion. Patients included were men < 70 years old admitted for unstable angina with > 75% stenosis in at least one epicardial coronary artery.

Exclusion. Patients excluded had acute myocardial infarction, atypical chest pain, a previous myocardial infarction within 3 months, previous CABG, normal coronary arteries or left main coronary artery disease, LVEF < 30%, or other serious illness.

End Points. Criteria for end points were mortality and nonfatal myocardial infarction.

RESULTS
The mean age of patients was 56 years, with 18% having one-vessel, 35% having two-vessel, and 47% having three-vessel coronary artery disease. At 5-year follow-up, no significant difference in mortality between surgical and medical therapy was observed among all patients or subgroups of patients defined by type I, type II, or left ventricular function. Surgical therapy significantly reduced mortality only in the subgroup of patients with triple-vessel disease (11% surgical vs. 24% medical, P < 0.02).

After 8 years of follow-up, overall mortality was similar between CABG and medical therapy (29% CABG vs. 28% medical, P = NS). A further subgroup of patients with type II unstable angina and impaired

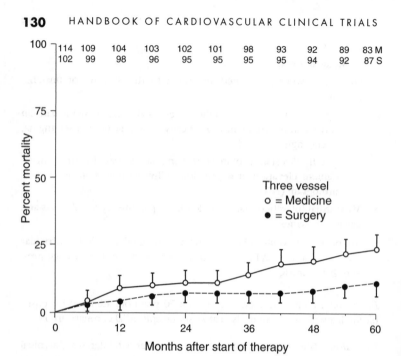

Figure 2-3. The cumulative mortality for medical and surgical patients with three-vessel disease. (From Parisi et al.,[8] with permission.)

left ventricular function had significantly reduced mortality with surgical therapy (13% CABG vs. 46% medical, P = 0.04). This subgroup, however, had no significant difference in the incidence of nonfatal myocardial infarction between the two treatment strategies. All patients with type I unstable angina and type II unstable angina with normal left ventricular function had similar mortality and incidence of nonfatal myocardial infarction between surgical and medical therapy. No analysis of mortality outcome according to the number of diseased vessels was performed at 8-year follow-up (Figs. 2-3 and 2-4).

CONCLUSIONS

Treatment with CABG in men with unstable angina prolongs survival only in the subgroups of patients with triple-vessel disease at 5-year follow-up and those with severe rest angina and impaired left ventricular function at 8-year follow-up compared to medical therapy. No significant

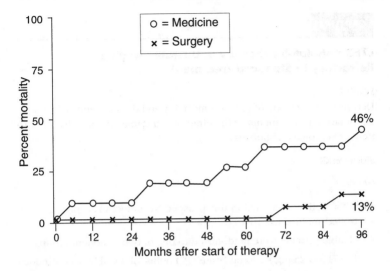

Figure 2-4. The cumulative mortality for medical and surgical patients with type II unstable angina and abnormal left ventricular function. (From Sharma et al.,[9] with permission.)

difference in the incidence of myocardial infarction was observed among any subgroups.

(5-year follow-up data from Parisi et al.[8]; 8-year follow-up data from Sharma et al.[9]) ∎

CAPTURE

c7E3 Antiplatelet Therapy in Unstable Angina Refractory to Standard Treatment

PURPOSE

Determine the effects of c7E3 on mortality and the incidence of myocardial infarction in patients with refractory unstable angina scheduled to undergo coronary angioplasty.

STUDY DESIGN

General

- 1,266 patients enrolled in this prospective, randomized, placebo-controlled, multicenter trial.

- Eligible patients were randomized to one of two treatment groups:

  1. c7E3: 0.25-mg/kg intravenous (IV) bolus followed by a continuous infusion of 10 µg/min

  2. Placebo

- Study medications were started 24 hr before the coronary intervention and continued for 1 hr after the intervention.

- All patients received aspirin, heparin, and nitrates.

Inclusion. Patients included had refractory unstable angina with recurrent pain and electrocardiogram changes compatible with myocardial ischemia despite treatment with aspirin, heparin, and nitrates.

End Points. The criteria for the combined end point was death, myocardial infarction, or urgent revascularization at 30 days.

RESULTS

The Data Safety Monitoring Committee recommended early termination of the trial after analysis of the first 1,050 enrolled patients. Treatment with c7E3 significantly reduced the combined 30-day end point of death, myocardial infarction, or urgent revascularization by 34% compared to placebo (10.8% c7E3 vs. 16.4% placebo, $P < 0.05$). The use of c7E3 reduced the individual end points of death (1.0% c7E3 vs. 1.5% placebo), myocardial infarction by 53% (4.4% c7E3 vs. 9.4% placebo), and urgent revascularization by 32% (6.9% c7E3 vs. 10.2% placebo). However, an increased incidence of major bleeding was observed with c7E3 treatment (2.9% c7E3 vs. 1.7% placebo).

CONCLUSIONS

In patients with refractory unstable angina, treatment with c7E3 starting 24 hr before and continued for 1 hr after percutaneous transluminal coronary angioplasty reduced the combined 30-day end point of death, myocardial infarction, or urgent revascularization at a cost of an increased incidence of major bleeding events.

(Data courtesy of James J. Ferguson, M.D.; presented at the 1996 Annual Meeting of the American College of Cardiology.)   ■

c7E3 IN UNSTABLE ANGINA

Pilot Study

PURPOSE

Determine the effects of c7E3, a Fab antibody fragment directed against the platelet glycoprotein IIb/IIIa integrin, on acute ischemic events in patients undergoing angioplasty for refractory unstable angina.

STUDY DESIGN

General

- 60 patients enrolled in this prospective, randomized, double-blinded, placebo-controlled, multicenter trial.

- Eligible patients with a single culprit coronary lesion amenable to percutaneous transluminal coronary angioplasty (PTCA) in whom the angioplasty procedure could be delayed 18 to 24 hr after the initial angiogram were randomized to one of two treatment groups:

    1. c7E3: 0.25-mg/kg intravenous (IV) bolus starting within 4 hr after completion of the first angiogram followed by a continuous infusion of 10 μg/min until 1 hr after the PTCA procedure, which was scheduled between 18–24 hr after the bolus dose

    2. Placebo

- Patients with severe refractory angina were allowed to have urgent PTCA.

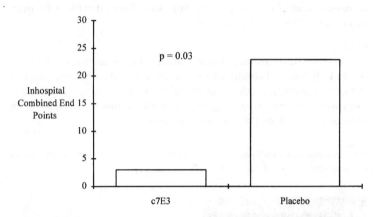

Figure 2-5. The incidence of in-hospital combined end points of death, myocardial infarction, and recurrent ischemia requiring urgent intervention.

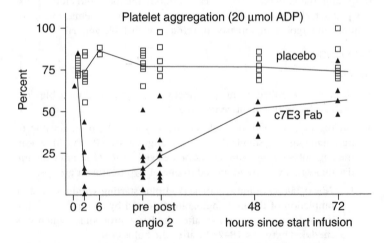

Figure 2-6. Platelet aggregation to 20 μmol adenosine diphosphate in patients receiving c7E3 compared to placebo. (From Simoons et al.,[10] with permission.)

- All patients received nitroglycerin IV 50–200 μg/min, aspirin 250-mg initial dose followed by ≥ 80 mg/day, and heparin IV titrated to maintain the partial thromboplastin time (PTT) 2.0–2.5 × control.
- Other medications were left to the discretion of each physician.

Inclusion. Patients included were 21–75 years old with one or more episodes of angina with associated dynamic ST-T-segment changes despite bed rest and medical treatment with aspirin, IV heparin, and IV nitroglycerin.

Exclusion. The criteria for exclusion were ongoing ischemia requiring immediate intervention, prior PTCA of the same coronary segment within 6 months, Q-wave myocardial infarction within 7 days, women of childbearing potential, recent major trauma or surgery within 6 weeks, bleeding diathesis, or autoimmune disorders.

End Points. The criteria for the combined end point was death, myocardial infarction, and recurrent ischemia requiring urgent intervention.

RESULTS

Treatment with c7E3 produced a trend toward less ischemia during infusion of the study drug compared to placebo (30.0% c7E3 vs. 53.3% placebo, P = 0.06) with no significant difference in the development of ischemia observed after PTCA (30.0% c7E3 vs. 20.0% placebo). Significantly fewer in-hospital combined end points occurred in patients treated with c7E3 compared to placebo (3.0% c7E3 vs. 23% placebo, P = 0.03).

Quantitative coronary analysis showed no significant difference in minimal luminal diameter or reduction in the percentage diameter of stenosis between the two study groups. Platelet function studies in patients receiving c7E3 demonstrated > 90% blockade of glycoprotein IIb/IIIa receptors, > 90% reduction in platelet aggregation to adenosine diphosphate, and a significantly prolonged bleeding time exceeding twice the baseline. There were no differences in bleeding complications between c7E3 and placebo (Figs. 2-5 and 2-6).

CONCLUSIONS

In patients undergoing angioplasty for refractory unstable angina, the use of c7E3 significantly reduced the in-hospital combined incidence of death, myocardial infarction, and recurrent ischemia requiring urgent intervention without increasing bleeding complications compared to placebo.

(Data from Simoons et al.[10]) ∎

Reactivation of Unstable Angina After Abrupt Discontinuation of Heparin: Montreal Heart Institute

PURPOSE

Study the reactivation of unstable angina and the occurrence of myocardial infarction after the discontinuation of heparin in patients during the acute phase of unstable angina.

STUDY DESIGN

General

- 479 patients enrolled in this prospective, randomized, double-blinded, placebo-controlled trial.

- Eligible patients were randomized to one of four treatment groups:

  1. Aspirin/heparin
  2. Aspirin alone
  3. Heparin alone
  4. Placebo

- Aspirin: initial dose of 650 mg given immediately, then 325 mg PO bid.

- Heparin: 5,000-U intravenous (IV) bolus, then continuous infusion of 1,000 U/hr titrated to maintain partial thromboplastin time (PTT) 1.5–2.0 × control.

- Medications other than antiplatelet and anticoagulant drugs were left to the discretion of the treating physician.

- Coronary arteriography was performed a mean of 6 days after enrollment.

- Study medications were discontinued when the patient returned from coronary angiography with the option of further treatment left to the discretion of the treating physician.

- All study medications were stopped abruptly, without tapering.

Inclusion. Patients included were < 75 years old presenting within 24 hr of symptom onset with a history of an accelerating pattern of chest pain occurring at rest or with minimal exertion or chest pain lasting ≥ 20 min. Serum creatine kinase levels were less than twice w the upper limit of normal on admission. Electrocardiogram changes compatible with myocardial ischemia were required.

Exclusion. The criteria for exclusion were the pre-existing use of aspirin, other active platelet drugs, or warfarin; percutaneous transluminal coronary angioplasty within the previous 6 months, coronary artery bypass graft within the past year, identifiable precipitating cause of angina, or contraindications to aspirin or heparin.

End Points. The criteria for end points were death, nonfatal myocardial infarction, and refractory recurrent angina.

RESULTS

Overall reactivation of disease (recurrent unstable angina, myocardial infarction, or both) occurred in 7.2% of patients during the first 96 hr after cessation of the study drugs. There was a significant excess of reactivation events in the heparin alone group (13%) compared to the other three groups combined (5.0% aspirin alone, 4.6% aspirin/heparin, 5.7% placebo, P < 0.01). The reactivation was more likely to be clinically severe (requiring urgent intervention) in the heparin-alone group (11 patients heparin alone vs. 2 patients in the other three groups combined, P < 0.01) and occurred earlier after cessation of study medication in the heparin alone group (9.5 hr in the heparin-alone groups vs. 28 hr in the other three groups combined, P < 0.05). A logistic regression analysis identified therapy with heparin alone as the most powerful predictor of reactivation after cessation of treatment (P = 0.009).

CONCLUSIONS

In patients with acute unstable angina, the abrupt discontinuation of heparin after an average of 6 days of treatment with heparin alone resulted in a significantly higher incidence of reactivation of disease (recurrent unstable angina, myocardial infarction, or both) compared to the other three study groups. This clinical reactivation was not observed when aspirin was administered concurrently with heparin.

(Data from Théroux et al.[11]) ■

References

1. Cairns JA, Gent M, Singer J et al: Aspirin, sulfinpyrazone, or both in unstable angina—results of a Canadian multicenter trial. N Engl J Med 313:1369, 1985
2. Serruys PW, Herrman JR, Simon R et al: A comparison of hirudin with heparin in the prevention of restenosis after coronary angioplasty. N Engl J Med 333:757, 1995

3. Gold HK, Torres FW, Garabedian HD et al: Evidence for a rebound coagulant phenomenon after cessation of a 4 hour infusion of a specific thrombin inhibitor in patients with unstable angina pectoris. J Am Coll Cardiol 21:1039, 1993

4. Freeman MR, Langer A, Wilson RF et al: Thrombolysis in unstable angina: randomized double-blind trial of t-PA and placebo. Circulation 85:150, 1992

5. Nicklas JM, Topol EJ, Kander N et al: Randomized, double-blind, placebo-controlled trial of tissue plasminogen activator in unstable angina. Am J Cardiol 13:434, 1989

6. Théroux P, Quimet H, McCans J et al: Aspirin, heparin, or both to treat acute unstable angina. N Engl J Med 319:1105-11, 1988

7. Lewis DH Jr, Davis JW, Archibald DG et al: Protective effects of aspirin against acute myocardial infarction and death in men with unstable angina: results of a Veterans Administration Cooperative Study. N Engl J Med 309:396-403, 1983

8. Parisi AF, Khuri S, Deupree RH et al: Medical compared with surgical management of unstable angina: 5-year mortality and morbidity in the Veterans Administration Study. Circulation 80:1176-89, 1989

9. Sharma GVRK, Deupree RH, Khuri SF et al: Coronary bypass surgery improves survival in high-risk unstable angina: results of a Veterans Administration Cooperative Study with an 8-year follow-up. Circulation 84(suppl III):III-260-7, 1991

10. Simoons ML, de Boer MJ, van den Brand MJ et al: Randomized trial of a GPIIb/IIIa platelet receptor blocker in refractory unstagle angina. Circulation 89:596-603, 1994

11. Théroux P, Waters D, Lam J et al: Reactivation of unstable angina after the discontinuation of heparin. N Engl J Med 327:141-5, 1992

CHAPTER 3

Antithrombotic Trials

OVERVIEW

The current approach to treatment of coronary thrombosis uses antiplatelet agents, antithrombin agents, and thrombolytic agents. Clinical trials studying thrombolytic agents are discussed in Chapter 1, "Myocardial Infarction Trials." The most widely used antiplatelet agents, aspirin, and more recently, ticlopidine, have proven efficacy in treating ischemic coronary syndromes. Aspirin, however, has some variability in its ability to inhibit platelet function, especially when local catecholamine concentration is increased, which may limit the effectiveness of aspirin in preventing coronary thrombosis. Aspirin acts by inhibiting cyclo-oxygenase-dependent production of thromboxane A_2, a potent activator of platelets. In addition to thromboxane A_2, however, there are many other activators of platelets including serotonin, platelet-activating factor, collagen, thrombin, epinephrine, and adenosine diphosphate (ADP). Since aspirin has no effect on these other platelet activators, many pathways for platelet activation remain intact with aspirin therapy alone (Fig. 3-1).

Glycoprotein IIb/IIIa Receptor Blockers

Recent attention has focused on the glycoprotein (GP) IIb/IIIa integrin, which represents the final common pathway for platelet activation. Inhibiting the GP IIb/IIIa integrin prevents the aggregation of platelets and fibrinogen to form the platelet–fibrin thrombus, regardless of the initiating stimulus for platelet activation. Several GP IIb/IIIa receptor blockers are currently undergoing intense investigation, including c7E3 (monoclonal antibody against the GP IIb/IIIa receptor), Integrelin (cyclic heptapeptide antagonist to the GP IIb/IIIa receptor), and MK-383 (a selective nonpeptide platelet GP IIb/IIIa receptor antagonist).

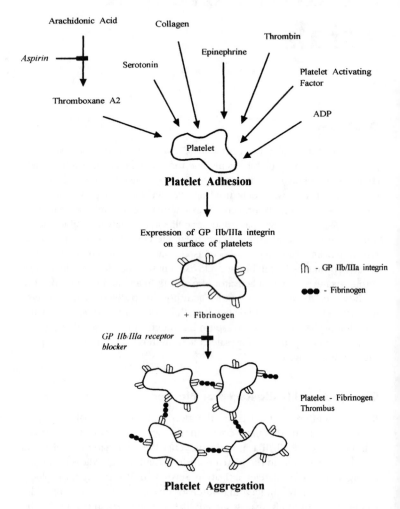

Figure 3-1. Mechanisms of platelet activation.

c7E3

c7E3 is a chimeric monoclonal antibody consisting of a mouse-derived variable region with high affinity for the platelet GP IIb/IIIa integrin linked to a constant region derived from human IgG immunoglobulin. Using a human-derived constant region provides this recombinant antibody with very low immunogenicity. c7E3 potently inhibits platelet adhesion and aggregation to all known platelet agonists with an effective half-life of greater than 6 hours.

The Evaluation of c7E3 for the Prevention of Ischemic Complications (EPIC) trial randomized 2,099 patients undergoing coronary angioplasty at high risk for abrupt vessel closure (within 12 hours of acute myocardial infarction, refractory unstable or postinfarction angina, or high angiographic risk) to treatment with c7E3 bolus plus sustained infusion, c7E3 bolus only, or placebo. All patients received daily aspirin and at least 12 hours of intravenous heparin. At 1-month follow-up, the use of c7E3 bolus plus infusion resulted in a significant 35% reduction in the incidence of ischemic complications compared to placebo. However, the c7E3 bolus plus infusion produced a substantial increase in the incidence of major bleeding at groin puncture sites and in the need for transfusions. The c7E3 bolus-only group demonstrated a nonsignificant trend toward reduced ischemic complications. At 6-month follow-up, a significant 23% reduction in the need for repeat target-vessel revascularization was observed for the c7E3 bolus plus infusion group compared to placebo. This long-term effect of c7E3 raises speculation about a possible role of c7E3 in reducing restenosis.

A small pilot study examined the effect of c7E3 bolus plus infusion compared to placebo in 60 patients undergoing angioplasty for unstable angina.[1] All patients received aspirin, intravenous heparin, and intravenous nitroglycerin. The administration of c7E3 resulted in a trend toward less ischemic events before angioplasty, and a significantly reduced combined incidence of in-hospital deaths, myocardial infarction, and recurrent ischemia requiring urgent intervention after angioplasty compared to placebo. The Chimeric 7E3 Antiplatelet Therapy in Unstable Angina Refractory to Standard Treatment (CAPTURE) trial randomized 1,266 patients with refractory unstable angina scheduled to undergo percutaneous transluminal coronary angioplasty (PTCA) to treatment with c7E3 bolus plus sustained infusion or placebo administered 18 to 24 hours before PTCA and continuing for 1 hour after PTCA. This trial was terminated early because of a significant benefit in the combined end point of death, myocardial infarction, or need for urgent intervention with c7E3 treatment compared to placebo at 30-day follow-up. The final results of CAPTURE should be published in 1996.

The Evaluation of PTCA to Improve Long-Term Outcome by c7E3 GP IIb/IIIa Receptor Blocker (EPILOG) trial evaluated the effect of c7E3 in reducing ischemic complications after low- and high-risk angioplasty. A total of 2,793 patients were randomized to standard-dose heparin and c7E3 bolus plus sustained infusion, low-dose heparin and c7E3 bolus plus sustained infusion, or standard-dose heparin and placebo. This trial was terminated early because of a significant reduction in the combined 30-day end point of death, myocardial infarction, and urgent revascularization in the c7E3 arms. The incidence of "major" bleeds was similar between the c7E3 arms and placebo. The final results of EPILOG should be published in 1996.

Integrelin

Integrelin is a synthetic cyclic heptapeptide antagonist with high affinity and specificity for the platelet GP IIb/IIIa integrin. A bolus plus continuous infusion of Integrelin leads leads to profound reversible inhibition of platglelet aggregation. Compared to c7E3, Integrelin has a much shorter half-life of platelet inhibition, which may allow for a lower incidence of bleeding complications.

The Integrelin to Manage Platelet Aggregation to Prevent Coronary Thrombosis (IMPACT 1) trial randomized 150 patients undergoing elective angioplasty or directional atherectomy to Integrelin bolus plus 4-hour infusion, Integrelin bolus plus 12-hour infusion, or placebo. All patients received aspirin and intravenous heparin. The incidence of ischemic complications (death, nonfatal myocardial infarction, urgent repeat revascularization for refractory ischemia, or stent implantation) was reduced from 12% in the placebo group to 4% in the Integrelin bolus plus 12-hour infusion group, although the difference was not statistically significant. No significant difference in "major" bleeds or intracranial hemorrhage was observed among any group.

The IMPACT 2 trial is currently examining the effect of Integrelin in 4,010 patients undergoing either high-risk or elective angioplasty. Preliminary results at 3-month follow-up demonstrated that Integrelin reduced the combined end point of death, myocardial infarction, or urgent revascularization at 24-hour follow-up but had no significant effect by 30 days.

Six-month angiographic follow-up failed to demonstrate a beneficial effect of Integrelin on restenosis. The final results of IMPACT 2 should be published in 1996.

MK-383

MK-383 (Tirofiban) appears to be well tolerated and is currently undergoing clinical investigations in patients with acute coronary syndromes.

Antithrombins

Fibrinogen acts as an adhesive molecule to bridge the GP IIb/IIIa receptor on activated platelets. Once the fibrinogen–platelet complex begins to form in the acute phase of thrombosis, thrombin converts fibrinogen to fibrin, resulting in a fibrin meshwork, which constitutes an integral structure of the platelet fibrin thrombus. Heparin, along with its cofactor antithrombin III, acts to inhibit activation of factor X, which is responsible for converting inactive prothrombin to active thrombin. By reducing the formation of thrombin, heparin slows the progression of developing thrombus. Disadvantages of heparin, in addition to its dependence on the cofactor antithrombin III, include its inability to inactivate clot-bound thrombin, and its susceptibility to inactivation by heparinase and platelet factor IV.

Direct thrombin inhibitors, which bind to the active catalytic site and to the substrate recognition site of thrombin, include hirudin, hirulog, and argatroban. Because these agents inactivate free circulating and clot-bound thrombin, do not require cofactors, and do not have any known natural inhibitors, they have theoretical advantages over heparin in patients with acute thrombotic coronary syndromes.

Hirudin

The prototype of the direct thrombin inhibitors is hirudin, which was discovered in 1894 from the salivary glands of the European leech, *Hirudo medicinalis*. Hirudin is currently available as a recombinant product that lacks a sulfate residue on tyrosine 63 (desulfatohirudin) but maintains the anticoagulant profile of natural hirudin. Hirudin binds near the active center of thrombin at the substrate recognition site with extraordinary affinity and inhibits all known functions of thrombin. Recombinant hirudin produces the clinical effects of prolonging the activated prothrombin time and especially the thrombin time with an effective half-life of 2 hours in healthy individuals.

The Thrombolysis in Myocardial Infarction (TIMI 5) trial compared the effect of hirudin with heparin in 240 patients with acute myocardial infarction treated with front-loaded tissue plasminogen activator (t-PA) and aspirin. Treatment with hirudin resulted in significantly better coronary flow at the 18- to 36-hour angiography compared to heparin. No significant difference in TIMI grade 3 flow, the primary prespecified end point, was observed at the 90-minute or 18- to 36-hour angiography between the treatment groups. Hirudin also substantially reduced the incidence of reinfarction and produced a trend toward reduced in-hospital mortality. "Major" bleeding events were similar between hirudin and heparin.

The TIMI 6 trial studied the safety profile of hirudin compared with heparin in 193 patients with acute myocardial infarction treated with streptokinase and aspirin. Hirudin was equivalent to heparin regarding the incidence of major hemorrhage and the incidence of "combined unsatisfactory outcomes." No angiographic data were obtained in this trial.

The Hirudin in a European Trial vs. Heparin in the Prevention of Restenosis After PTCA (HELVETICA) trial[2] compared the effect of hirudin with heparin on the prevention of restenosis among 1,141 patients with unstable angina who were scheduled for angioplasty. The administration of hirudin was associated with a significant reduction in early cardiac events compared to heparin. Event-free survival at 7 months and mean minimal luminal diameter at 6-month angiography were not meaningfully different between the treatment groups. Bleeding events were similar among heparin- and hirudin-treated groups. Thus, hirudin reduced early cardiac events, although no substantial reduction in restenosis was observed.

The Global Utilization of Streptokinase and t-PA for Occluded Arteries (GUSTO 2A) and TIMI 9A trials evaluated the effect of hirudin compared with heparin in patients with acute coronary syndromes and as a conjunctive therapy to thrombolytic agents and aspirin in patients with acute myocardial infarction, respectively. Both trials dosed hirudin as a 0.6-mg/kg intravenous bolus followed by a 0.2 mg/kg/hr continuous infusion titrated only if the partial thromboplastin time (PTT) > 150 and heparin as a 5,000-U intravenous bolus followed by weight-adjusted continuous infusions to maintain a PTT of 60 to 90 seconds. Both trials were terminated early because of an excess of intracranial hemorrhage and "major" hemorrhage in the hirudin and heparin groups. These excess bleeding complications were possibly a result of the high levels of anticoagulation obtained by the administered doses of hirudin and heparin. These trials were redesigned as GUSTO 2B and TIMI 9B with lower doses of hirudin (0.1-mg/kg bolus plus 0.1-mg/kg/hr infusion) and heparin (5,000-U bolus plus 1,000 μ/hr without weight adjustment) titrated to maintain a slightly lower PTT of 55 to 85 seconds. The results of GUSTO 2B and TIMI 9B should more clearly define the role of hirudin in acute coronary syndromes.

Hirulog

Hirulog is a 20-amino-acid peptide with structural similarities to the C-terminus and N-terminus of hirudin. Hirulog has a shorter half-life (40 minutes) compared to hirudin because thrombin can slowly cleave a Pro-ARg bond in the hirulog molecule. The mechanism of binding to thrombin and the clinical effects of hirulog are similar to that of hirudin.

The Hirulog Angioplasty Study Investigation (HASI) trial examined the role of hirulog to prevent ischemic complication in 4,098 patients undergoing coronary angioplasty for unstable or postinfarction angina. No significant difference was observed in the incidence of acute or 6-month ischemic complications between hirulog and heparin. However, in the subgroup of patients with postinfarction angina, a meaningful reduction in the incidence of myocardial infarction and combined ischemic complications was observed with hirulog treatment. In addition, treatment with hirulog resulted in significantly fewer transfusions and "major" hemorrhages compared to heparin.

Argatroban

Argatroban is a nonpeptide arginine derivatinve that reversibly binds to the catalytic site of thrombin with intermediate affinity. The effective half-life or argatroban is approximately 30 minutes.

Two clinical trials, the Myocardial Infarction Using Novastan (argatroban) and t-PA (MINT) and Argatroban Myocardial Infarction (AMI) trials are currently in progress.

Conclusions

The most widely used antiplatelet and antithrombin agents, aspirin and heparin, respectively, both have theoretical limitations to their effectiveness in treating coronary ischemic syndromes. New antiplatelet agents, such as the GP IIb/IIIa receptor blockers, have generated intense investigation. c7E3 significantly reduces ischemic complications and the need for repeat target-vessel revascularization compared to placebo (aspirin and heparin) at the expense of increased bleeding events in patients undergoing high-risk angioplasty. c7E3 has also been shown to reduce ischemic complications in patients undergoing low- and high-risk PTCA and in patients with refractory unstable angina. Integrelin has demonstrated the potential to reduce ischemic complications after elective angioplasty but does not appear to reduce 6-month restenosis. MK-383 is being evaluated.

Direct thrombin inhibitors like hirudin, hirulog, and argatroban have potential advantages over heparin in the treatment of thrombotic coronary syndromes. Hirudin may result in improved coronary flow after successful thrombolysis compared to heparin in patients with acute myocardial infarction. In patients with unstable angina undergoing angioplasty, treatment with hirudin reduces early cardiac events but does not reduce 6-month restenosis compared to heparin. At high doses, however, hirudin increases the incidence of intracranial hemorrhage and "major" bleeds. The concern is to find a clinically effective dose of hirudin that does not increase intracerebral hemorrhage risk. Hirulog reduces the incidence of ischemic complications after angioplasty in patients with postinfarction angina. Argatroban is being evaluated but appears to be safe. These new antithrombotic agents are currently being investigated in larger clinical trials to more precisely define their role in the treatment of ischemic coronary syndromes.

EPIC

Evaluation of c7E3 for the Prevention of Ischemic Complications

PURPOSE

Determine the effect of c7E3, a monoclonal antibody Fab fragment directed against the platelet glycoprotein IIb/IIIa integrin, on clinical outcome in patients undergoing high-risk coronary angioplasty.

STUDY DESIGN

General

- 2,099 patients enrolled in this prospective, randomized, double-blinded, placebo-controlled, multicenter trial.

- Eligible patients were randomized to one of three treatment groups:
  1. c7E3 bolus only
  2. c7E3 bolus and infusion
  3. Placebo

     c7E3 bolus: 0.25 mg/kg infused over 5 min at least 10 min before the procedure

     c7E3 infusion: 10 µg/min infused continuously over 12 hr

- All patients were treated with aspirin 325 mg at least 2 hr before the procedure and then daily, and heparin 10,000–12,000 U intravenous (IV) bolus with additional boluses if needed to achieve an activated clotting time (ACT) 300–350 sec during the procedure followed by a continuous infusion to maintain the partial thromboplastin time (PTT) 1.5–2.5 × control for at least 12 hr.

- Vascular sheaths were removed ≥ 6 hr after the end of the c7E3 continuous infusion.

Inclusion. Patients included were < 80 years old scheduled to undergo coronary angioplasty or directional atherectomy if they were considered high risk for abrupt-vessel closure defined as at least one of following criteria:

1. Acute evolving myocardial infarction within 12 hr of symptom onset requiring rescue percutaneous intervention
2. Early postinfarction angina or unstable angina despite medical therapy
3. Clinical or angiographic characteristics indicating high risk according to criteria of the American Heart Association or American College of Cardiology

Exclusion. Criteria for exclusion were bleeding diathesis, major surgery within the previous 6 weeks, or stroke within the previous 2 years.

End Points. The criteria for end points were as follows:

- 1 month: Composite end point of mortality, nonfatal myocardial infarction, coronary artery bypass graft (CABG) or repeat percutaneous intervention for acute ischemia, requirement for endovascular stent because of procedural failure, or placement of an intra-aortic balloon pump (IABP) for refractory ischemia.

- 6 month: Composite end point of mortality, nonfatal myocardial infarction, or CABG or repeat percutaneous intervention for acute ischemia.

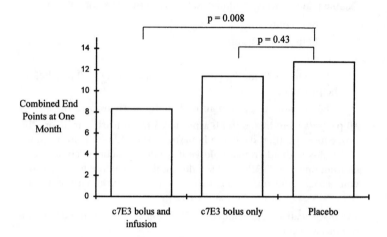

Figure 3-2. A significant reduction in combined end points at 1 month with c7E3 bolus plus infusion compared to placebo.

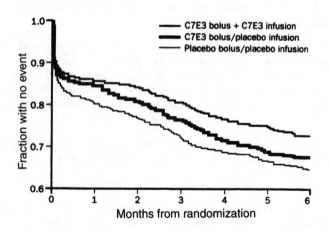

Figure 3-3. Kaplan-Meier curves of combined end points. (From Topol et al.,[4] with permission.)

RESULTS

One-Month Outcome. The use of c7E3 bolus and infusion resulted in a significant reduction in combined end points by 35% compared to placebo (8.3% c7E3 bolus plus infusion vs. 12.8% placebo, P = 0.008). The c7E3 bolus-only group showed a 10% reduction in combined end points, although this difference was not statistically significant (11.4% c7E3 bolus only vs. 12.8% placebo, P = 0.43). This graded effect was also observed for each of the most important individual end points relating to ischemia and nonfatal reinfarction. The use of c7E3 markedly delayed the onset of post-procedure ischemic events and the timing of repeat angioplasty.

Patients treated with c7E3 bolus and infusion had a significantly higher incidence of major bleeding (14% c7E3 bolus plus infusion vs. 7% placebo, P = 0.001) and need for transfusions (15% c7E3 bolus plus infusion vs. 7% placebo, P , 0.001) compared to placebo. No difference was found in the incidence of intracranial hemorrhage between the three groups.

Six-Month Outcome. The use of c7E3 bolus and infusion resulted in a 23% reduction in the combined end points (27.0% c7E3 bolus plus infusion vs. 35.1% placebo, P = 0.001) and a 26% reduction in the need for repeat target-vessel revascularization (16.5% c7E3 bolus plus infusion vs. 22.3% placebo, P = 0.007). The c7E3 bolus-only group was not significantly different from placebo (Figs. 3-2 to 3-4).

CONCLUSIONS

The use of c7E3 bolus and infusion in patients undergoing high-risk angioplasty resulted in a significant reduction in combined end points (mortality, nonfatal reinfarction, emergency CABG or percutaneous transluminal coronary angioplasty (PTCA), and requirement for stent or IABP) but at a cost of significantly more major bleeds and transfusions compared to placebo at 1 month. At 6-month follow-up, c7E3 bolus and infusion significantly reduced the combined end point (mortality, nonfatal reinfarction, or emergency CABG or PTCA) and the need for repeat target-vessel revascularization compared to placebo. The c7E3 bolus-only group was not significantly different from placebo at 1- and 6-month follow-up.

(One-month follow-up data from the Epic Investigators[3]; 6-month follow-up data from Topol et al.[4]) ■

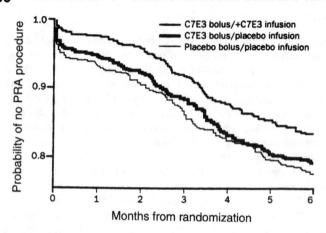

Figure 3-4. Need for subsequent target-vessel revascularization. (From Topol et al.,[4] with permission.)

Evaluation of PTCA to Improve Long-Term Outcome by c7E3 GP IIb/IIIa Receptor Blocker

PURPOSE

Determine the effect of c7E3 in reducing mortality and the incidence of reinfarction in patients undergoing coronary angioplasty or directional atherectomy.

STUDY DESIGN

General.

- 2,793 patients enrolled in this prospective, randomized, placebo-controlled, multicenter trial.
- Eligible patients were randomized to one of three treatment groups:
  1. c7E3 plus standard-dose weight-adjusted heparin
  2. c7E3 plus low-dose weight-adjusted heparin
  3. Placebo plus standard-dose weight-adjusted heparin

Standard-dose weight-adjusted heparin: 100-U/kg intravenous (IV) bolus plus additional boluses titrated to an activated clotting time (ACT) of 300–350 sec, followed by a 10-U/kg/hr continuous infusion during the procedure.

Low-dose weight-adjusted heparin: 70-U/kg IV bolus plus additional boluses titrated to an ACT of 200 sec, followed by a 7-U/kg/hr continuous infusion during the procedure.

- All patients received aspirin.
- Heparin was administered only during the procedure.
- Vascular sheaths were removed when the ACT was < 175 sec during the c7E3 infusion (typically within 6 hr of completion of the procedure).

Inclusion. Patients included were undergoing high- and low-risk coronary angioplasty or atherectomy.

Exclusion. Patients excluded had unstable angina with accompanying electrocardiogram changes or acute myocardial infarction within the preceding 24 hr.

End Points. The criteria for the combined end point were all-cause mortality, myocardial infarction, and urgent revascularization at 30 days.

RESULTS

The Data Safety Monitoring Committee recommended early termination of the trial after analysis of the first 1,500 enrolled patients. Treatment with c7E3 significantly reduced the combined end point of death, myocardial infarction, and urgent revascularization by 53% in the c7E3 plus standard-dose heparin ($P < 0.05$) and by 68% in the c7E3 plus low-dose heparin ($P < 0.05$) compared to placebo (3.8% c7E3 plus standard-dose heparin, 2.6% c7E3 plus low-dose heparin, 8.1% placebo plus standard-dose heparin). Treatment with c7E3 significantly reduced the primary end point in subgroups of patients with high- and low-risk interventions. The incidence of major bleeding episodes was not significantly different between the three treatment groups (3.5% c7E3 plus standard-dose heparin, 1.4% c7E3 plus low-dose heparin, 3.1% placebo plus standard-dose heparin) (Fig. 3-5).

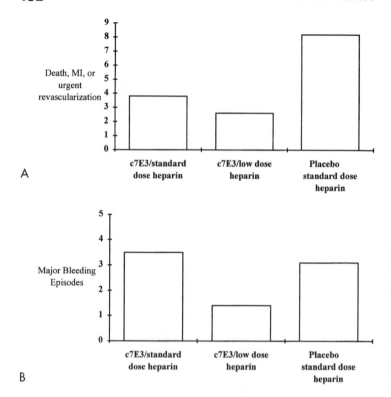

Figure 3-5. (A & B) Significantly reduced combined clinical end point for both c7E3 groups compared to placebo with no significant increase in major bleeding events.

CONCLUSIONS

Among patients undergoing high- and low-risk coronary angioplasty or atherectomy, treatment with c7E3 significantly reduced the combined incidence of death, myocardial infarction, or urgent revascularization without producing an increase in bleeding complications at 30-day follow-up compared to placebo. The use of weight-adjusted low-dose heparin with c7E3 appears to provide the lowest incidence of bleeding complications.

(Data courtesy of James J. Ferguson, M.D.; presented at the 1996 American College of Cardiology Meeting.) ∎

HASI

Hirulog Angioplasty Study Investigators

PURPOSE
Compare the effect of hirulog with heparin on the incidence of ischemic complications in patients undergoing coronary angioplasty for unstable or postinfarction angina.

STUDY DESIGN

General

- 4,098 patients enrolled in this prospective, randomized, double-blinded, multicenter trial.
- Eligible patients were randomized to one of two treatment groups:
  1. Hirulog: 1.0-mg/kg intravenous (IV) bolus, then 2.5-mg/kg infusion over 4 hr, then 0.2-mg/kg infusion over 14–20 hr
  2. Heparin: 175-U/kg IV bolus, then 15-U/kg continuous infusion for 18–24 hr
- Activated clotting time (ACT) was maintained ≥ 350 sec during the procedure in heparin-treated patients.
- Aspirin 300–325 mg was given to all patients.
- Other medical therapy was left to the discretion of each physician.

Inclusion. Patients included were > 21 years old who were urgently scheduled to undergo angioplasty for unstable angina or for postinfarction angina < 2 weeks after myocardial infarction (MI).

Exclusion. Criteria for exclusion were patients scheduled for a staged angioplasty procedure; the use of atherectomy, stents, or laser angioplasty;

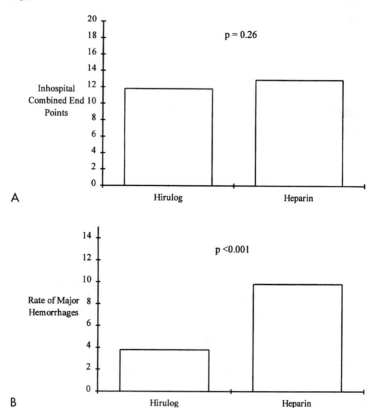

Figure 3-6. (A & B) Similar incidence of in-hospital combined end points. Hirulog therapy resulted in less major bleeding compared to heparin.

contraindication to aspirin or heparin; concern about pregnancy; creatinine > 3.0 mg/dl, or use of thrombolytic therapy within the past 24 hr.

End Points. The criteria for the combined end point were death, MI, abrupt vessel disclosure, emergency coronary artery bypass graft (CABG), the need for intra-aortic balloon pump (IABP), or repeat angioplasty.

RESULTS

No significant difference was observed in the in-hospital combined end point between hirulog and heparin (11.8% hirulog vs. 12.9% heparin, P = 0.26). Specifically, there were similar incidences of in-hospital death, MIs, and emergency CABG. Subgroup analysis of patients with postinfarction angina treated with hirulog revealed a significant reduction in the incidence of MI (2.0% hirulog vs. 5.1% heparin, P = 0.04) and combined end points (9.1% hirulog vs. 14.2% heparin, P = 0.04). In the subgroup of patients with unstable angina without recent MI, there were no significant differences in any of the clinical end points. Treatment with hirulog also resulted in a substantial reduction in the incidence of retroperitoneal hemorrhage (0.2% hirulog vs. 0.7% heparin, P = 0.02), need for transfusion (3.7% hirulog vs. 8.6% heparin, P = 0.02), and major hemorrhage (3.8% hirulog vs. 9.8% heparin, P < 0.001). At 6 months, the incidence of death, MI, repeat revascularization, and clinical restenosis was similar among both treatment groups (Fig. 3-6).

CONCLUSIONS

In patients undergoing urgent angioplasty for unstable angina or postinfarction angina, no significant difference was found in the incidence of acute or 6-month ischemic complications between hirulog and heparin treatment. In the subgroup of patients with postinfarction angina treated with hirulog, a significant reduction in the incidence of MI and combined acute ischemic complications was observed compared with heparin. Hirulog was associated with a significantly lower rate of bleeding.

(Data from Bittl et al.[5]) ■

IMPACT 1

Integrelin to Manage Platelet Aggregation to Prevent Coronary Thrombosis

PURPOSE

Determine if treatment with Integrelin, a synthetic cyclic heptapeptide antagonist to the platelet glycoprotein IIb/IIIa integrin, improves clinical outcome in patients undergoing elective coronary angioplasty or directional coronary atherectomy.

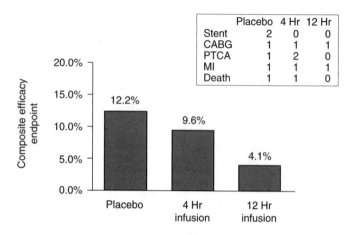

Figure 3-7. Composite outcomes to 30 days. (From Tcheng,[6] with permission.)

STUDY DESIGN

General

- 150 patients enrolled in this prospective, randomized, double-blind, placebo-controlled, multicenter trial.

- Eligible patient were randomized to one of three treatment groups:

  1. Integrelin: bolus of 90 µg/kg, followed by 1.0 µg/kg/min infusion for 4 hr

  2. Integrelin: bolus of 90 µg/kg, followed by 1.0-µg/kg/min infusion for 12 hr

  3. Placebo

- All patients received aspirin 325 mg PO at least 2 hr before the procedure and then daily, heparin 10,000-U bolus to achieve an activated clotting time (ACT) of > 300 sec during the procedure followed by a continuous infusion to maintain a partial thromboplastin time (PTT) of 2.0–3.0 × control.

- Vascular sheaths were removed the following day, 4–6 hr after discontinuation of heparin.

- A subset of patients underwent serial measurements of platelet aggregation studies and bleeding times.

Inclusion. Patients undergoing elective, routine, high- and low-risk percutaneous coronary angioplasty or atherectomy.

Exclusion. The criteria for exclusion were bleeding diathesis, recent gastrointestinal bleeding, major surgery within 6 weeks, history of stroke or other central nervous system structural abnormality, severe hypertension, pregnancy, baseline prothrombin time > 1.2 × control, hematocrit < 30%, platelet count < 100,000/μl, or serum creatinine > 4.0 mg/dl.

End Points. The criteria for composite end point at 30 days follow-up were death, nonfatal myocardial infarction, urgent or emergent coronary intervention, stent implantation, or coronary artery bypass graft (CABG) for ischemia.

RESULTS

The incidence of composite end points at 30 days was 4.1% for the 12-hr infusion of Integrelin, 9.6% for the 4-hr infusion of Integrelin, and 12.2% for placebo, which shows a graded trend toward better clinical outcome

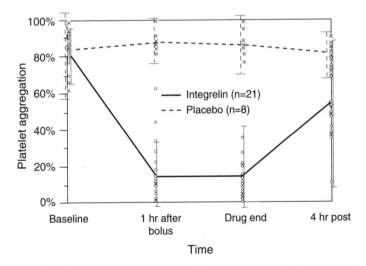

Figure 3-8. Inhibition of platelet aggregation to 20 μmol adenosine diphosphate. (From Tcheng et al.,[6] with permission.)

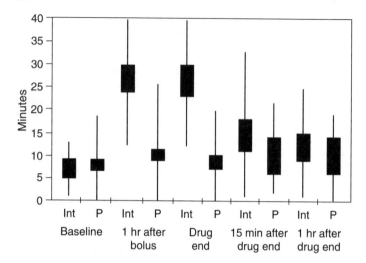

Figure 3-9. Bleeding times after study drug administration demonstrate rapid return to baseline after discontinuation of the drug infusion. (From Tcheng et al.[6] with permission.)

with administration of Integrelin. The results, however, were not statistically significant (4-hr infusion vs. placebo, P = 0.67; 12-hr infusion vs. placebo, P = 0.13). Analysis of angiographic results revealed a significant reduction in coronary dissection with Integrelin (P = 0.015) but no difference in postprocedure stenosis, TIMI grade 1 flow, or acute thrombus formation. Minor bleeding occurred more often with Integrelin (40%) compared to placebo (14%), with no difference in major bleeds or intracranial hemorrhage. Integrelin caused rapid and profound inhibition of platelet function during drug infusion with subtotal recovery at 4 hr after drug infusion (Figs. 3-7 to 3-9).

CONCLUSIONS

In this pilot study, the use of Integrelin, along with aspirin and heparin, in patients undergoing routine, elective percutaneous angioplasty or atherectomy had a favorable trend toward lowering composite end points (death, nonfatal myocardial infarction, repeat intervention, stent, or CABG for refractory ischemia) compared to placebo at 1-month follow-up without an excessive risk of major bleeding.

(Data from Tcheng et al.[6]) ∎

IMPACT 2

Integrelin to Manage Platelet Aggregation to Prevent Coronary Thrombosis

PURPOSE

Determine the effect of Integrelin, a platelet glycoprotein IIb/IIIa receptor antagonist, on reducing ischemic complications in patients undergoing coronary angioplasty or atherectomy.

STUDY DESIGN

General

- 4,010 patients enrolled in this prospective, randomized, double-blinded, placebo-controlled, multicenter trial.
- Eligible patients were randomized to one of three treatment groups:
  1. Low-dose Integrelin: 135-μg/kg intravenous (IV) bolus followed by a continuous infusion of 0.50 μg/kg/min for up to 24 hr
  2. High-dose Integrelin: 135-μg/kg IV bolus followed by a continuous infusion of 0.75-μg/kg/min for up to 24 hr
  3. Placebo
- All patients received aspirin 325 mg before the procedure and weight-adjusted heparin titrated to an activated clotting time (ACT) of 300–350 sec during the procedure.
- Patients were stratified as high-risk (acute myocardial infarction or unstable angina) or as elective at the time of enrollment.

Inclusion. Patients included were undergoing coronary angioplasty or atherectomy.

End Points. The criteria for the combined end point were death, myocardial infarction, or urgent revascularization at 30 days.

RESULTS

At 24-hr follow-up, treatment with Integrelin at both high and low doses significantly reduced the combined primary end point of death, myocardial infarction, and urgent revascularization compared to placebo (7.0% high-dose Integrelin, 6.8% low-dose Integrelin, 9.3% placebo, P < 0.01 for either Integrelin dose vs. placebo). At 30 days follow-up, however, there was no significant difference between the three treatment groups. Angiographic data from 617 patients at baseline and 6 months revealed no difference in minimal luminal diameter or restenosis between Integrelin and placebo treatment. Major bleeding events were similar among the three treatment groups. Clinical follow-up at 6 months for the entire population has not been reported.

CONCLUSIONS

Treatment with Integrelin significantly reduced ischemic complications compared to placebo in patients undergoing coronary angioplasty or atherectomy at 24-hr follow-up. By 30-day follow-up, however, there was no significant difference between Integrelin and placebo treatment, and at 6-month follow-up, there was no difference in the incidence of restenosis.

(Data courtesy of James J. Ferguson, M.D.; presented at the 1995 European Society of Cardiology Meeting.) ∎

References

1. Simoons ML, Jan de Boer M, van der Brand M et al: Randomized trial of a glycoprotein IIb/IIIa platelet receptor blocker in refractory unstable angina. Circulation 89:595, 1994
2. Serruys PW, Herrman JR, Simon R et al: A comparison of hirudin with heparin in the prevention of restenosis after coronary angioplasty. N Engl J Med 333:757, 1995
3. The Epic Investigators: Use of a monoclonal antibody directed against the platelet glycoprotein IIb/IIIa receptor in high-risk coronary angioplasty. N Engl J Med 330:956–61, 1994
4. Topol EJ, Califf RM, Weisman HF et al: Randomised trial of coronary intervention with antibody against platelet IIb/IIIA integrin for reduction of clinical restenosis: results at six months. Lancet 343:881–6, 1994
5. Bittl JA, Strony J, Brinker JA et al: Treatment with bivalirudin (Hirulog) as compared with heparin during coronary angioplasty for unstable or postinfarction angina. N Engl J Med 333:764–9, 1995
6. Tcheng JE, Harrington RA, Kottke-Marchant K et al: Multicenter, randomized, double-blind, placebo-controlled trial of the platelet integrin glycoprotein IIb/IIIa blocker Integrelin in elective coronary intervention. Circulation 91:2151–7, 1995

β-Blocker Trials

OVERVIEW

β-Adrenoreceptor-blocking agents reduce myocardial workload and oxygen consumption through reductions in heart rate, systolic blood pressure, and contractility. The application of β-blockers to ischemic coronary syndromes has therefore generated considerable interest. During the past 30 years, numerous clinical trials have examined the effects of β-blockers in patients with acute myocardial infarction. Earlier trials in the 1960s and 1970s, which were small and used low doses of β-blockers for short follow-up periods, did not clearly show a beneficial effect on total mortality. In the early 1980s, several large well-designed trials conclusively established significant 25% to 40% reductions in overall mortality with the use of β-blockers after myocardial infarction.

Chronic Administration of β-Blockers After Myocardial Infarction

The first large clinical trial to clearly demonstrate a survival benefit for treatment with β-blockers after myocardial infarction was the Goteborg Metoprolol Trial, which evaluated the effect of metoprolol administered immediately in 1,395 patients with suspected myocardial infarction. The use of metoprolol significantly reduced total mortality by 36% at 3 months. Following the results of Goteborg, several other large trials were reported confirming the advantage of β-blockers after myocardial infarction. The β-Blocker Heart Attack Trial (BHAT) randomly assigned 3,837 patients with acute myocardial infarction to treatment with propranolol started 5 to 21 days after admission or placebo. BHAT was terminated early because of the 26% reduction in total mortality observed with propranolol treatment at 25-month follow-up. The Norwegian Timolol Trial randomized 1,884 patients with acute myocardial infarction to treatment with timolol started on day 6 to 27 after admission or placebo. After 33-month follow-up, treatment with timolol reduced total mortality by 40% and the rate of reinfarction by 28% compared to placebo.

These three landmark trials convincingly demonstrated a 25% to 40% decrease in mortality from chronic β-blocker therapy in patients with acute myocardial infarction. The agents used in these trials, propranolol, metoprolol, and timolol, are selective and nonselective β-blockers that do not have intrinsic sympathomimetic activity (ISA). ISA is a partial adrenergic stimulating effect (agonist effect) seen with certain β-blockers. Pooled data on β-blockers with ISA, like practolol and alprenolol, have shown no significant effect on mortality in patients after myocardial infarction.

Immediate Administration of β-Blockers After Myocardial Infarction

The issue of when to initiate β-blockers after myocardial infarction, immediately within hours of admission or after several days, has been studied in clinical trials. The International Study of Infarct Survival (ISIS 1) examined the effects of atenolol administered immediately and continued for 1 week in 16,027 patients with suspected myocardial infarction. The use of atenolol significantly reduced 1-week vascular mortality by 15%, with all of the benefit occurring on day 0 to 1 after myocardial infarction. The Metoprolol in Acute Myocardial Infarction (MIAMI) trial randomized 5,778 patients with suspected myocardial infarction to immediate intravenous metoprolol or placebo. Mortality at 15 days was reduced by 13% with metoprolol treatment, although the difference was not statistically different (P = 0.29). Thus, immediate administration of atenolol or metoprolol to patients with suspected myocardial infarction reduced early mortality by 13% to 15%. The MIAMI trial failed to attain statistical significance, which is likely due to its relatively small number of patients.

ISIS 1 and MIAMI were performed in the early 1980s, before the effects of thrombolytic agents and aspirin were known. As a result, patients did not receive thrombolytic agents, and only 5% received antiplatelet therapy. The Thrombolysis in Myocardial Infarction (TIMI 2B) trial examined the effect of immediate vs. delayed (starting on day 6) administration of metoprolol in 1,434 patients with acute myocardial infarction who were all treated with tissue plasminogen activator (t-PA), aspirin, and heparin. Mortality was virtually identical between the two groups at 6 days (2.4%), 6 weeks (3.4%), and 1 year (4.9).

Immediate treatment with metoprolol did significantly reduce the incidence of nonfatal reinfarction and recurrent ischemia compared to delayed therapy. The disparity between the results of TIMI 2B and the results of ISIS 1 and MIAMI may be due to the difference in the use of thrombolytic agents and aspirin. In ISIS 1 and MIAMI, β-blockers were the only effective therapy received by the patients, and hence a reduction in mortality was observed. In TIMI 2B, the routine use of t-PA and aspirin already provided approximately a 50% reduction in early mortality, such that the additive effects of immediate β-blockade on short-term mortality were negligible.

β-Blockers in Sudden Cardiac Death

Long-term treatment with β-blockers is unequivocally associated with a reduction in the incidence of sudden cardiac death. The BHAT trial demonstrated a 28% reduction in the incidence of sudden cardiac death (P < 0.05) among patients treated with propranolol after myocardial infarction over a 2-year follow-up period. The Goteborg Metoprolol Trial showed a reduction in the in-hospital incidence of ventricular fibrillation (P = 0.03) and the requirement for lidocaine (P < 0.01) among postinfarction patients treated with metoprolol compared to placebo. The Norwegian Propranolol Study demonstrated a 51% reduction in sudden cardiac death (P = 0.04) and a significant reduction in premature ventricular contractions and nonsustained ventricular tachycardia among high-risk survivors of acute myocardial infarction treated with propranolol over a 1-year follow-up period. Finally, in the Norwegian Timolol Trial, sudden cardiac death was reduced by 45% (P = 0.0001) with timolol treatment for 3 years in patients surviving acute myocardial infarction. Thus, chronic administration of select β-blockers to patients after myocardial infarction substantially decreases the incidence of sudden cardiac death.

Conclusions

The benefit of β-blockers, administered to patients after myocardial infarction, has been well documented in randomized clinical trials. Specific agents proven to reduce the risk of recurrent myocardial infarction or death are timolol, metoprolol, propranolol, and atenolol. These agents also substantially decreased the incidence of sudden cardiac death and nonfatal ventricular dysrhythmias. Chronic administration of propranolol, metoprolol, and timolol significantly reduces long-term mortality by 25% to 40% in patients with acute myocardial infarction who do not receive thrombolytic agents or aspirin. The effect of chronically administered β-blockers, used adjunctively with thrombolytic agents and aspirin, has not been clearly evaluated. The immediate administration of metoprolol reduces recurrent ischemia and the risk of nonfatal myocardial infarction, without meaningfully improving survival, compared to delayed therapy in patients treated with t-PA, heparin, and aspirin. β-Blockers with intrinsic sympathomimetic activity, as a class, do not appear to provide a reduction in the incidence of death or reinfarction.

BHAT

β-Blocker Heart Attack Trial

PURPOSE

Determine the effect of propranolol on reducing mortality in patients with acute myocardial infarction.

STUDY DESIGN

General

- 3,837 patients enrolled in this prospective, randomized, double-blinded, placebo-controlled, multicenter trial.

- Eligible patients were randomized 5–21 days after hospital admission for acute myocardial infarction to one of two treatment groups:

  1. Propranolol: 20 mg PO initially, then 40 mg PO every 8 hr for 2 days, with a final dose adjusted to 180 mg or 240 mg/day according to serum levels of propranolol (82% of patients received 180 mg/day)

  2. Placebo

- Other medical therapy was left to the discretion of each physician.

Inclusion. Patients included were men and women from age 30 to 69 who were hospitalized with an acute myocardial infarction documented by appropriate symptoms, electrocardiogram changes, and enzymatic changes.

Exclusion. The criteria for exclusion were contraindications to or clear indications for propranolol, a history of severe congestive heart failure or asthma, previous coronary artery bypass graft, other serious illness, or previous the use of β-blockers at time of enrollment.

End Points. The criterion for end point was total mortality.

RESULTS

BHAT was ended 8 months earlier than scheduled because of the significant benefit of propranolol. At 25.1-month average follow-up, total mor-

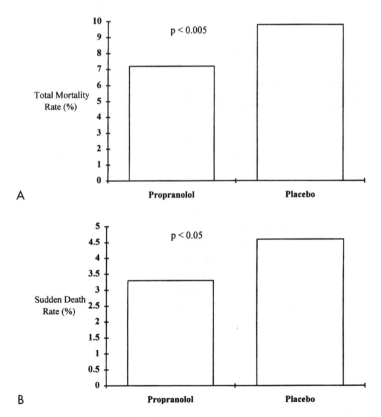

Figure 4-1. *(A & B)* A significant reduction in 2-year mortality and sudden death rate with propanolol therapy compared to placebo.

tality was significantly reduced in the propranolol group by 26% compared to placebo (7.2% propranolol vs. 9.8% placebo, P < 0.005). Cause-specific mortality analysis showed that propranolol significantly reduced mortality that was due to cardiovascular disease (6.6% propranolol vs. 8.9% placebo, P < 0.01), arteriosclerotic heart disease (6.2 propranolol vs. 8.5% placebo, P < 0.01), and sudden death (3.3% propranolol vs. 4.6% placebo, P < 0.05) (Fig. 4-1).

CONCLUSIONS

Propranolol administered 5–21 days after acute myocardial infarction significantly reduced mortality by 26% compared to placebo during the 2-year follow-up period.

(Data from β-Blocker Heart Attack Trial Research Group.[1]) ■

GOTEBORG METOPROLOL TRIAL

PURPOSE

Determine the effect of early administration of metoprolol on mortality in the setting of definite or suspected acute myocardial infarction.

STUDY DESIGN

General

- 1,395 patients enrolled in this prospective, randomized, double-blinded, placebo-controlled, multicenter trial.
- Eligible patients were randomized to one of two treatment groups:
  1. Metoprolol: 5 mg intravenously (IV) q 2 min × 3 (total 15 mg) given immediately, then after 15 min 50 mg PO q 6 hr for 48 hr, then 100 mg PO q 12 hr continued for 90 days
  2. Placebo
- After 90 days, all patients were openly treated with metoprolol if appropriate.
- The use of other medications was left to the discretion of each physician.

Inclusion. Patients included were 40–74 years old with chest pain of acute onset lasting 30 min or electrocardiogram signs of acute myocardial infarction with onset of infarction within the previous 48 hr.

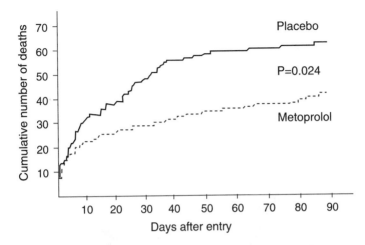

Figure 4-2. Cumulative number of deaths in all patients. (From Hjalmarson et al.,[2] with permission.)

Exclusion. The criteria for exclusion were contraindications to or clear indications for β-blockade, other serious illness, psychiatric disorder, chronic atrial fibrillation, permanent pacemaker, previous coronary artery bypass graft, or the use of calcium channel blockers at entry.

End Points. The criterion for end point was 3-month mortality.

RESULTS

A definite myocardial infarction was confirmed in 58.0% of patients; 42.0% of patients did not meet criteria for myocardial infarction. Metoprolol significantly reduced 3-month mortality by 36% compared to placebo (5.7% metoprolol vs. 8.9% placebo, P < 0.03). This reduction in mortality remained significant in the subgroups of patients aged 40–64 and 65–74 years, patients with confirmed myocardial infarction, patients with or without previous myocardial infarction, and patients with or without chronic β-blockade therapy before entry into the trial. The use of metoprolol also significantly reduced the incidence of ventricular fibrillation (0.9% metoprolol vs. 2.4% placebo, P = 0.033) and the requirement for lidocaine (2.3% metoprolol vs. 5.5% placebo, P < 0.01) (Figs. 4-2 and 4-3).

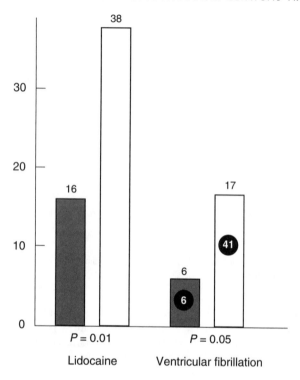

Figure 4-3. Number of patients treated with lidocaine and of patients with ventricular fibrillation according to treatment with metoprolol (hatched bars) or placebo (open bars). (From Rydén et al.,[3] with permission.)

CONCLUSIONS

Metoprolol treatment started immediately after admission and continued for 3 months significantly reduced total mortality by 36% and the incidence of ventricular fibrillation in patients with definite or suspected myocardial infarction at 3 months follow-up compared to placebo.

(Data from Hjalmarson et al.[2] and Rydén et al.[3]) ■

Metoprolol in Acute Myocardial Infarction

PURPOSE

Determine the effects of early administration of metoprolol on short-term (15-day) morbidity and mortality in the setting of acute myocardial infarction.

STUDY DESIGN

General

- 5,778 patients enrolled in this prospective, randomized, double-blinded, placebo-controlled, multicenter trial.
- Eligible patients were randomized to one of two treatment groups:
  1. Metoprolol: 5 mg intravenously (IV) q 2 min × 3 doses administered immediately on arrival to the coronary care unit, then 50 mg PO q 6 hr × 2 days, then 100 mg PO q 12 hr at least through day 15
  2. Placebo
- After 15 days, all patients were openly treated with metoprolol if appropriate.
- Other medical treatment of acute myocardial infarction was left to the discretion of the physician.

Inclusion. Patients included were < 75 years old with chest pain of acute onset at least 15 min in duration occurring within the past 24 hr with a suspicion of myocardial infarction or electrocardiogram (ECG) signs of acute myocardial infarction.

Exclusion. Criteria for exclusion were current treatment with β-blockers or calcium channel blockers, heart rate < 65 bpm, systolic blood pressure < 105 mmHg, left ventricular failure, first-degree atrioventricular block, chronic obstructive pulmonary disease, permanent pacemaker, cardiopulmonary resuscitation, and other serious illness.

End Points. The criteria for end points were 15-day mortality and morbidity.

RESULTS

A definite myocardial infarction was confirmed in 71.4% of patients. Cumulative 15-day mortality was slightly lower in the metoprolol-treated group compared to placebo, although the results were not statistically significant (4.3% metoprolol vs. 4.9% placebo, P = 0.29). A trend toward a lower reinfarction rate was observed with metoprolol treatment (3.0% metoprolol vs. 3.9% placebo, P = 0.08). There was no significant difference in the incidence of ventricular fibrillation or ventricular tachycardia requiring electrical cardioversion between metoprolol and placebo. In a retrospective subgroup analysis, metoprolol significantly reduced 15-day mortality by 29% in a high-mortality risk group defined as three or more of the following: age > 60 years, abnormal ECG at entry, history of previous myocardial infarction, angina pectoris, congestive heart failure, hypertension, diabetes, and chronic or acute treatment with diuretics of digoxin before randomization (6.0% metoprolol vs. 8.5% placebo, P = 0.033). Metoprolol did result in less need for antianginal medications, less supraventricular tachycardia, and less use of digoxin and other antiarrhythmics (Figs. 4-4 and 4-5).

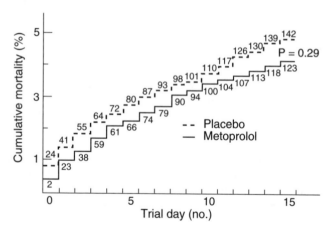

Figure 4-4. Cumulative mortality rate in all patients. (From The Miami Trial Research Group,[4] with permission.)

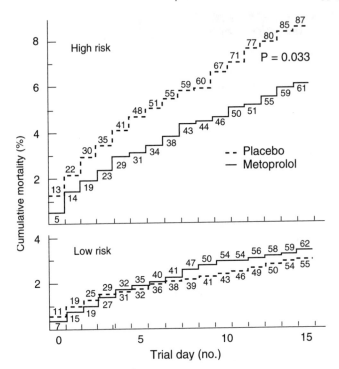

Figure 4-5. Cumulative mortality rates in low- and high-risk groups. (From The Miami Trial Research Group,[4] with permission.)

CONCLUSIONS

Early administration of metoprolol to patients with acute myocardial infarction produced a trend toward a lower 15-day mortality and reinfarction rate compared to placebo, although the results were not statistically significant. The incidence of ventricular fibrillation or ventricular tachycardia requiring cardioversion were similar between metoprolol and placebo. Metoprolol did result in less supraventricular tachycardia, need for antianginal medications, and use of digoxin and other antiarrhythmics.

(Data from The Miami Trial Research Group.[4])   ∎

NORWEGIAN PROPRANOLOL STUDY

PURPOSE

Determine the effect of propranolol on sudden cardiac death at 1 year in high-risk patients surviving acute myocardial infarction.

STUDY DESIGN

General

- 560 patients enrolled in this prospective, randomized, double-blinded, placebo-controlled trial.

- Eligible patients were randomized within 4–6 days after acute myocardial infarction to one of two treatment groups:

  1. Propranolol: 40 mg PO qid continued for 1 year
  2. Placebo

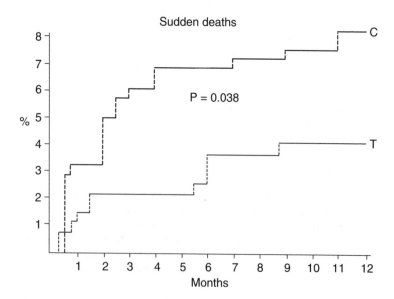

Figure 4-6. The incidence of sudden cardiac death in propranolol vs. control groups. C, control; T, treatment. (From Hansteen,[5] with permission.)

• Other medical therapy was left to the discretion of each physician.

Inclusion. Patients included were 35–70 years old with definite acute myocardial infarction diagnosed by World Health Organization criteria who were at high risk of sudden cardiac death defined as follows:

> Group 1: patients treated for ventricular fibrillation, prolonged ventricular tachycardia, or asystole
>
> Group 2: patients treated for ventricular tachycardia of short duration or complex premature ventricular contraction (PVC), new-onset atrial fibrillation or flutter, persistent sinus tachycardia (heart rate > 120 bpm), or left ventricular failure

Exclusion. Patients excluded had severe heart failure (cardiogenic shock or pulmonary edema) and general contraindications to or clear indications for β-blocker therapy.

End Points. The criteria for end points were sudden cardiac death at 1 year and total mortality and nonfatal reinfarction.

RESULTS

The incidence of sudden cardiac death at 1-year follow-up was significantly lower in the propranolol group compared to the placebo group (4.0% pro-

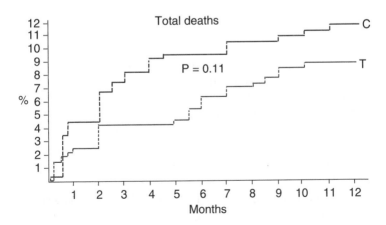

Figure 4-7. The total mortality rate in propranolol vs. control groups. C, control; T, treatment. (From Hansteen,[5] with permission.)

pranolol vs. 8.2% placebo, P = 0.038). Total mortality (9.0% propranolol vs. 13.1% placebo, P = 0.11) and nonfatal reinfarction rates (5.7% propranolol vs. 7.5% placebo, P = not significant) showed a trend in favor of propranolol treatment, but these results were not statistically significant. Propranolol significantly reduced the incidence of complex PVC and short runs of ventricular tachycardia during the first 4 days of treatment (9.8% propranolol vs. 36.6% placebo, P < 0.01) and also produced a favorable trend of reducing complex PVC at 2 months (Figs. 4-6 and 4-7).

CONCLUSIONS

Treatment with propranolol for 1 year after a recent myocardial infarction in selected high-risk patients significantly reduced the risk of sudden cardiac death by 52% and produced a trend toward lower total mortality compared to placebo.

───────────

(Data from Hansteen.[5]) ∎

NORWEGIAN TIMOLOL TRIAL

PURPOSE

Determine the effect of timolol on mortality in patients surviving acute myocardial infarction.

STUDY DESIGN

General

- 1,884 patients enrolled in this prospective, randomized, double-blinded, placebo-controlled trial.
- Patients who were clinically stable from day 6–27 after acute myocardial infarction were randomly assigned to one of two treatment groups:
  1. Timolol: started 7–28 days after the myocardial infarction given as 5 mg PO bid for 2 days, then 10 mg PO bid
  2. Placebo
- Other medical therapy was left to the discretion of each physician.
- Clinical follow-up every 6 months.

Inclusion. Patients included were 20–75 years old with acute myocardial infarction diagnosed by at least two of the following:

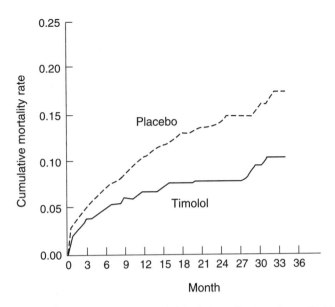

Figure 4-8. Life-table cumulated rates of death from all causes. (From The Norwegian Multicenter Study Group,[6] with permission.)

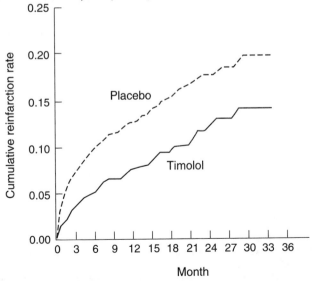

Figure 4-9. Life-table cumulated rates of first reinfarction. (From The Norwegian Multicenter Study Group,[6] with permission.)

1. Central anterior chest pain of more than 15-min duration, acute pulmonary edema, or cardiogenic shock
2. Electrocardiogram (ECG) changes with development of pathologic Q waves or ST-segment elevation followed by T-wave inversion in at least two leads
3. Two separate aspartate aminotransferase (AST) values increased above upper normal limits or one such value accompanied by an elevated lactic dehydrogenase level

Exclusion. Criteria for exclusion were contraindication to β-blockade on the day of enrollment; concurrent other serious illness; clear indication for β-blockade; any indication for antiarrhythmics; lipid-lowering agents, salicylates, or anticoagulants expected to be continued for more than 3 months.

End Points. The criterion for end point was total mortality at 33 months.

RESULTS

Cumulative mortality rates at 33 months were 10.6% for timolol and 17.5% for placebo, demonstrating that timolol significantly reduced mortality by 39.4% (P = 0.0005). The use of timolol also significantly reduced the rate of sudden cardiac death (7.7% timolol vs. 13.9% placebo, P = 0.0001) and the rate of reinfarction (14.4% timolol vs. 20.1% placebo, P = 0.0006) at 33 months compared to placebo (Figs. 4-8 and 4-9).

CONCLUSIONS

Long-term treatment with timolol in patients surviving acute myocardial infarction significantly reduced total mortality by 39.4%, sudden death by 44.6%, and the rate of reinfarction by 28.4% compared to placebo during a 33-month follow-up period.

(Data from The Norwegian Multicenter Study Group.[6])   ■

References

1. β-Blocker Heart Attack Trial Research Group: A randomized trial of propranalol in patients with acute myocardial infarction. I. Mortality results. JAMA 247:1707–14, 1982
2. Hjalmarson A, Elmfeldt D, Herlitz J et al: Effect on mortality of metroprolol in acute myocardial infarction: a double-blind randomised trial. Lancet 2:823–7,

1981
3. Rydén L, Ariniego R, Arnman K et al: A double-blind trial of metoprolol in acute myocardial infarction: effects on ventricular tachyarrhythmias. N Engl J Med 308:614-8, 1983
4. The MIAMI Trial Research Group: Metoprolol in acute myocardial infarction (MIAMI): a randomised placebo-controlled international trial. Eur Heart J 6:199-266, 1985
5. Hansteen V: Beta blockade after myocardial infarction: the Norwegian Propranolol Study in high-risk patients. Circulation 67(suppl. I):57-60, 1983
6. The Norwegian Multicenter Study Group: Timolol-induced reduction in mortality and reinfarction in patients surviving acute myocardial infarction. N Engl J Med 304:801-7, 1981

CHAPTER 5

Calcium Channel Blocker Trials

OVERVIEW

Calcium is an obligatory intracellular cation required for initiating actin–myosin interactions leading to muscular contraction and for propagating action potentials used for electrical conduction. Calcium channel blockers act by slowing calcium transport into the cell. In the cardiovascular system, verapamil, and to a lesser extent diltiazem, decrease myocardial contractility and slow conduction through the sinoatrial and atrioventricular nodes. Diltiazem also causes coronary smooth muscle relaxation leading to coronary vasodilatation. Nifedipine has potent vasodilator effects, resulting in reduced systemic vascular resistance and coronary vasodilatation, without negative inotropic effects. Since calcium channel blockers, as a class, reduce afterload and contractility, thereby reducing oxygen demand, and increase coronary flow, thereby increasing oxygen supply, their application to ischemic coronary syndromes has generated considerable interest. In addition, agents that reduce afterload, like nifedipine and amlodipine, have potential use in the treatment of left ventricular dysfunction and regurgitant valvular disease.

Calcium Channel Blockers in Ischemic Heart Disease

The Danish Group on Verapamil in Myocardial Infarction Trial (DAVIT) studied the effect of verapamil on survival and the incidence of reinfarction in patients with acute myocardial infarction. The DAVIT 1 trial, which randomized approximately 3,500 patients with acute myocardial infarction to immediate administration of verapamil or placebo, revealed no significant difference in total mortality or the incidence of reinfarction between the two treatment groups at 12-month follow-up. The use of verapamil, however, was associated with an increased incidence of heart failure and atrioventricular block. The DAVIT 2 trial examined the effect of late administration of verapamil in patients with acute myocardial infarction. Among the 1,800 patients randomized to verapamil or placebo starting on day 7 to 15 after myocardial infarction, there was no significant difference in 18-month mortality or the incidence of reinfarction. However, in a retrospective analysis, the subgroup of patients without heart failure who were treated with verapamil had a significant 34% reduction in mortality and a 26% reduction in the incidence of reinfarction at 18 months.

The Diltiazem Reinfarction Study (DRS) randomized 576 patients with non-Q-wave myocardial infarction to early treatment with diltiazem or placebo. The use of diltiazem significantly reduced the incidence of reinfarction by 51% compared to placebo at 14-day follow-up. No difference was observed in total mortality of the incidence of postinfarction angina. The Multicenter Diltiazem Postinfarction Trial (MDPIT) examined the effect of diltiazem administration to patients after acute myocardial infarction. The use of diltiazem among all patients resulted in no significant difference in mortality or cardiac events compared to placebo at 25-month follow-up. The effect of diltiazem appeared to depend on the presence of pulmonary congestion. In the subgroup of patients without pulmonary congestion, treatment with diltiazem reduced mortality and cardiac events compared to placebo, whereas in patients with pulmonary congestion, diltiazem increased mortality and cardiac events.

The Secondary Prevention Reinfarction Israeli Nifedipine Trial (SPRINT) examined the effect of nifedipine in patients with acute myocardial infarction. SPRINT 1, which administered nifedipine or placebo from days 7 to 21 after myocardial infarction to 2,200 patients, and SPRINT 2, which administered nifedipine or placebo immediately to 1,000 patients with acute myocardial infarction, both revealed no significant difference in mortality or the incidence of reinfarction at 8-month follow-up. SPRINT 2 was terminated early due because of a trend toward increased mortality with use of nifedipine.

Thus, treatment with verapamil, diltiazem, or nifedipine after myocardial infarction does not reduce overall mortality. Retrospective analyses suggest that verapamil and diltiazem may be beneficial in patients without pulmonary congestion. Diltiazem reduces the incidence of recurrent myocardial infarction in patients with non-Q-wave myocardial infarction.

Meta-analysis of Short-Acting Nifedipine in Ischemic Heart Disease

Data from the SPRINT trials and several other randomized trials have raised a suspicion of increased mortality with the use of short-acting nifedipine in patients with ischemic heart disease. To help clarify this issue, Furberg et al.[1] performed a meta-analysis examining the dose-related effect of nifedipine on mortality in patients with coronary heart disease. Data were analyzed from 16 randomized secondary prevention clinical trials to include approximately 8,350 patients. Twelve trials examined patients after myocardial infarction, three trials included patients with unstable angina, and one trial included patients with stable angina. Overall, the use of nifedipine was associated with a statistically significant increase in mortality (risk ratio = 1.6, 95% confidence interval [CI] 1.01–1.33). Further analysis according to the administered daily dose of nifedipine revealed a dose–response relationship to mortality. For daily doses of 30 to 50 mg, the relative risk for total mortality was 1.06 (95% CI 0.89–1.27), whereas for daily doses of 60 and 80 mg, the relative risks were 1.18 (95% CI 0.93–1.50) and 2.83 (95% CI 1.35–5.93), respectively (Fig. 5-1).

Postulated mechanisms for the increase in mortality associated with use of large doses of relatively short-acting nifedipine include proischemic effects associated with tachycardia and hypotension, possible proarrhythmic effects, and potential prohemorrhagic effects that are due to the antiplatelet and vasodilatory properties of nifedipine. Held and Yusuf[2] and Yusuf et al.[3] have reported similar increases in mortality in separate meta-analyses of trials of short-acting nifedipine.

Nifedipine in Regurgitant Valvular Heart Disease

The use of afterload-reducing agents in asymptomatic patients with severe aortic regurgitation has generated considerable interest. Vasodilator therapy with nifedipine has been shown to be superior to hydralazine in this population of patients due to a greater reduction in left ventricular volume, increase in ejection fraction, and reduction in left ventricular mass at 12-month follow-up. Scognamiglio et al. reported the long-term effects of nifedipine compared to digoxin on the incidence and timing of aortic valve replacement (AVR) in asymptomatic patients with severe aortic regurgitation and normal ejection fraction. Over a 6-year follow-up period, the use of nifedipine reduced the need for AVR by 56%, as only 15% of

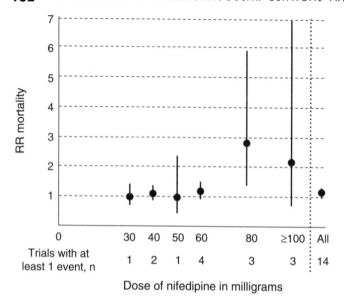

Figure 5-1. Mortality risk according to the daily dose of nifedipine. (From Furberg et al.,[1] with permission.)

patients treated with nifedipine required AVR compared to 34% of patients treated with digoxin who required AVR (P < 0.001). In addition, the rate of progression to AVR was significantly slower with use of nifedipine compared to digoxin. The effect of other vasodilators, such as angiotensin-converting enzyme inhibitors, in asymptomatic patients with severe aortic regurgitation or severe mitral regurgitation needs to be evaluated in randomized clinical trials.

Calcium Channel Blockers in Congestive Heart Failure

The use of calcium channel blockers in the treatment of patients with congestive heart failure is common practice. In the Studies of Left Ventricular Dysfunction (SOLVD) trials, which enrolled 6,800 patients with a left ventricular ejection fraction (LVEF) less than 35%, approximately 30% of patients were being treated with calcium channel blockers at the time of enrollment. However, from the results of clinical trials, first-generation calcium channel blockers appear to have no beneficial effect and may actually worsen symptoms and increase mortality in patients with congestive heart failure. Long-term nifedipine therapy has been shown to increase pulmonary capillary wedge pressure, worsen symptoms, and increase hospitalizations for congestive heart failure in two small randomized trials.[4,5] The Multicenter Diltiazem Postinfarction Trial (MDPIT) demonstrated that treatment with diltiazem increased the incidence of "cardiac events" among the subgroup of patients with pulmonary congestion after myocardial infarction compared to placebo. Furthermore, treatment with diltiazem increased the development of chronic heart failure among patients with acute pulmonary congestion, anterolateral Q-wave myocardial infarction, and reduced left ventricular function (LVEF less than 40%). Treatment with verapamil in patients with congestive heart failure after acute myocardial infarction resulted in no significant improvement in mortality compared to placebo in the DAVIT trials.

Second-generation agents, like nicardipine, amlodipine, and felodipine, which have pure vasodilator effects with negligible negative inotropic effects, may have an advantage over the first-generation agents. Nicardipine, however, was shown in a small randomized trial of patients with moderate-to-severe congestive heart failure concurrently treated with captopril to worsen symptoms of congestive heart failure in 60% of patients compared to 20% of patients receiving placebo.[6] The PRAISE and Veterans Administration Cooperative Vasodilator–Heart Failure (VHEFT 3) trials are currently in progress, evaluating the effects of amlodipine and felodipine, respectively, in patients with congestive heart failure.

Conclusions

The use of verapamil or diltiazem in patients with acute myocardial infarction did not reduce mortality or the incidence of reinfarction. A subgroup of patients after myocardial infarction without evidence of left ventricular dysfunction may derive a reduction in mortality with use of these agents. Diltiazem appears to reduce the risk of reinfarction after non-Q-wave myocardial infarction. The administration of nifedipine to patients after myocardial infarction produced a trend toward increased mortality with no reduction in the incidence of reinfarction. Meta-analyses examining the effect of nifedipine in patients with ischemic heart disease have revealed a significant increase in total mortality with use of short-acting nifedipine, especially when the daily dose exceeds 60 mg. In asymptomatic patients with severe aortic regurgitation and normal left ventricular function, the chronic administration of nifedipine significantly delays and reduces the need for aortic valve replacement compared to digoxin therapy over a 6-year follow-up period. First-generation calcium channel blockers provide no beneficial effects and appear to be detrimental in patients with congestive heart failure. The effect of second-generation agents with pure vasodilatory properties, such as amlodipine and felodipine, are currently being examined in large clinical trials of patients with congestive heart failure.

DAVIT 1

Danish Study Group on Verapamil in Myocardial Infarction

PURPOSE
Determine the effect of early administration of verapamil on total mortality and rate of reinfarction in patients with acute myocardial infarction.

STUDY DESIGN

General

- 3,498 patients enrolled in this prospective, randomized, double-blinded, placebo-controlled, multicenter trial.
- Eligible patients were randomized to one of two treatment groups:
  1. Verapamil: 0.1 mg/kg intravenously (IV) and 120 mg PO immediately after admission to the coronary care unit, then 120 mg PO tid for 6 months
  2. Placebo
- Other medical therapy was left to the discretion of each physician.

Inclusion. Patients included were < 75 years old with verified acute myocardial infarction by history, electrocardiogram changes, and serum enzyme elevation according to World Health Organization criteria.

Exclusion. The criteria for exclusion were cardiogenic shock, systolic blood pressure < 90 mmHg, heart failure, cardiac arrest before admission,

PR interval > 300 msec, second- and third-degree atrioventricular block, sinoatrial block, heart rate < 45 bpm, QRS interval > 110 msec, valvular or congenital heart disease, treatment with calcium antagonists or β-blockers on admission, or serious other illness.

End Points. The criteria for end points were total mortality and reinfarction.

RESULTS

No significant difference in total mortality was observed between verapamil and placebo at 12-month follow-up (15.2% verapamil vs. 16.4% placebo, P = NS). The incidence of reinfarction was similar among verapamil and placebo treatments (7.0% verapamil vs. 8.3% placebo, P = NS). Treatment with verapamil was associated with a significantly increased incidence of heart failure and atrioventricular block; however, the incidence of atrial fibrillation was significantly reduced (Fig. 5-2).

CONCLUSIONS

Verapamil administered early and continued for 6 months after acute myocardial infarction had no benefit in reducing 12-month total mortality or the incidence of reinfarction compared to placebo.

(Data from The Danish Study Group on Verapamil in Myocardial Infarction.[7]) ■

DAVIT 2

Danish Study Group on Verapamil in Myocardial Infarction

PURPOSE

Determine the effect of late administration of verapamil on total mortality and major events (death or reinfarction) in patients with acute myocardial infarction.

STUDY DESIGN

General

- 1,775 patients enrolled in this prospective, randomized, double-blinded, placebo-controlled, multicenter trial.

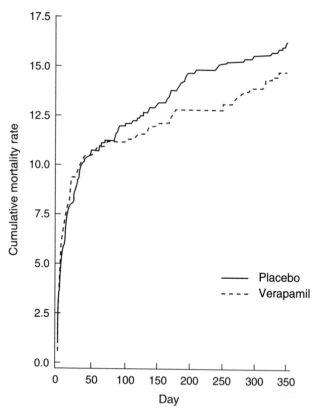

Figure 5-2. Cumulative mortality rate for verapamil and placebo groups. (From The Danish Study Group on Verapamil in Myocardial Infarction,[7] with permission.)

- Eligible patients were randomized between 7 and 15 days after acute myocardial infarction to one of two treatment groups:
    1. Verapamil: 120 mg PO tid continued for 12–18 months
    2. Placebo
- Other medical therapy was left to the discretion of each physician.

Inclusion. Patients included were < 76 years old with verified acute myocardial infarction by history, electrocardiogram changes, and serum enzyme elevation according to World Health Organization criteria.

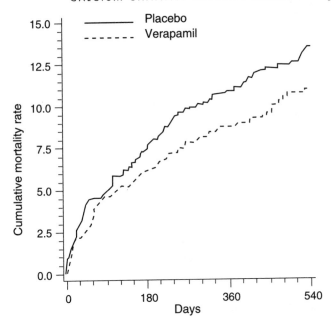

Figure 5-3. Cumulative mortality rate for verapamil and placebo groups. (From The Danish Study Group on Verapamil in Myocardial Infarction,[8] with permission.)

Exclusion. The criteria for exclusion were heart failure not stabilizing even with furosemide ≤ 160 mg/day, systolic blood pressure < 90 mmHg, second- or third-degree atrioventricular block or sinoatrial block after day 3, treatment with calcium antagonists or β-blockers, contraindication to calcium antagonists, or other serious illness.

End Points. The criteria for end points were total mortality and major events (death and reinfarction).

RESULTS

After 18-month follow-up, no significant difference in total mortality was observed between verapamil and placebo treatment (11.1% verapamil vs. 13.8% placebo, P = 0.11). Verapamil did significantly reduce the incidence of reinfarction compared to placebo (11.0% verapamil vs. 13.2% placebo, P = 0.04). The subgroup of patients without heart failure treated with verapamil had significant reductions in total mortality (7.8% verapamil vs. 11.8% placebo, P = 0.02) and first reinfarction (9.4% verapamil vs. 12.7% placebo, P = 0.02) (Fig. 5-3).

CONCLUSIONS

Late administration of verapamil in patients with acute myocardial infarction had no significant effect on total mortality but did significantly reduce the incidence of reinfarction by 17% compared to placebo over the 18-month follow-up period. The subgroup of patients without heart failure treated with verapamil had significant reductions in both total mortality and reinfarction compared to placebo.

(Data from The Danish Study Group on Verapamil in Myocardial Infarction.[8]) ■

DRS

Diltiazem Reinfarction Study

PURPOSE

Determine the effect of diltiazem on the incidence of reinfarction in patients with non-Q-wave myocardial infarction.

STUDY DESIGN

General

- 576 patients enrolled in this prospective, randomized, double-blinded, placebo-controlled, multicenter trial.
- Eligible patients were randomized to one of two treatment groups:
  1. Diltiazem: titration up to 90 mg PO q 6 hr started within 1–3 days of randomization and continued for up to 14 days
  2. Placebo
- Concurrent treatment with other calcium channel blockers was prohibited.
- Other medical therapy was left to the discretion of each physician.

Inclusion. Patients included were < 75 years with an acute non-Q-wave myocardial infarction documented by elevated MB creatine kinase and ischemic chest pain ≥ 30-min duration or new ST-segment elevation or depression of ≥ 0.1 mV or T-wave inversion.

Exclusion. The criteria for exclusion were Q-wave myocardial infarction, conduction disturbance that would mask the development of Q-waves, heart rate < 50 bpm, second- or third-degree atrioventricular block, cardiogenic shock or systolic blood pressure < 100 mmHg, coronary artery bypass graft within 3 months, or other serious illness.

End Points. The criteria for end points were reinfarction, recurrent angina, and mortality during the 14-day treatment period.

RESULTS

The use of diltiazem significantly reduced the incidence of reinfarction by 51% compared to placebo at 14-day follow-up (6.3% diltiazem vs. 12.9% placebo, P = 0.003). No significant difference was observed in the incidence of postinfarction angina (41% diltiazem vs. 44% placebo, P = not significant [NS]) or total mortality (3.8% diltiazem vs. 3.1% placebo, P = NS) (Fig. 5-4).

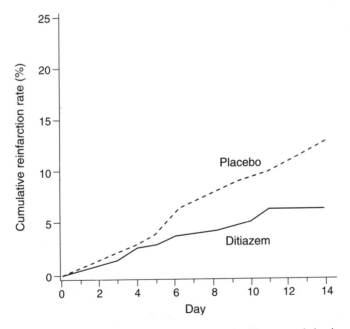

Figure 5-4. Life table cumulative reinfarction rates for diltiazem and placebo groups. (From Gibson et al.,[9] with permission.)

CONCLUSIONS

Treatment with diltiazem significantly reduced the incidence of reinfarction compared to placebo in patients with non-Q-wave myocardial infarction at 14-day follow-up. Diltiazem treatment had no significant effect on postinfarction angina or total mortality.

(Data from Gibson et al.[9]) ■

MDPIT

Multicenter Diltiazem Postinfarction Trial

PURPOSE

Determine the effect of diltiazem on reducing mortality and reinfarction in patients after acute myocardial infarction.

STUDY DESIGN

General

- 2,466 patients enrolled in this prospective, randomized, double-blinded, placebo-controlled, multicenter trial.
- Eligible patients were randomized between days 3 and 15 after acute myocardial infarction to one of two treatment groups:
  1. Diltiazem: initial dose of 60 mg PO qid, but dosage could be reduced to bid schedule if deemed necessary
  2. Placebo
- Other medical therapy was left to the discretion of each physician.
- Baseline chest x-ray, radionuclide ventriculography, and Holter monitor were obtained.

Inclusion. Patients included were 25–75 years old and within 15 days of an acute myocardial infarction.

Exclusion. The criteria for exclusion were cardiogenic shock or symptomatic hypotension, pulmonary hypertension with right ventricular failure, second- or third-degree atrioventricular block, heart rate < 50 bpm,

Wolff-Parkinson-White syndrome, likely need for coronary artery bypass graft, clear indication for or contraindication to diltiazem, or other serious illness.

End Points. The criteria for end points were total mortality, cardiac mortality, and nonfatal reinfarction.

RESULTS

Total mortality was similar among patients treated with diltiazem and placebo at a mean 25-month follow-up (13.4% diltiazem vs. 13.5% placebo, P = NS). No significant difference in cardiac events (death and nonfatal reinfarction) was observed between diltiazem and placebo. A subgroup of patients with pulmonary congestion treated with diltiazem

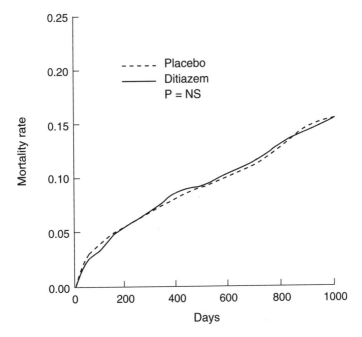

Figure 5-5. Cumulative total mortality rate for diltiazem and placebo groups. (From The Multicenter Diltiazem Postinfarction Trial Research Group,[10] with permission.)

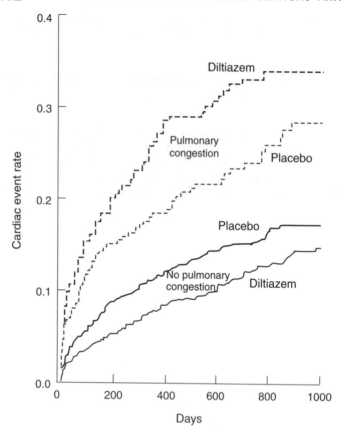

Figure 5-6. Cumulative rate of first recurrent cardiac event according to treatment in patients with and without pulmonary congestion. (From The Multicenter Diltiazem Postinfarction Trial Research Group,[10] with permission.)

had higher cumulative rates of mortality and cardiac events than placebo; whereas patients without pulmonary congestion treated with diltiazem had lower rates of mortality and cardiac events compared to placebo (Figs. 5-5 and 5-6).

CONCLUSIONS

The use of diltiazem after acute myocardial infarction did not reduce total mortality or cardiac events (death and reinfarction) compared to placebo at 25-month follow-up. A retrospective subgroup analysis of patients without pulmonary congestion had lower rates of mortality and cardiac events with diltiazem compared to placebo.

(Data from The Multicenter Diltiazem Postinfarction Trial Research Group.[10]) ■

NIFEDIPINE IN AORTIC REGURGITATION

Nifedipine in Asymptomatic Patients With Severe Aortic Regurgitation and Normal Left Ventricular Function

PURPOSE

Compare the effects of nifedipine with digoxin on delaying and reducing the need for aortic valve replacement (AVR) in asymptomatic patients with severe aortic regurgitation and normal left ventricular function.

STUDY DESIGN

General

- 143 Patients enrolled in this prospective, randomized trial.
- Patients were randomized to one of two treatment groups:
    1. Nifedipine: 20 mg PO bid
    2. Digoxin: 0.25 mg PO qd
- All measurements of left ventricular function and severity of aortic regurgitation were made by echocardiography, which was repeated every 6 months.
- Severity of aortic regurgitation (AR) was graded by the ratio of the height of the regurgitant jet to the diameter of the left ventricular outflow tract in the parasternal long axis view (45%–60% graded as 3+ AR, > 65% graded as 4+ AR).
- Criteria for AVR replacement were
    1. Development of left ventricular ejection fraction (LVEF) < 50% confirmed by a repeat echocardiogram 1 month later

2. Development of symptoms defined as an increase to New York Heart Association functional class II or higher, the development of angina, or both

3. Left ventricular dilatation defined as an increase in the left ventricular end-diastolic volume index (LVEDVI) by $\geq$ 15% confirmed by repeat echocardiogram 1 month later

- The use of an angiotensin-converting enzyme inhibitor was not allowed.

Inclusion. Patients included were asymptomatic, with isolated chronic severe aortic regurgitation (grade 3+ or 4+) and normal left ventricular systolic function with LVEF $\geq$ 50%.

Exclusion. The criteria for exclusion were patients with recent development or worsening of aortic regurgitation (within 6 months); diastolic blood pressure > 90 mmHg; history of coronary artery disease; mixed aortic stenosis with valve gradient $\geq$ 20 mmHg and aortic regurgitation; other valvular or congenital heart disease; LVEF < 50% by echocardiogram; or poor-quality echocardiographic images.

End Points. The criteria for end points were AVR and timing of AVR over 6 years.

RESULTS

The causes of severe aortic regurgitation were rheumatic (61%), bicuspid aortic valve (22%), and aortic valve prolapse (17%). The rate of progression to AVR was significantly lower in the nifedipine group at all times after the first year of follow-up. At 2 years, there were no valve replacements in the nifedipine group compared to a 9% incidence of valve replacement in the digoxin group. At 6-year follow-up, treatment with nifedipine significantly reduced the need for AVR by 56% compared to treatment with digoxin (15% AVR with nifedipine vs. 34% AVR with digoxin, P < 0.001). At the end of follow-up or at the time of AVR, the use of nifedipine substantially reduced the LVEDVI (112 ml/M^2 nifedipine vs. 140 ml/M^2 digoxin, P = 0.003), reduced the left ventricular end-systolic volume index (51 ml/M^2 nifedipine vs. 56 ml/M^2 digoxin, P = 0.004), reduced the left ventricular mass (108 g/M^2 nifedipine vs. 142 g/M^2 digoxin, P = 0.002) and increased the LVEF (62% nifedipine vs. 58% digoxin, P = 0.03) compared to digoxin therapy (Fig. 5-7).

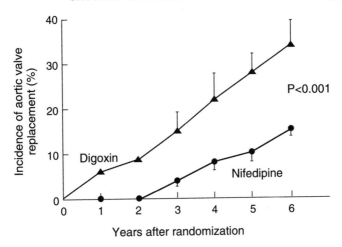

Figure 5-7. Cumulative incidence of progression to aortic valve replacement in nifedipine and placebo groups. (From Scognamiglio et al.,[11] with permission.)

CONCLUSIONS

In asymptomatic patients with chronic severe aortic regurgitation and normal LVEF, treatment with nifedipine significantly delayed and reduced the need for AVR compared to treatment with digoxin at 6-year follow-up. Nifedipine therapy decreased left ventricular dilatation and left ventricular mass and improved left ventricular function.

(Data from Scognamiglio et al.[11]) ■

SPRINT 1

Secondary Prevention Reinfarction Israeli Nifedipine Trial

PURPOSE

Determine the effect of nifedipine on reducing mortality and morbidity in patients with acute myocardial infarction.

STUDY DESIGN

General

- 2,276 patients enrolled in this prospective, randomized, double-blinded, placebo-controlled multicenter trial.

- Eligible patients were randomized between days 7 and 21 after acute myocardial infarction to one of two treatment groups:

  1. Nifedipine: 30 mg PO daily continued for 1 year
  2. Placebo

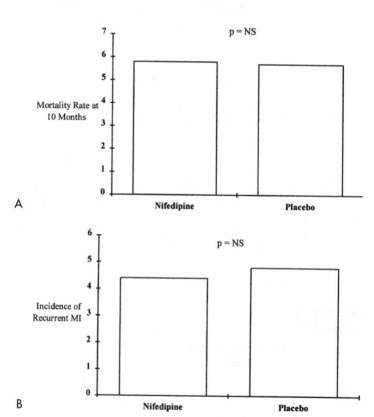

Figure 5-8. *(A & B)* Bar graphs showing no difference in 10-month mortality rate or incidence of recurrent myocardial infarction in nifedipine and placebo groups.

- Other medical therapy was left to the discretion of each physician.

Inclusion. Patients included were 30–74 years of age and within 3 weeks of an acute myocardial infarction.

Exclusion. The criteria for exclusion were clear indication or contraindication to calcium antagonist, Prinzmetal's variant angina, noncoronary heart disease, previous cardiac surgery or pacemaker implantation, severe pulmonary hypertension, uncontrollable severe congestive heart failure preceding the myocardial infarction, persistent hypotension with systolic blood pressure < 90 mmHg, left bundle branch block, Wolff-Parkinson-White syndrome, previous stroke, or other serious illness.

End Points. The criteria for end points were total mortality and nonfatal recurrent myocardial infarction.

RESULTS
During the average 10-month follow-up, total mortality rates were similar between nifedipine and placebo (5.8% nifedipine vs. 5.7% placebo, P = not significant [NS]). No significant difference in the incidence of nonfatal recurrent myocardial infarction was observed between nifedipine and placebo (4.4% nifedipine vs. 4.8% placebo, P = NS) (Fig. 5-8).

CONCLUSIONS
Nifedipine (30 mg daily) administered prophylactically to survivors of acute myocardial infarction had no significant effect on reducing mortality or recurrent myocardial infarction compared to placebo at 10-month follow-up.

(Data from The Israeli Sprint Study Group.[12]) ∎

SPRINT 2

Secondary Prevention Reinfarction Israeli Nifedipine Trial

PURPOSE
Determine the effect of early administration of nifedipine on reducing mortality in patients with suspected acute myocardial infarction (MI).

STUDY DESIGN

General

- 1,006 patients enrolled in this prospective, randomized, double-blinded, placebo-controlled multicenter trial.
- Eligible patients were randomized to one of two treatment groups:
  1. Nifedipine: initiated usually within 3 hr of hospital admission with dosage individually titrated up to 60 mg/day PO by day 6 continued for 6 months
  2. Placebo
- Other medical therapy was left to the discretion of each physician.

Inclusion. Patients included were 50–79 years of age with typical anginal pain at rest lasting $\geq$ 20 min with or without diagnostic electrocardiogram changes for acute (MI). Any one of the following high-risk indicators had to be present by day 4 in order for the patient to be continued in the long-term phase: previous MI, anginal syndrome during previous month, history of hypertension, New York Heart Association functional class $\geq$ 2, anterior site of presenting MI, maximal lactic dehydrogenase $\geq$ 3 $\times$ upper limits of normal.

Exclusion. The criteria for exclusion were a clear indication or contraindication to calcium antagonist, noncoronary heart disease, previous cardiac surgery or pacemaker implantation, left bundle branch block or Wolff-Parkinson-White syndrome, persistent hypotension with systolic blood pressure < 90 mmHg, or other serious illness.

End Points. The criteria for end points were total mortality and nonfatal recurrent MI.

RESULTS

The Data Monitoring Board recommended early termination of the study after 8 months. Total mortality rates among all enrolled patients revealed a nonsignificant trend toward higher mortality with nifedipine compared to placebo (18.7% nifedipine vs. 15.6% placebo). The subgroup of patients considered to be high risk had similar mortality rates with nifedipine and placebo (9.5% nifedipine vs. 9.3% placebo). Subgroup

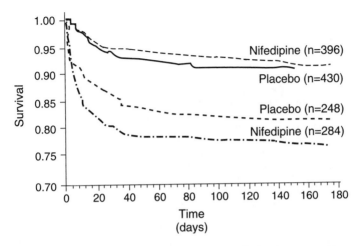

Figure 5-9. Kaplan-Meyer survival curves for 826 high-risk patients with myocardial infarction whle receiving study medication (top two curves) and 532 patients discontinuing medication during the 4-day titration period (bottom two curves.) (From Goldbourt et al.,[13] with permission.)

analysis according to the presence or absence of congestive heart failure did not reveal any significant benefit for nifedipine. No difference in the incidence of nonfatal recurrent MI (4.4% nifedipine vs. 4.8% placebo) or incidence of anginal attacks (36.0% nifedipine vs. 34.8% placebo) was observed between nifedipine and placebo (Fig. 5-9).

CONCLUSIONS

The early administration of nifedipine (60 mg daily) to patients with suspected high-risk acute MI resulted in no significant improvement in overall mortality, incidence of recurrent MI, or incidence of angina during an 8-month follow-up period.

(Data from Goldbourt et al.[13]) ■

References

1. Furberg CD, Psaty BM, Meyer JV: Nifedipine: dose-related increase in mortality in patients with coronary heart disease. Circulation 92:1326, 1995

2. Held PH, Yusuf S: Calcium antagonists in the treatment of ischemic heart disease: myocardial infarction. Coron Artery Dis 5:21, 1994
3. Yusuf S, Held PH, Furberg C: Update of effects of calcium antagonists in myocardial infarction or angina in light of the second Danish Verapamil Infarction Trial (DAVIT II) and other recent studies. Am J Cardiol 67:1295, 1991
4. Elkayam U, Amin J, Mehra A et al: A prospective, randomized, double-blind, crossover study to compare the efficacy and safety of chronic nifedipine therapy with that of isosorbide dinitrate and their combination in the treatment of chronic congestive heart failure. Circulation 82:1954, 1990
5. Agostone PG, DeCesane N, Doria E et al: Afterload reduction: a comparison of captopril and nifedipine in dilated cardiomyopathy. Br Heart J 55:391, 1986
6. Gheorghiade M, Hall V, Goldberg D et al: Long-term clinical and neurohormonal effects of nicardipine in patients with severe heart failure on maintenance therapy with angiotensin converting enzyme inhibitors. J Am Coll Cardiol 17(suppl.A):274A, 1991
7. The Danish Study Group on Verapamil in Myocardial Infarction: Verapamil in acute myocardial infarction. Eur Heart J 5:516-28, 1984
8. The Danish Study Group on Verapamil in Myocardial Infarction: Effect of verapamil on mortality and major events after acute myocardial infarction (The Danish Verapamil Infarction Trial II—DAVIT II). Am J Cardiol 66:779-85, 1990
9. Gibson RS, Boden WE, Théroux P et al: Diltiazem and reinfarction in patients with non-Q-wave myocardial infarction: results of a double-blind, randomized, multicenter trial. N Engl J Med 315:423-9, 1986
10. The Multicenter Diltiazem Postinfarction Trial Research Group: The effect of diltiazem on mortality and reinfarction after myocardial infarction. N Engl J Med 319:385-92, 1988
11. Scognamiglio R, Rahimtoola SH, Fasoli G et al: Nifedipine in asymptomatic patients with severe aortic regurgitation and normal left ventricular function. N Engl J Med 331:689-94, 1994
12. The Israeli Sprint Study Group: Secondary Prevention Reinfarction Israeli Nifedipine Trial (SPRINT): a randomized intervention trial of nifedipine in patients with acute myocardial infarction. Eur Heart J 9:354-64, 1988
13. Goldbourt U, Behar S, Reicher-Reiss H et al: Early administration of nifedipine in suspected acute myocardial infarction: the Secondary Prevention Reinfarction Israel Nifedipine Trial 2 Study. Arch Intern Med 153:345-53, 1993

CHAPTER 6

Congestive Heart Failure Trials

OVERVIEW

Heart failure is a clinical syndrome characterized by effort intolerance, dyspnea, fluid retention, and decreased longevity that is physiologically related to an identifiable abnormality of cardiac function. Effort intolerance results from an inadequate cardiac output that fails to meet the metabolic demands of the body. Fluid retention results from heart failure in which abnormalities in ventricular performance cause elevated left and/or right atrial pressures resulting in pulmonary congestion and/or dependent edema. Heart failure can be further differentiated as right vs. left sided, low output vs. high output, or systolic vs. diastolic dysfunction. Patients with severely impaired left ventricular systolic function have substantially increased mortality risks that correlate with the degree of left ventricular failure (i.e., left ventricular ejection fraction [LVEF]) and severity of congestive symptoms (i.e., New York Heart Association functional class) (Fig. 6-1).

Low cardiac output results in inadequate tissue perfusion, which leads to several compensatory mechanisms aimed at restoring perfusion to vital organs. In the kidneys, the juxtaglomerular apparatus responds to hypoperfusion and low tubular flow by increasing secretion of renin. Elevated plasma renin leads to increased production of angiotensin II, a potent vasoconstrictor, and increased secretion of aldosterone, a mineralocorticoid, which causes sodium retention. Tissue hypoperfusion also produces greatly enhanced catecholamine levels due to norepinephrine release from the sympathetic nervous system and epinephrine secretion from the adrenal medulla. Finally, the posterior pituitary gland increases secretion of arginine vasopressin (AVP) as a response to increased serum

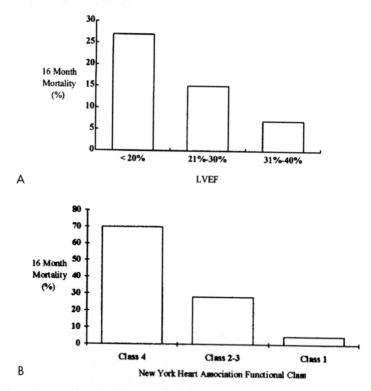

Figure 6-1. The effect of *(A)* LVEF and *(B)* New York Heart Association functional class on 16-month survival in patients with congestive heart failure.

angiotensin II and perhaps as a result of decreased sensitivity of atrial stretch receptors, which normally inhibit AVP release. The increased serum AVP causes potent vasoconstriction and water retention. Collectively, these compensatory mechanisms should act to increase contractility, increase systemic vascular resistance, and increase sodium and water retention. In the normal heart, these actions increase cardiac output and systolic blood pressure, thereby restoring tissue perfusion. In the failing heart, however, these actions may lead to a decrease in cardiac output (due to elevated systemic vascular resistance), development of congestive symptoms (which is due to sodium and water retention), and potential stimulation of fatal dysrhythmias (which is possibly due to high serum cate-cholamines).

Vasodilator Therapy in Congestive Heart Failure

The use of vasodilators to decrease systemic vascular resistance and thereby increase cardiac output has generated considerable interest in the treatment of patients with congestive heart failure. The Veterans Administration Cooperative Vasodilator–Heart Failure Trial (VHEFT 1) was the first large randomized trial to study the effects of vasodilators in patients with left ventricular systolic dysfunction. A total of 642 patients with predominantly New York Heart Association (NYHA) functional class III and IV congestive heart failure were randomized to treatment with combination hydralazine-isosorbide dinitrate, prazosin (an α_1-adrenergic antagonist), or placebo. During a 2.3-year follow-up, treatment with hydralazine-isosorbide dinitrate significantly reduced mortality by 23% compared to placebo. Prazosin therapy had no sustained beneficial effect.

The Cooperative North Scandinavian Enalapril Survival Study (CONSENSUS 1) reported the results of enalapril therapy in patients with severe congestive heart failure (NYHA IV) shortly after VHEFT 1 was published. This trial was terminated early by the Ethical Review Committee, due to the substantial 31% reduction in mortality observed with enalapril treatment compared to placebo at 12-month follow-up. The reduction in mortality with enalapril was due to reduced progression of heart failure. Improvement in NYHA functional class occurred in 42% of patients receiving enalapril therapy.

VHEFT 2 compared enalapril with combination hydralazine-isosorbide dinitrate in patients with chronic congestive heart failure. At 2-year follow-up, treatment with enalapril significantly reduced mortality by 28% compared to hydralazine-isosorbide dinitrate therapy. The mortality reduction with enalapril therapy persisted throughout the study; however, at the 5-year end point, the difference was not statistically different from the hydralazine-isosorbide group.

The Studies of Left Ventricular Dysfunction (SOLVD) examined the effect of enalapril on mortality in patients with LVEFs less than 35% who were symptomatic (treatment trial) and in those who were asymptomatic (prevention trial). The treatment trial, which enrolled 2,569 patients, demonstrated a significant 11% reduction in mortality and a 30% reduction in the incidence of hospitalization for congestive heart failure with enalapril treatment compared with placebo over a 41-month follow-up. The prevention trial, which enrolled 4,228 patients, demonstrated that treatment with enalapril significantly reduced the development of clinical congestive heart failure by 31% and the incidence of hospitalization for congestive heart failure compared to placebo. No significant difference in mortality was observed between the two treatment groups in the asymptomatic population.

The Hydralazine vs. Captopril in Advanced Heart Failure (HY-C) trial examined the effect of captopril compared to hydralazine in patients referred for cardiac transplantation. This population of patients had severe congestive heart failure with a mean LVEF of 20% and an NYHA functional class IV in 80% of patients. Survival at 1 year for patients treated with captopril was 81%, which was significantly better than the 51% survival rate for hydralazine treatment. The survival benefit of captopril occurred mostly in patients with pulmonary capillary wedge pressures greater than 16 mmHg. Captopril also reduced the incidence of sudden cardiac death compared to hydralazine.

The effect of angiotensin-converting enzyme (ACE) inhibitors in patients with impaired left ventricular function after myocardial infarction has been studied in the Acute Infarction Ramipril Efficacy (AIRE) trial, the Survival and Ventricular Enlargement (SAVE) trial, and the Trandolapril Cardiac Evaluation (TRACE) trial.[1] The AIRE trial—which examined the effect of ramipril compared to placebo administered 3 to 10 days after myocardial infarction in 2,006 patients with clinical congestive heart failure—demonstrated a significant 27% reduction in mortality with ramipril therapy over a 15-month follow-up. The SAVE trial evaluated the effect of captopril compared to placebo administered 3 to 16 days after myocardial infarction in 2,231 patients with impaired LVEFs less than 40% but without clinical heart failure. Treatment with captopril significantly reduced mortality by 20%, the need for hospitalizations for congestive heart failure, and the incidence of reinfarction compared to placebo over a 42-month follow-up period. The TRACE trial randomized 1,750 patients with left ventricular failure (LVEF less than 35%) 3 to 7 days after myocardial infarction to trandolapril or placebo. Treatment with trandolapril produced a significant reduction in overall mortality, cardiovascular mortality, sudden cardiac death, and the development of severe congestive heart failure compared to placebo over a 4-year follow-up.

Collectively, these trials demonstrate the substantial beneficial effects of afterload-reducing agents in patients with impaired left ventricular function. Specifically, treatment with ACE inhibitors significantly reduces mortality, slows the progression of symptoms, prevents the development of symptoms in asymptomatic patients, and reduces the need for subsequent hospitalization for the treatment of congestive heart failure. Combination hydralazine-isosorbide dinitrate therapy also reduces total mortality but is not as effective as ACE inhibitors.

Digoxin in Congestive Heart Failure

Although digoxin has been used for more than two centuries, its role in the treatment of congestive heart failure has been controversial. The Randomized Assessment of Digoxin on Inhibitors of the Angiotensin Converting Enzyme (RADIANCE) trial examined the effect of withdrawal of digoxin from patients with chronic congestive heart failure who were clinically stable while receiving digoxin, diuretics, and an ACE inhibitor. One hundred seventy eight patients were randomly separated into a group that continued digoxin therapy or a group that had digoxin withdrawn for placebo. The withdrawal of digoxin for 3 months significantly worsened the clinical severity of heart failure, the patients' subjective assessment of their progress, and the LVEF and left ventricular end-diastole dimension compared to patients continued on digoxin. The effect of withdrawal of digoxin on mortality could not be assessed, because of the small size and short follow-up of this study.

The Prospective Randomized Study of Ventricular Failure and the Efficacy of Digoxin (PROVED) trial[2] was performed with identical methodology to RADIANCE, except the 88 enrolled patients were not receiving ACE inhibitors. Patients withdrawn from digoxin therapy developed decreased exercise tolerance, an increased incidence of treatment failures, and a lower LVEF compared to patients continuing to receive digoxin. These two withdrawal trials provide evidence for a beneficial effect of digoxin therapy on functional status in patients with congestive heart failure.

A recently completed trial by Gorlin and Garg et al.[3] reported the effects of digoxin on mortality in patients with congestive heart failure and normal sinus rhythm. A total of 7,788 patients with symptoms of congestive heart failure and LVEF less than 45% were randomly assigned to treatment with digoxin or placebo. Patients were also treated with diuretics and ACE inhibitors if indicated. The mean LVEF was 32%, with 84% of patients in NYHA functional class III or IV. During a mean follow-up of 37 months, overall mortality was essentially identical between digoxin- and placebo-treated patients. Thus, treatment with digoxin in patients with congestive heart failure improves functional status and LVEF but does not significantly improve survival.

β-Blockers in Congestive Heart Failure

The use of β-blockers in patients with congestive heart failure has been perceived to be contraindicated because of the negative inotropic properties of these agents. However, recent understanding of the interactions of the neuroendocrine system in patients with left ventricular failure has focused attention on the potential benefit of β-blockers in congestive heart failure. Patients with left ventricular failure have high circulating levels of catecholamines, particularly norepinephrine, which are induced by low cardiac output and tissue hypoperfusion. It is hypothesized that high levels of norepinephrine cause cardiac muscle β-receptor downregulation. A paucity of β-receptors makes the heart less responsive to the positive inotropic effects of catecholamines, which may result in blunted left ventricular function. In addition, high levels of catecholamines may precipitate harmful ventricular dysrhythmias, which might be attenuated with β-blocker therapy.

The Metoprolol in Dilated Cardiomyopathy (MDC) trial randomized 383 patients with symptomatic idiopathic dilated cardiomyopathy and LVEF less than 40% already optimally treated with digoxin, diuretics, and ACE inhibitor to treatment with metoprolol or placebo. The majority of patients had NYHA II (45%) or III (49%) functional capacity. The addition of metoprolol significantly reduced the need for heart transplantation and significantly improved LVEF, hemodynamics, exercise capacity, and NYHA functional class compared to placebo over an 18-month follow-up period. Treatment with metoprolol did not meaningfully reduce overall mortality

The. U.S. Carvedilol Heart Failure Study Group has reported the effect of carvedilol, a new type of vasodilator β-blocker with antioxidant properties, in 1,052 patients with congestive heart failure. Patients were required to have NYHA functional class II to IV and an LVEF less than 35%. After 25-month follow-up, this trial was terminated early by the Data Safety Monitoring Board. Treatment with carvedilol significantly reduced total mortality by 65%. This improvement in survival was consistent among the subgroups of patients with NYHA functional class II, III, and IV, ischemic cardiomyopathies, and nonischemic cardiomyopathies.

In other trials, carvedilol has been shown to improve the quality of life and NYHA functional class, increase the LVEF, and reduce the incidence of worsening congestive heart failure compared to placebo.

Myocarditis

Myocarditis is a condition in which an inflammatory process involves the heart, often leading to left ventricular dysfunction. The major causes of myocarditis include infectious disorders, most commonly viruses, drugs, autoimmune disorders, metabolic disorders, transplant rejection, and idiopathic processes. The use of immunosuppressive agents has been controversial; most published reports are retrospective or anecdotal, studying small numbers of patients. The Myocarditis Treatment Trial (MTT) examined the effect of immunosuppressive therapy in 111 patients with histologically proven myocarditis and an LVEF less than 45%. The treatment arms consisted of azathioprine and prednisone, cyclosporine and prednisone, and control. Over a 2-year follow-up, the use of immunosuppressive agents produced no significant benefit on LVEF or mortality compared to control. Although this trial did not reveal an advantage to immunosuppressive therapy, a larger scale randomized clinical trial would be helpful to definitively prove or disprove the benefit of immunosuppression in patients with myocarditis.

Inotropic Agents

The chronic administration of positive inotropic agents, like phosphodiesterase inhibitors and β_2-receptor agonists, has been evaluated in clinical trials. The Prospective Randomized Milrinone Survival Evaluation (PROMISE) trial randomized 1,088 patients with severe congestive heart failure despite conventional therapy to treatment with milrinone or placebo. Over a 6-month follow-up, the use of milrinone significantly increased mortality by 25% compared to placebo, prompting early termination of the trial. The Prospective Randomized Flosequinan Longevity Evaluation (PROFILE) trial[4] reported similar results of increased mortality with the use of flosequinan in patients with heart failure. Smaller trials using other phosphodiesterase inhibitors like indolidan and imazodan have reported no beneficial effects.[5,6] The chronic administration of β-agonists like dobutamine or isoproterenol also appears to increase mortality.[7,8] Collectively, these trials demonstrate that chronic stimulation of a failing heart with positive inotropic agents may be harmful.

Conclusions

Normal compensatory mechanisms to low cardiac output and tissue hypoperfusion may be harmful to the failing heart in the long term. Vasodilator therapy with ACE inhibitors or combination hydralazine-isosorbide dinitrate significantly reduces mortality in symptomatic patients with congestive heart failure. ACE inhibitors provide better clinical outcomes compared to combination hydralazine-isosorbide dinitrate. Furthermore, ACE inhibitors reduce the progression to congestive heart failure and the need for hospitalizations in asymptomatic patients with impaired LVEF. The use of ACE inhibitors in patients with impaired LVEF after myocardial infarction also substantially reduces mortality and the need for hospitalization for congestive heart failure compared to placebo. The withdrawal of digoxin from stable patients with congestive heart failure worsens the NYHA functional classification, the patients' subjective assessment of their progress, and LVEF compared to patients continuing on digoxin therapy. Chronic digoxin therapy in patients with congestive heart failure and normal sinus rhythm does not appear to prolong survival. In selected patients with congestive heart failure, metoprolol improves exercise capacity and NYHA functional class without significantly affecting mortality. Carvedilol reduces overall mortality and improves NYHA functional class, LVEF, and quality of life in patients with congestive heart failure. Immunosuppressive therapy in patients with myocarditis and impaired LVEF appear to offer no clinical benefit, but larger trials are needed to assess the role of immunosuppression definitively in myocarditis. The chronic administration of inotropic agents appears to increase mortality in patients with congestive heart failure.

AIRE

Acute Infarction Ramipril Efficacy Study

PURPOSE

Determine the effect of ramipril on mortality in patients with clinical congestive heart failure after acute myocardial infarction.

STUDY DESIGN

General

- 2,006 patients enrolled in this prospective, randomized, double-blind, placebo-controlled, multicenter trial.
- Eligible patients were randomized from day 3 to 10 after acute myocardial infarction to one of two treatment groups:
  1. Ramipril: initial dose of 2.5 mg PO bid for 2 days, then titrated up to 5 mg PO bid
  2. Placebo
- Patients could receive any medication by their physician except other ACE inhibitors.
- Clinical heart failure after acute myocardial infarction could be transient and not necessarily present at the time of randomization.

Inclusion. Patients included were > 18 years old admitted to the coronary care unit with a definite Q-wave or non-Q-wave acute myocardial infarction and clinical evidence of heart failure at any time after the index myocardial infarction. Randomization occurred between day 3–10 after the myocardial infarction.

Exclusion. The criteria for exclusion were severe heart failure (New York Heart Association functional class IV), heart failure of primary valvular or congenital cause, unstable angina, or contraindications to angiotensin-converting enzyme inhibitor therapy.

End Points. The criteria for end points were total mortality with the combined end point of death, progression to severe resistant heart failure, reinfarction or stroke.

RESULTS

During the average 15-month follow-up, total mortality was significantly reduced by 27% with use of ramipril compared to placebo (17% ramipril vs. 23% placebo, P = 0.002). Ramipril also substantially reduced the combined end point (death, reinfarction, stroke, or resistant heart failure) by 19% compared to placebo (28% ramipril vs. 34% placebo, P = 0.008) (Fig. 6-2).

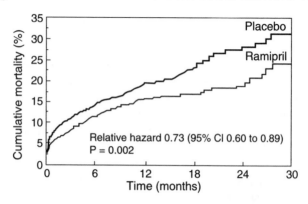

Figure 6-2. Cumulative all-cause mortality for ramipril and placebo groups. (From The Acute Infarction Ramipril Efficacy [AIRE] Study Investigators,[9] with permission.)

CONCLUSIONS

Ramipril, administered on the third to tenth day after acute myocardial infarction to patients with clinical evidence of heart failure, resulted in a significant 27% reduction in total mortality compared to placebo during a 15-month follow-up period.

(Data from The Acute Infarction Ramipril Efficacy [AIRE] Study Investigators.[9]) ■

CARVEDILOL HEART FAILURE STUDY GROUP

PURPOSE

Determine the effect of carvedilol, a vasodilatory β-blocker with antioxidant properties, on survival and the risk of hospitalization for cardiovascular causes in patients with chronic heart failure.

STUDY DESIGN

General

- 1,094 patients enrolled in this prospective, randomized, double-blind, placebo-controlled, multicenter trial.

- Eligible patients were randomized to one of two treatment groups:
    1. Carvedilol: initial dose of 6.25 mg PO bid, titrated up to 25–50 mg PO bid as tolerated
    2. Placebo
- A 2-week open-label run-in period was used to exclude patients who could not tolerate carvedilol 6.25 mg bid because of worsening heart failure or death (these events were not included in the final results).
- All patients were treated with diuretics and an angiotensin-converting enzyme (ACE) inhibitor.
- Treatment with digoxin, hydralazine, or nitrates was permitted but not required.
- All nontrial medications were kept constant during the study protocol.
- Patients were stratified into mild, moderate, or severe heart failure protocols based on their performance in a 6-min corridor-walk test.

Inclusion. Patients included had symptoms of heart failure for at least 3 months with left ventricular ejection fraction (LVEF) ≤ 35% despite at least 2 months of therapy with diuretics and ACE inhibitors.

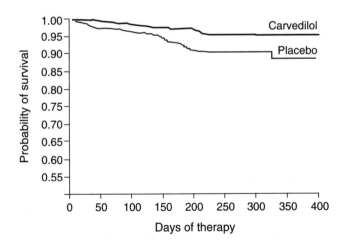

Figure 6-3. Kaplan-Meier survival curves for carvedilol and placebo groups. (From Packer et al.,[10] with permission.)

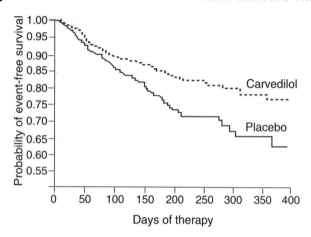

Figure 6-4. Kaplan-Meier event-free survival curves for carvedilol and placebo groups. (From Packer et al.,[10] with permission.)

Exclusion. The criteria for exclusion were a major cardiovascular event or major surgical procedure within 3 months; uncorrected primary valvular disease; active myocarditis; refractory sustained ventricular tachycardia; advanced heart block not controlled with a pacemaker; systolic blood pressure > 160 mmHg or < 85 mmHg or diastolic blood pressure > 100 mmHg; baseline heart rate < 68 bpm; hepatic or renal dysfunction; therapy with calcium channel blockers, α- or β-adrenergic agonists or antagonists, or class IC or III antiarrhythmics; hospitalization with heart failure; or other serious illness.

End Points. The criteria for end points were overall mortality and hospitalizations for cardiovascular causes.

RESULTS

The mean LVEF was 23% with New York Heart Association functional class II, III, and IV occurring in 53%, 44%, and 3% of patients, respectively. The mean dose of carvedilol was 45 mg daily. The Data Safety Monitoring Board recommended early termination of the trial after an average of 6.5-month follow-up. Overall mortality was significantly reduced by 65% with carvedilol treatment compared to placebo (3.2% carvedilol vs. 7.8%

placebo, P < 0.001). This reduction in mortality with carvedilol treatment was evident regardless of age, sex, cause of heart failure (ischemic or nonischemic), LVEF, or exercise tolerance. In addition, carvedilol therapy significantly reduced the incidence of hospitalization for cardiovascular causes (14.1% carvedilol vs. 19.6% placebo, P = 0.036). Worsening heart failure occurred more commonly in the placebo group (2.3%) compared to the carvedilol group (1.6%) (Figs. 6-3 and 6-4).

CONCLUSIONS

Treatment with carvedilol significantly reduced overall mortality by 65% and reduced the risk of hospitalizations for cardiovascular causes compared to placebo in symptomatic patients with congestive heart failure who were receiving conventional therapy with digoxin, diuretics, and an ACE inhibitor during a mean follow-up of 6.5 months.

(Data from Packer et al.[10]) ■

CONSENSUS 1

Cooperative North Scandinavian Enalapril Survival Study

PURPOSE

Determine the effect of enalapril on mortality in patients with severe congestive heart failure who are already receiving conventional medical therapy.

STUDY DESIGN

General

- 253 patients enrolled in this prospective, randomized, double-blind, placebo-controlled, multicenter trial.
- Eligible patients were randomized to one of two treatment groups:
  1. Enalapril: initial dose 5 mg PO bid titrated up to 20 mg PO bid as tolerated.
  2. Placebo.
- All patients had severe congestive heart failure (New York Heart Association [NYHA] functional class IV).

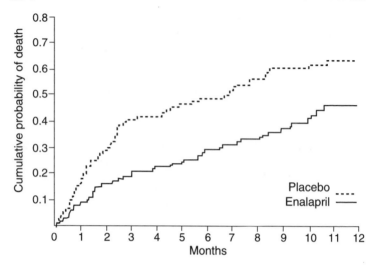

Figure 6-5. Cumulative probability of death for enalapril and placebo groups. (From The CONSENSUS Trial Study Group,[11] with permission.)

- Patients received optimal treatment with diuretics and digitalis.
- Use of other vasodilators (nitrates, prazosin, hydralazine) was permitted except for other angiotensin-converting enzyme inhibitors.

Inclusion. Patients included had a clinical diagnosis of severe congestive heart failure (NYHA functional class IV) with a heart size determined radiographically of more than 600 ml/M^2 in men and 550 ml/M^2 in women. Measurements of myocardial function were not required.

Exclusion. The criteria for exclusion were acute pulmonary edema, hemodynamically important aortic or mitral valve stenosis, myocardial infarction within the previous 2 months, unstable angina pectoris, planned cardiac surgery, cor pulmonale, and serum creatinine > 300 μmol/l.

End Points. The criteria for end points were 6- and 12-month mortality.

RESULTS

The Ethical Review Committee recommended early termination of the study. The overall mortality at 6 months was significantly reduced by 40% with enalapril treatment compared to placebo (26% enalapril vs. 44% placebo, P = 0.002). At 12 months, mortality was substantially reduced by 31% in patients receiving enalapril (36% enalapril vs. 52% placebo, P = 0.001). The entire mortality benefit from enalapril was due to reduced progression of heart failure, not to reduced sudden cardiac death. Improvement in NYHA functional class was observed in 42% of patients receiving enalapril compared to 22% of patients receiving placebo (P = 0.001) (Fig. 6-5).

CONCLUSIONS

The addition of enalapril to conventional therapy in patients with severe congestive heart failure (NYHA functional class IV) significantly reduced 1-year mortality by 31% and improved NYHA functional class compared to placebo.

(Data from The CONSENSUS Trial Study Group.[11]) ∎

HY-C

Hydralazine vs. Captopril in Advanced Heart Failure

PURPOSE

Compare the effect of captopril with hydralazine on mortality in patients with advanced congestive heart failure referred for cardiac transplantation.

STUDY DESIGN

General

- 117 patients enrolled in this prospective, randomized, multicenter trial.
- Eligible patients were randomized to one of two treatment groups:
  1. Captopril: initial dose of 6.25 mg PO q 6 hr, titrated up to 100 mg PO every 6 hr as tolerated.

2. Hydralazine: initial dose of 25 mg PO q 6 hr, titrated up to 150 mg PO q 6 hr as tolerated.

- Isosorbide dinitrate was given to all patients receiving hydralazine and to patients receiving captopril if pulmonary capillary wedge pressure (PCWP) remained >20 mmHg as an initial dose of 10 mg PO q 6 hr, titrated up to 80 mg PO q 6 hr as tolerated.

- After placement of a pulmonary artery catheter in all patients, treatment was initiated with nitroprusside infusion and intravenous furosemide to keep PCWP ≤ 15 mmHg, systemic vascular resistance ≤ 1,200 dynes-sec/cm^5, and systolic blood pressure ≥ 80 mmHg.

- Patients were discharged on study drug, digoxin, and a flexible regimen of loop diuretic and metolazone if needed to keep their weight within 2 lb of discharge weight.

- Left ventricular ejection fraction was measured by radionuclide ventriculography.

- Patients with high-grade asymptomatic ventricular arrhythmias on Holter monitor were started on amiodarone 200 mg PO per day after a loading schedule.

Inclusion. Patients included had severe congestive heart failure (New York Heart Association [NYHA] functional class III or IV) with marked left ventricular dilatation and impaired systolic function referred for cardiac transplantation.

Exclusion. The criteria for exclusion were myocardial infarction within the previous 2 months, unstable angina, cor pulmonale, restrictive cardiomyopathy, serum creatinine > 2.5 mg/dl, other serious illness, or contraindication to study drugs.

End Points. The criterion for end point was mortality.

RESULTS
Mean left ventricular ejection fraction was 20%; NYHA functional class IV heart failure was present in 80% of patients. After a mean follow-up of 8 months, the actuarial 1-year survival rate was 81% for captopril treatment compared to 51% for hydralazine treatment (P = 0.05), which is a 37% reduction in mortality for captopril-treated patients. Subgroup analysis revealed that most of the survival benefit for captopril occurred in

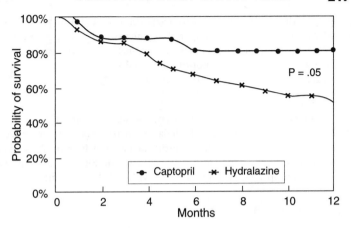

Figure 6-6. Kaplan-Meier survival curves for captopril and hydralazine-isosorbide dinitrate groups. (From Fonarow et al.,[12] with permission.)

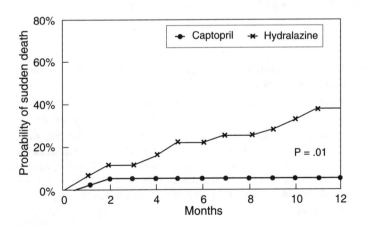

Figure 6-7. Kaplan-Meier curves of sudden death for captopril and hydralazine-isosorbide dinitrate groups. (From Fonarow et al.,[12] with permission.)

patients with a PCWP > 16 mmHg (82% survival captopril vs. 18% survival hydralazine, P = 0.01) compared to patients with PCWP ≤ 16 mmHg (P = NS). The incidence of sudden cardiac death was significantly lower for patients treated with captopril compared to hydralazine (7% captopril vs. 28% hydralazine, P = 0.01) (Figs. 6-6 and 6-7).

CONCLUSIONS
When added to conventional therapy, captopril significantly reduced mortality by 37% compared to hydralazine in patients with severe congestive heart failure (mean left ventricular ejection fraction 20%) who were being evaluated for cardiac transplantation. Most of the survival benefit of captopril occurred in patients with PCWP > 16 mmHg.

(Data from Fonarow et al.[12])   ■

MDC

Metoprolol in Dilated Cardiomyopathy Trial

PURPOSE
Determine the effect of metoprolol on overall survival and morbidity in patients with idiopathic dilated cardiomyopathy.

STUDY DESIGN

General

- 383 patients enrolled in this prospective, randomized, placebo-controlled, multicenter trial.
- If patients tolerated a test dose of metoprolol 5 mg PO bid for 2–7 days, they were randomized to one of the following two groups:
  1. Metoprolol: initial dose of 10 mg/day for 1 week, then titrated up as follows: 15 mg/day during week 2, 30 mg/day during week 3, 50 mg/day during week 4, 75 mg/day during week 5, 100 mg/day during week 6, and 150 mg/day during week 7. Daily doses were divided bid or tid. Mean dose of metoprolol was 108 mg/day.
  2. Placebo.
- All patients had achieved a state of optimally compensated heart failure through the use of digitalis, diuretics, nitrates, and angiotensin-converting enzyme inhibitors before randomization.

- Systolic blood pressure had to be ≥ 90 mmHg and heart rate ≥ 45 bpm.

- Symptom-limited exercise testing, right heart catheterization, and measurement of left ventricular ejection fraction (LVEF) by radionuclide ventriculography were performed at baseline and at 6 and 12 months.

Inclusion. Patients included were 16–75 years old with symptomatic idiopathic dilated cardiomyopathy and LVEF < 40%.

Exclusion. The criteria for exclusion were treatment with β-blockers, calcium channel blockers, inotropic agents (except digitalis), or high doses of tricyclic antidepressants; significant coronary artery disease; ongoing myocarditis; chronic obstructive pulmonary disease; alcoholism or substance abuse; insulin-dependent diabetes mellitus; pheochromocytoma; thyroid disease; or other serious illness.

End Points. The criteria for primary end points were mortality and clinical deterioration requiring cardiac transplantation. The criteria for secondary end points were cardiac function, exercise capacity, quality of life, and New York Heart Association (NYHA) functional class.

RESULTS

Mean left ventricular ejection fraction was 22% in both groups; most patients had NYHA functional class II (45%) or class III (49%). Total mortality was not significantly different between metoprolol and placebo during the 18-month follow-up (11.8% metoprolol vs. 10.1% placebo, $P = 0.69$). The use of metoprolol significantly reduced the need for heart transplantation compared to placebo (1.0% metoprolol vs. 10.0% placebo, $P = 0.0001$). In addition, patients receiving metoprolol had a significantly greater increase in ejection fraction (% increase in LVEF: 55% metoprolol vs. 27% placebo, $P < 0.0001$), improved quality of life ($P = 0.01$), improved exercise capacity on treadmill testing ($P = 0.046$), improved hemodynamics (lower pulmonary capillary wedge pressure, $P = 0.01$), increased systolic blood pressure ($P = 0.03$), increased cardiac index ($P = 0.05$), and improved NYHA functional class ($P = 0.01$) (Fig. 6-8).

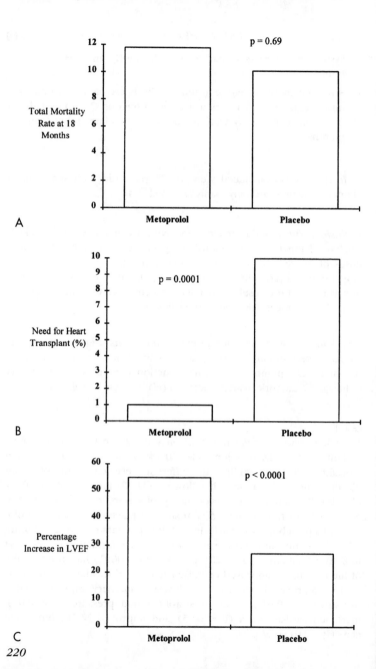

Figure 6-8. *(A–C)* The reduced need for heart transplantation and increased LVEF with metoprolol treatment compared to placebo. Total mortality was not significantly different.

CONCLUSIONS

The addition of metoprolol to patients with symptomatic idiopathic dilated cardiomyopathy receiving optimal heart failure therapy did not significantly decrease total mortality but did significantly reduce the need for heart transplantation and improved the LVEF, hemodynamics, exercise capacity, and NYHA functional class compared to placebo at 18-month follow-up.

(Data from Waagstein et al.[13]) ■

MTT

Myocarditis Treatment Trial

PURPOSE

Determine the effect of immunosuppressive therapy on left ventricular function and mortality in patients with a histopathologic diagnosis of myocarditis and left ventricular ejection fraction (LVEF) < 45%.

STUDY DESIGN

General

- 111 patients enrolled in this prospective, randomized, controlled, multicenter trial.

- Eligible patients were randomized to one of three treatment groups:

  1. Azathioprine and prednisone
  2. Cyclosporine and prednisone
  3. Control

     Azathioprine: 1 mg/kg PO bid for 24 weeks
     Prednisone
       Week 1: 1.25 mg/kg/day in divided doses

Week 2–12: Taper dose by 0.08 mg/kg/week until dose was 0.33 mg/kg/day

Week 13–20: Continue 0.33 mg/kg/day

Week 21–24: Taper dose by 0.8 mg/kg/week, then discontinue drug after 24 weeks

Cyclosporine

Week 1: 5 mg/kg PO bid titrated to maintain serum levels of 200–300 µg/ml

Week 2–4: Dose tapered to keep levels 100–200 µg/ml

Week 5–24: Dose tapered to keep levels 60–150 µg/ml, then discontinued after 24 weeks

Inclusion. Patients included had an onset of congestive heart failure during the 2 years preceding enrollment but without coronary artery disease or another specific cause who had histopathologic evidence of myocarditis on endomyocardial biopsy and an LVEF < 45%.

End Points. The criteria for end points were LVEF and mortality at 28 weeks.

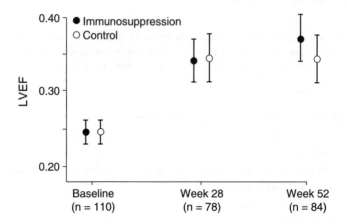

Figure 6-9. Mean LVEF in immunosuppression and control groups. (From Mason et al.,[14] with permission.)

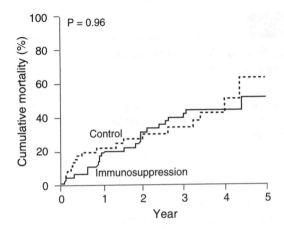

Figure 6-10. Actuarial mortality curves for immunosuppression and control groups. (From Mason et al.,[14] with permission.)

RESULTS

Only 10% of screened patients with clinical myocarditis had a positive endomyocardial biopsy. Mean LVEF was 24% in all three groups. No significant difference in the LVEF was observed between immunosuppressive therapy and control at baseline ($P = 0.97$), at week 28 ($P = 0.95$), or at week 52 ($P = 0.45$). Pulmonary capillary wedge pressure was also not different between the three groups up to 52-week follow-up. Actuarial mortality, defined as deaths and cardiac transplants, did not differ significantly between control and immunosuppressive groups at 1 year ($P = 0.62$) or throughout the entire follow-up period ($P = 0.96$) (Figs. 6-9 and 6-10).

CONCLUSIONS

Immunosuppressive therapy did not have a significant effect on LVEF or mortality compared to control in patients with histopathologically confirmed myocarditis and LVEF < 45% during the 1-year follow-up.

(Data from Mason et al.[14])   ■

Prospective Randomized Milrinone Survival Evaluation

PURPOSE

Determine the effect of oral milrinone on mortality in patients with severe congestive heart failure who remain symptomatic despite conventional therapy.

STUDY DESIGN

General

- 1,088 patients enrolled in this prospective, randomized, double-blind, placebo-controlled, multicenter trial.

- Eligible patients were randomized to one of two treatment groups:

  1. Milrinone: initial dose of 10 mg PO qid with titration allowed between 5 and 15 mg PO qid, depending on the clinical response
  2. Placebo

- All patients received digoxin, diuretics, and an angiotensin-converting enzyme inhibitor for at least 4 weeks before randomization. The doses were determined by each physician.

- Treatment with nitrates, hydralazine, prazosin, and other vasodilatory drugs was allowed.

Inclusion. Patients included had chronic congestive heart failure, New York Heart Association (NYHA) functional class III or IV for at least 3 months. Their symptoms remained severe despite conventional therapy. Congestive heart failure was defined as dyspnea or fatigue at rest or with exertion associated with a left ventricular ejection fraction (LVEF) $\leq 35\%$ assessed by radionuclide ventriculography.

Exclusion. The criteria for exclusion were heart failure that was due to obstructive valvular disease; active myocarditis; hypertrophic or amyloid cardiomyopathy; uncorrected thyroid disease; malfunctioning mechanical heart valves; serious ventricular arrhythmias; severe angina pectoris; myocardial infarction within the previous 3 months; systolic blood pressure < 85 mmHg; the need for β-blockers, calcium channel blockers,

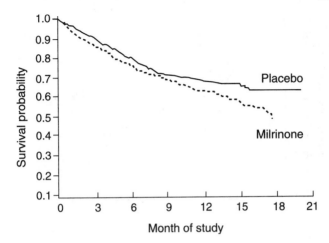

Figure 6-11. Kaplan-Meier cumulative rates of survival in all patients. (From Packer et al.,[15] with permission.)

disopyramide, flecainide, encainide, levodopa, dopamine, or dobutamine: or other serious illness.

End Point. The criterion for end point was mortality.

RESULTS

After an average of 6 months of follow-up, the Data and Safety Monitoring Board recommended early termination of the study. Use of milrinone resulted in a significant increase in total mortality by 25% (30% milrinone vs. 24% placebo, P = 0.04) and cardiac mortality by 26% (29% milrinone vs. 23% placebo, P = 0.016) compared to placebo. The increase in mortality was also evident in the subgroup of patients with low ejection fraction (LVEF < 21%) and NYHA functional class IV (53% increase in mortality). No significant difference in symptoms or functional classification was observed between milrinone and placebo (Figs. 6-11 and 6-12).

CONCLUSIONS

The use of oral milrinone in patients with severe congestive heart failure who remain symptomatic despite conventional heart failure therapy resulted in a significant 28% increase in total mortality compared to

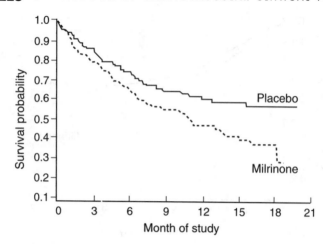

Figure 6-12. Kaplan-Meier cumulative rates of survival in patients with NYHA class IV heart failure. (From Packer et al.,[15] with permission.)

placebo with no difference in symptoms or functional capacity over a 6-month follow-up period.

(Data from Packer et al.[15]) ∎

RADIANCE

Randomized Assessment of Digoxin on Inhibitors of the Angiotensin-Converting Enzyme

PURPOSE

Evaluate the effect of the withdrawal of digoxin from patients with chronic heart failure who were clinically stable while receiving digoxin, diuretics, and an angiotensin-converting enzyme (ACE) inhibitor.

STUDY DESIGN

General

- 178 patients enrolled in this prospective, randomized, double-blind, placebo-controlled, withdrawal trial.

- There was an initial 8-week run-in period during which heart failure therapy was optimized: The digoxin dose was adjusted to keep serum levels 0.9–2.0 ng/ml, the dose of diuretic was adjusted to maintain optimal fluid balance, and the dose of the ACE inhibitor was adjusted to at least 25 mg captopril or 5 mg enalapril per day.

- After patients were stabilized on optimal heart failure therapy, they were randomly assigned to one of two treatment groups:

  1. Continue digoxin.
  2. Discontinue digoxin and receive placebo.

- The study protocol was continued for 3 months.

- New York Heart Association (NYHA) functional class, Minnesota Living with Heart Failure questionnaire, chest x-ray, echocardiography, radionuclide ventriculography, and exercise treadmill testing were serially performed.

Inclusion. Patients included were ≥ 18 years old with chronic congestive heart failure defined as dyspnea and fatigue on exertion in association with a left ventricular ejection fraction (LVEF) ≤ 35% by radionuclide ventriculography and a left ventricular end-diastole (LVED) dimension of ≥ 60 mm (or 34 mm/M²) by echocardiography. Subjective and objective evidence for reduced exercise capacity and normal sinus rhythm were required.

Exclusion. The criteria for exclusion were supraventricular or sustained ventricular arrhythmias; uncorrected primary valvular disease; active myocarditis; cardiomyopathy of obstructive, hypertrophic, or restrictive type; systolic blood pressure ≥ 160 mmHg or < 90 mmHg; diastolic blood pressure > 95 mmHg; exercise limited by angina, lung disease, or claudication; angina pectoris; myocardial infarction within the past 3 months or stroke within the past 12 months; or other serious illness.

End Points. The criteria for end points were rate and time of withdrawal from the study as a result of worsening heart failure and changes in exercise tolerance.

RESULTS

During the 3-month study period, clinical severity of heart failure worsened enough to require therapeutic intervention (change in the baseline therapy, visit to the emergency department or hospitalization for heart failure) in 23 patients receiving placebo compared to 4 patients continuing to receive digoxin (P < 0.001). Patients receiving placebo developed worsening exercise tolerance on treadmill testing defined as an exercise duration 43 sec less than those continuing to receive digoxin (P = 0.033). Deterioration in NYHA functional class was reported in 27% of patients receiving placebo compared to 10% of those continuing to receive digoxin (P = 0.019). Patients' subjective assessment of their overall progress was significantly worse in those receiving placebo. LVEF and LVED dimension worsened moderately but significantly in patients receiving placebo (Fig. 6-13).

CONCLUSIONS

The withdrawal of digoxin for 3 months from patients who were clinically stable while receiving optimal doses of digoxin, diuretics, and ACE inhibitors significantly worsened the clinical severity of heart failure,

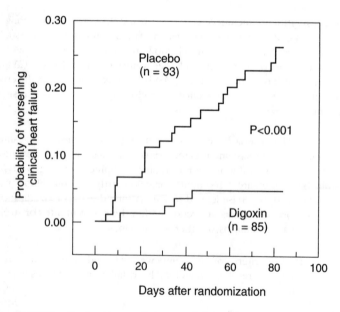

Figure 6-13. Kaplan-Meier cumulative probability of worsening heart failure in patients continuing to receive digoxin and those switched to placebo. (From Packer et al.,[16] with permission.)

NYHA functional class, patients' subjective assessment of their prognosis, and LVEF and LVED dimension compared to patients continuing to receive digoxin.

(Data from Packer et al.[16]) ■

SAVE

Survival and Ventricular Enlargement Trial

PURPOSE

Determine the efficacy of captopril on reducing mortality and morbidity in patients with left ventricular dysfunction after acute myocardial infarction.

STUDY DESIGN

General

- 2,231 patients enrolled in this prospective, randomized, double-blinded, placebo-controlled, multicenter trial.
- Eligible patients were randomized to one of two treatment groups:
    1. Captopril: initial dose 12.5 mg PO tid titrated up to 50 mg PO tid as tolerated
    2. Placebo
- Treatment was started from 3–16 days after myocardial infarction.
- Revascularization, if deemed necessary, had to be performed before the patient underwent randomization.
- Clinical follow-up was every 4 months and repeat radionuclide ventriculography at 36 months.

Inclusion. Patients included were 21–80 years old presenting within 16 days of acute myocardial infarction with left ventricular ejection fraction ≤ 40% measured by radionuclide ventriculography but without overt heart failure.

Exclusion. The criteria for exclusion were failure to undergo randomization within 16 days after myocardial infarction, contraindication to or clear indication for angiotensin-converting enzyme inhibitors, serum creatinine > 2.5 μg/dl, or other serious illness.

End Points. The criteria for end points were mortality, development of severe congestive heart failure, and recurrent myocardial infarction.

RESULTS

Mean radionuclide left ventricular ejection fraction was 31% in both groups. After an average of 42-month follow-up, the use of captopril significantly reduced total mortality by 20% (20% captopril vs. 25% placebo, P = 0.019) and cardiovascular mortality by 20% (17% captopril vs. 21% placebo, P = 0.014) compared to placebo. Patients taking captopril also had significantly less need for hospitalization for congestive heart failure (14% captopril vs. 17% placebo, P = 0.019) and had a reduced incidence of recurrent myocardial infarction (12% captopril vs. 15.2% placebo, P = 0.015) (Figs. 6-14 and 6-15).

CONCLUSIONS

Treatment with captopril in survivors of acute myocardial infarction with asymptomatic depressed left ventricular ejection fraction (≤P 40%) resulted in significantly reduced total and cardiovascular mortality, reduced incidence of hospitalization for severe congestive heart failure,

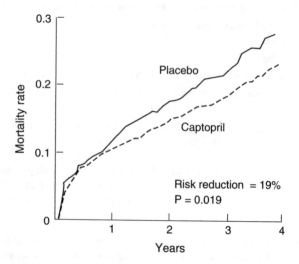

Figure 6-14. Cumulative all-cause mortality for captopril and placebo groups. (From Pfeffer et al.,[17] with permission.)

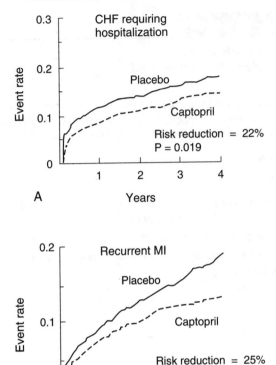

Figure 6-15. *(A & B)* Life tables for cumulative nonfatal cardiovascular events. (From Pfeffer et al.,[17] with permission.)

and reduced rate of recurrent myocardial infarction compared to placebo at 42-month follow-up.

(Data from Pfeffer et al.[17]) ∎

Studies of Left Ventricular Dysfunction—Prevention Trial

PURPOSE

Determine the effect of enalapril on mortality, development of congestive heart failure, and hospitalization for congestive heart failure among patients with asymptomatic left ventricular dysfunction.

STUDY DESIGN

General

- 4,228 Patients enrolled in this prospective, randomized, double-blind, placebo-controlled, multicenter trial.

- Eligible patients were randomized to one of two treatment groups:

    1. Enalapril: initially 2.5 mg PO bid titrated up to 10 mg PO bid as tolerated

    2. Placebo

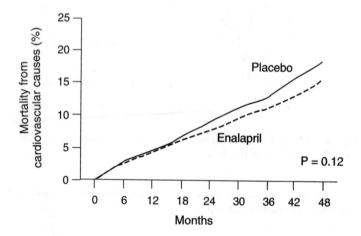

Figure 6-16. Mortality from cardiovascular causes. (From The SOLVD Investigators,[18] with permission.)

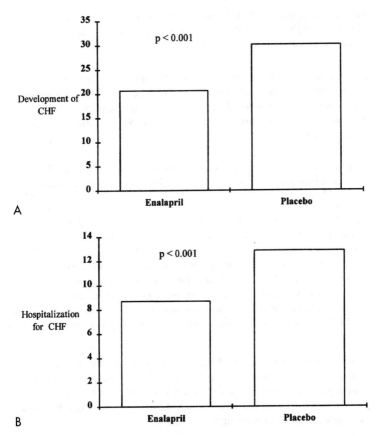

Figure 6-17. The reduced development of *(A)* congestive heart failure and *(B)* hospitalizations for congestive heart failure in patients receiving enalapril compared to placebo.

- Left ventricular ejection fraction (LVEF) was measured by radionuclide ventriculography, contrast angiography, and two-dimensional echocardiography.
- Patients were allowed to use diuretics for hypertension, digoxin for current or past atrial fibrillation, and/or nitrates for angina.
- Clinical follow-up was every 4 months.

Inclusion. Patients included had asymptomatic left ventricular dysfunction with LVEF ≤ 35% who were not receiving diuretics, digoxin, or vasodilators for the treatment of heart failure.

Exclusion. The criteria for exclusion were age > 80 years, hemodynamically serious valvular disease requiring surgery, unstable angina pectoris, angina severe enough to warrant revascularization, myocardial infarction during the previous 1 month, severe pulmonary disease, or other serious illness.

End Points. The criteria for end points were total and cardiovascular mortality, development of heart failure, and hospitalization for heart failure.

RESULTS

Mean baseline LVEF was 28.0% in both treatment groups. At an average of 37-month follow-up, total mortality was not significantly different between the enalapril and placebo groups (14.8% enalapril vs. 15.8% placebo, P = 0.30). Cardiovascular mortality was also not significantly different (P = 0.12). Use of enalapril did result in substantially lower incidence of development of clinical congestive heart failure (20.7% enalapril vs. 30.2% placebo, P < 0.001) and hospitalization for congestive heart failure (8.7% enalapril vs. 12.9% placebo, P < 0.001) (Figs. 6-16 and 6-17).

CONCLUSIONS

Enalapril significantly reduced the development of clinical heart failure and the need for hospitalization for heart failure compared to placebo among patients with asymptomatic left ventricular dysfunction (LVEF ≤ 35%) during a 37-month follow-up period. Enalapril treatment did not significantly reduce total mortality in this group.

(Data from The SOLVD Investigators.[18]) ■

SOLVD—TREATMENT

Studies of Left Ventricular Dysfunction—Treatment Trial

PURPOSE

Determine the effect of enalapril on mortality and the incidence of hospitalization for congestive heart failure in patients with overt chronic congestive heart failure and left ventricular ejection fractions (LVEFs) $\leq 35\%$.

STUDY DESIGN

General

- 2,569 patients enrolled in this prospective, randomized, double-blind, placebo-controlled, multicenter trial.
- Eligible patients were randomized to one of two treatment groups:
    1. Enalapril: initially 2.5 mg PO bid titrated up to 10 mg PO bid as tolerated
    2. Placebo
- LVEF was measured by radionuclide ventriculography, contrast angiography, and two-dimensional echocardiography.
- Clinical follow-up was every 4 months.
- In patients with worsening symptoms of congestive heart failure, increased dose of diuretics or addition of other vasodilators was attempted. If symptoms persisted, open-label treatment with an angiotensin-converting enzyme (ACE) inhibitor was allowed.

Inclusion. Patients included had congestive heart failure and LVEF $\leq 35\%$ and were already taking medications other than ACE inhibitors.

Exclusion. The criteria for exclusion were age > 80 years, hemodynamically serious valvular disease requiring surgery, unstable angina pectoris, angina severe enough to warrant revascularization, myocardial infarction during the previous 1 month, severe pulmonary disease, or other serious illness.

End Points. The criteria for end points were mortality and hospitalization for congestive heart failure.

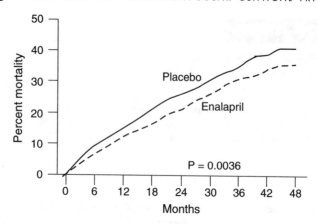

Figure 6-18. Mortality curves for enalapril and placebo groups. (From The SOLVD Investigators,[19] with permission.)

RESULTS

The mean baseline LVEF was 24.8% in both treatment groups. At an average of 41-month follow-up, treatment with enalapril significantly reduced the cumulative mortality rate by 11% compared to placebo (35.2% enalapril vs. 39.7% placebo, P = 0.0036). The causes of death were chiefly due to progressive heart failure, not arrhythmias. The number of patients hospitalized at least once for congestive heart failure was significantly lower in the enalapril group compared with placebo (25.8% enalapril vs. 36.6% placebo, P < 0.001) (Fig. 6-18).

CONCLUSIONS

Enalapril used with conventional therapy significantly reduced mortality and hospitalizations for heart failure compared to placebo at 41-month follow-up in patients with overt chronic congestive heart failure and left ventricular ejection fractions ≤ 35%.

(Data from The SOLVD Investigators.[19]) ■

VHEFT 1

Veterans Administration Cooperative Vasodilator–Heart Failure Trial

PURPOSE

Evaluate the effects of prazosin and combination hydralazine-isosorbide dinitrate on mortality in patients with chronic congestive heart failure.

STUDY DESIGN

General

- 642 patients enrolled in this prospective, randomized, double-blind, placebo-controlled, multicenter trial.
- Eligible patients were randomized to one of three treatment groups:
    1. Prazosin: 2.5 mg PO qid
    2. Hydralazine-isosorbide dinitrate combination: hydralazine 37.5 mg PO qid and isosorbide dinitrate 20 mg PO qid
    3. Placebo
- All doses could be doubled or halved according to patient tolerance (average doses used were prazosin 18.6 mg/day, hydralazine 270 mg/day, isosorbide dinitrate 136 mg/day).
- Digoxin (to achieve serum concentrations > 0.7 ng/ml) and diuretics were used as needed.
- Patients were stratified according to the presence or absence of coronary artery disease.

Inclusion. Patients included were men aged 18–75 years with chronic congestive heart failure with cardiac dilatation (cardiothoracic ratio on chest x-ray > 55% or left ventricular end-diastole diameter > 2.7 cm/M² by echocardiography) or left ventricular functional impairment (radionuclide left ventricular ejection fraction < 45%) associated with reduced exercise tolerance.

Exclusion. The criteria for exclusion were exercise tolerance limited by angina rather than by breathlessness or fatigue; myocardial infarction within the previous 3 months; substantial obstructive valvular or myocardial disease; other serious illness; contraindications to the study drugs; or the need for long-acting nitrates, calcium antagonists, β-blockers, or anti-hypertensive medications other than diuretics.

End Points. The criterion for end point was mortality.

RESULTS

During the mean follow-up of 2.3 years, the combination of hydralazine-isosorbide dinitrate significantly reduced mortality at 1, 2, and 3 years by 38%, 25% (P < 0.028), and 23% (P = 0.05) compared to placebo (mortality at 3 years: 36.2% hydralazine-isosorbide dinitrate vs. 46.9% placebo, P = 0.05). Prazosin had no significant effect on reducing mortality. The beneficial effect of hydralazine-isosorbide dinitrate on mortality reduction was similar among patients with and without coronary artery disease; however, mortality was significantly higher in patients with coronary heart disease. Left ventricular ejection fraction at 1 year increased by 4.2% with hydralazine-isosorbide dinitrate compared to a 0.1% decrease with placebo (P < 0.001) (Fig. 6-19).

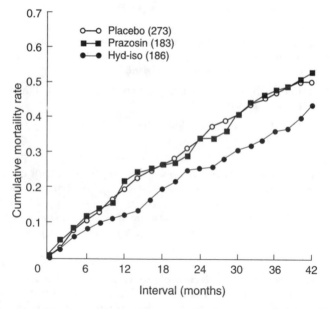

Figure 6-19. Cumulative mortality in the three treatment groups. (From Cohn et al.,[20] with permission.)

CONCLUSIONS

The combination of hydralazine and isosorbide dinitrate significantly improved survival and left ventricular ejection fraction compared to placebo at 3-year follow-up in patients with chronic congestive heart failure. Prazosin provided no significant benefit.

_____

(Data from Cohn et al.[20]) ∎

VHEFT 2

Veterans Administration Cooperative Vasodilator–Heart Failure Trial

PURPOSE

Compare the effects of enalapril with combination hydralazine-isosorbide dinitrate on mortality in men receiving digoxin and diuretics for chronic congestive heart failure.

STUDY DESIGN

General

- 804 men enrolled in this prospective, randomized, double-blind, placebo-controlled, multicenter trial.

- Eligible patients were randomized to one of two treatment groups:

    1. Enalapril: initial dose of 5 mg PO bid titrated up to 10 mg PO bid as tolerated

    2. Hydralazine-isosorbide dinitrate combination: hydralazine initial dose of 37.5 mg PO qid titrated up to 75 mg PO qid as tolerated; isosorbide dinitrate initial dose of 20 mg PO qid titrated up to 40 mg PO qid as tolerated

- Optimal therapy with digoxin and a diuretic was performed before randomization, and nonessential drugs were discontinued.

- Patients were asked not to take other vasodilatory or antihypertensive drugs.

- Exercise testing, radionuclide left ventricular ejection fraction (LVEF), and chest x-ray were serially obtained.

Inclusion. Patients included were men aged 18–75 years with chronic congestive heart failure who had cardiac dilatation (cardiothoracic ratio on chest x-ray > 55% or left ventricular end-diastole diameter > 2.7 cm/M^2 by echocardiography) or left ventricular functional impairment (radionuclide LVEF < 45%) associated with a reduced exercise tolerance.

Exclusion. The criteria for exclusion were exercise tolerance limited by angina rather than by breathlessness or fatigue, myocardial infarction or cardiac surgery within the previous 3 months, substantial obstructive valvular or myocardial disease, other serious illness, or contraindications to the study drugs.

End Points. The criterion for exclusion was mortality.

RESULTS

At 2-year follow-up, mortality in the enalapril group was significantly lower by 28% compared to the hydralazine-isosorbide dinitrate group (18% enalapril vs. 25% hydralazine-isosorbide dinitrate, P = 0.016). This trend continued throughout the study but did not attain statistical significance at 5 years of follow-up (48% enalapril vs. 54% hydralazine-isosorbide dinitrate, P = 0.08). The lower mortality in the enalapril arm was

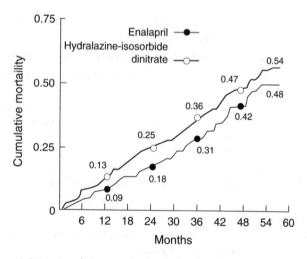

Figure 6-20. Cumulative mortality for enalapril and hydralazine-isosorbide dinitrate groups. (From Cohn et al.,[21] with permission.)

mostly due to reduction in the incidence of sudden cardiac death; death that was due to pump failure was not changed. Ejection fraction at 3 years improved similarly in both enalapril and hydralazine-isosorbide dinitrate groups (Fig. 6-20).

CONCLUSIONS

Enalapril substantially reduced mortality by 28% compared to hydralazine-isosorbide dinitrate in men with chronic congestive heart failure receiving digoxin and diuretics at 2-year follow-up. At 5-year follow-up, there was a trend toward reduced mortality with enalapril, but the results were not statistically significant.

(Data from Cohn et al.[21])   ■

References

1. Kober L, Torp-Pederson C, Carlsen J et al: A clinical trial of the angiotensin converting enzyme inhibitor trandolapril in patients with left ventricular dysfunction after myocardial infarction. N Engl J Med 333:1670, 1995

2. Uretsky BF, Young JB, Shahidi FE et al: Randomized study assessing the effect of digoxin withdrawal in patients with mild to moderate chronic congestive heart failure: results of the PROVED trial. J Am Coll Cardiol 22:955, 1993

3. Gorlin R, Garg R: Effects of digoxin on mortality in patients with congestive heart failure and normal sinus rhythm. Presented at the meeting of the American College of Cardiology, Orlando, CA, 1996

4. Flosequinan withdrawal (news). Lancet 342:235, 1993

5. Dies F, McNay JL, Andrejasich CM et al: Indolidan (a new phosphodiesterase inhibitor) in chronic heart failure. Circulation 80(suppl. II):11-175, 1989

6. Goldberg AD, Goldstein S, Nicklas J: Multicenter trial of imazodan in patients with chronic congestive heart failure. Circulation 82(suppl. III):III-673, 1990

7. Dies F, Krell MJ, Whitlow P et al: Intermittent dobutamine in ambulatory outpatients with chronic heart failure. Circulation 74(suppl. II):II-38, 1986

8. Yusuf S, Teo K: Inotropic agents increase mortality in patients with congestive heart failure. Circulation 82(suppl. III):III-673, 1990

9. The Acute Infarction Ramipril Efficacy (AIRE) Study Investigators: Effect of ramipril on mortality and morbidity of survivors of acute myocardial infarction with clinical evidence of heart failure. Lancet 342:821-8, 1993

10. Packer M, Bristow MR, Cohn JN et al: The effect of carvedilol on morbidity and mortality in patients with chronic heart failure. N Engl J Med 334:1349-55, 1996

11. The CONSENSUS Trial Study Group: Effects of enalapril on mortality in severe congestive heart failure: results of the Cooperative North Scandinavian Enalapril Survival Study (CONSENSUS). N Engl J Med 316:1429-35, 1987

12. Fonarow GC, Chelimsky-Fallick C, Stevenson LW et al: Effect of direct vasodilation with hydralazine versus angiotensin-converting enzyme inhibition with captopril on mortality in advanced heart failure: the Hy-C trial. J Am Coll Cardiol 19:842-50, 1992

13. Waagstein F, Bristow MR, Swedberg K et al: Beneficial effects of metoprolol in idiopathic dilated cardiomyopathy. Lancet 342:1441-6, 1993

14. Mason JW, O'Connell JB, Herskowitz A et al: A clinical trial of immunosuppressive therapy for myocarditis. N Engl J Med 333:269-75, 1995

15. Packer M, Carver JR, Rodeheffer RJ et al: Effect of oral milrinone on mortality in severe chronic heart failure. N Engl J Med 325:1468-75, 1991

16. Packer M, Gheorghiade M, Young JB et al: Withdrawal of digoxin from patients with chronic heart failure treated with angiotensin-converting-enzyme inhibitors. N Engl J Med 329:1-7, 1993

17. Pfeffer MA, Braunwald E, Moyé LA et al: Effect of captopril on mortality and morbidity in patients with left ventricular dysfunction after myocardial infarction. N Engl J Med 327:669-77, 1992

18. The SOLVD Investigators: Effect of enalapril on mortality and the development of heart failure in asymptomatic patients with reduced left ventricular ejection fraction. N Engl J Med 327:685-91, 1992

19. The SOLVD Investigators: Effect of enalapril in patients with reduced left ventricular ejection fractions and congestive heart failure. N Engl J Med 325:293-302, 1991

20. Cohn JN, Archibald DG, Ziesche S et al: Effect of vasodilator therapy on mortality in chronic congestive heart failure: results of a Veterans Administration Cooperative Study. N Engl J Med 314:1547-52, 1986

21. Cohn JN, Johnson G, Ziesche S et al: A comparison of enalapril with hydralazine-isosorbide dinitrate in the treatment of chronic congestive heart failure. N Engl J Med 325:313-10, 1991

CHAPTER 7

Antiarrhythmic Trials

OVERVIEW

Cardiac dysrhythmias, particularly ventricular tachycardia and fibrillation, contribute substantially to overall cardiac mortality and morbidity. Approximately 50% of all deaths from acute myocardial infarctions are due to sudden cardiac death from lethal ventricular dysrhythmias. It is estimated that more than 40% of patients with advanced congestive heart failure die of malignant dysrhythmias.

Drug treatment of cardiac dysrhythmias has been only modestly successful. A lack of uniformly successful agents along with a significant incidence of intolerable side effects has limited the effectiveness of pharmaceutical agents. More important is the serious potential for harmful proarrhythmias that are dysrhythmias actually caused by drug treatment. Torsade de pointes, associated with prolongation of the QT interval, is the classic proarrhythmia typically occurring with the administration of class Ia, Ic, and III agents. This rapid, often lethal form of ventricular tachycardia, is thought to account for the 8% incidence of syncopal spells associated with quinidine therapy, known as "quinidine syncope." A second form of proarrhythmia is incessant ventricular tachycardia, a form of ventricular tachycardia that is difficult or impossible to terminate and is associated with administration of the sodium channel blockers encainide, flecainide, and quinidine.

Invasive electrophysiologic (EP) testing is used to more clearly define the mechanism of dysrhythmia and then to test the effectiveness of rapidly administered pharmaceutical agents to customize drug therapy. Electrophysiologic testing has gained widespread acceptance despite a paucity of clinical evidence demonstrating an advantage of this procedure over noninvasive methods. The recent development of the automatic implantable cardioverter/defibrillator (AICD) may be a turning point in the treatment of dysrhythmias, because this device has real potential for reducing mortality from ventricular dysrhythmias. The AICD is currently being evaluated in randomized clinical trials.

Clinical Trials Demonstrating Proarrhythmia

The development of frequent premature ventricular contractions (PVCs) or nonsustained ventricular tachycardia (NSVT) after myocardial infarction is associated with a predisposition to sudden cardiac death. It is not clear whether these ventricular extrasystoles actually initiate and cause fatal ventricular dysrhythmias or simply serve as markers for hearts with more extensive ischemic damage that are independently at a high risk for fatal dysrhythmias. The Cardiac Arrhythmia Suppression Trials (CAST) were designed to determine if suppression of ventricular ectopy after myocardial infarction reduces the incidence of sudden cardiac death. CAST 1 randomized 1,498 patients with six or more PVCs per hour on Holter monitor after myocardial infarction to treatment with flecainide or encainide compared to placebo. After 10 months of follow-up, CAST 1 was terminated early because of a significant 2.6-fold increase in death or cardiac arrest in patients receiving flecainide or encainide therapy compared to patients receiving placebo. The use of flecainide or encainide increased mortality regardless of the left ventricular ejection fraction (LVEF) and also significantly increased nonarrhythmic deaths (acute myocardial infarction, congestive heart failure, postsurgical bypass). CAST 2 evaluated the effect of moricizine in 1,325 patients with ventricular ectopy after myocardial infarction. Again, a significant increase in mortality and cardiac arrests occurred in patients receiving moricizine compared to placebo during the 2-week run-in period, which resulted in early termination of the trial. The mechanisms underlying the results of the CAST trials are unclear; however, a proarrhythmic effect of drug therapy is the likely explanation for part of the increase in mortality associated with encainide, flecainide, and moricizine.

The International Mexilitine and Placebo Antiarrhythmic Coronary Trial (IMPACT) examined the effect of mexilitine compared to placebo in preventing dysrhythmias in 630 patients after myocardial infarction. These patients were not required to have frequent ventricular ectopy or dysrhythmias before enrollment. Patients receiving mexilitine had a significant reduction in the incidence of PVC and NSVT at 1 and 4 months compared to placebo, with no difference detected at 1 year. However, at 9 months, a trend toward increased mortality was observed in patients receiving mexilitine. Thus, although mexilitine therapy was effective initially in reducing the incidence of ventricular ectopy, this drug eventually produced a trend toward increased mortality compared to placebo.

In the 1970s, prophylactic treatment with lidocaine was standard practice in patients admitted with acute myocardial infarction. Lidocaine is a potent agent for suppressing ventricular dysrhythmias. The clinical effect of lidocaine has not been evaluated in large prospective randomized trials. Meta-analyses[1] have suggested that despite a reduction in primary ventricular fibrillation, the use of lidocaine results in a trend toward increased in-hospital mortality. Potential mechanisms explaining the apparent higher mortality include higher incidences of congestive heart failure and bradyarrhythmias, particularly asystole, associated with the use of lidocaine.

There is evidence that chronic quinidine therapy used in the treatment of atrial fibrillation increases mortality. Coplen et al.[2] performed a meta-analysis of six small randomized trials evaluating chronic quinidine therapy and found a significant 3.6-fold excess in mortality with use of quinidine compared to no antiarrhythmic therapy (2.9% mortality rate quinidine vs. 0..8% mortality rate control, $P < 0.05$). In addition, a retrospective analysis of the 1,330 patients enrolled in Stroke Prevention in Atrial Fibrillation (SPAF) 1[3] was performed to examine the effect of antiarrhythmic therapy on mortality. Among patients with a history of congestive heart failure, those given antiarrhythmic medications, most commonly quinidine, had a relative risk of cardiac death of 4.7 ($P < 0.001$) and a relative risk of arrhythmic death of 3.7 ($P = 0.01$) compared to patients not treated with antiarrhythmic medications. Patients without a history of congestive heart failure had no increase in mortality during antiarrhythmic drug therapy.

Collectively, these trials emphasize the potential for proarrhythmia and increased mortality associated with certain antiarrhythmic agents used in specific patient populations. Cautious use of antiarrhythmic agents with careful monitoring and close follow-up must be the rule to help minimize proarrhythmic complications. Clearly, further randomized clinical trials are required to define the safest and most effective antiarrhythmic agents.

Amiodarone Trials

Amiodarone has become the most widely used drug for treating ventricular dysrhythmias in Europe and is rapidly gaining acceptance in the

United States. The advantage of amiodarone over other antiarrhythmic drugs is due to its high efficacy in preventing ventricular dysrhythmias. The Basel Antiarrhtyhmic Study of Infarct Survival (BASIS) trial randomized 312 patients with complex ventricular dysrhythmias after myocardial infarction to amiodarone therapy, individualized therapy consisting mostly of quinidine or mexilitine, or control. Cumulative mortality after 12 months of follow-up was 5% for amiodarone therapy, 10% for individualized therapy, and 13% for control, which represents a 50% and 61% reduction in mortality with amiodarone over the individualized and control groups, respectively. Amiodarone also significantly reduced sudden death and sustained ventricular tachycardia or fibrillation compared to control. The Cardiac Arrest in Seattle—Conventional vs. Amiodarone Drug Evaluation (CASCADE) trial evaluated the effect of amiodarone therapy compared to conventional therapy (procainamide, quinidine, flecainide, and others) in 228 high-risk patients with sudden cardiac death not associated with acute myocardial infarction. At 6-year follow-up, amiodarone therapy significantly improved survival by 33% compared to conventional therapy. The combined end point of survival and the absence of sustained ventricular dysrhythmias was also significantly better with amiodarone therapy. Although these trials are relatively small, they provide evidence suggesting better survival and suppression of ventricular dysrhythmias with amiodarone therapy compared to conventional therapy in patients at high risk of malignant ventricular dysrhythmias.

AMIODARONE AFTER MYOCARDIAL INFARCTION

The prophylactic administration of amiodarone in survivors of acute myocardial infarction to prevent subsequent sudden cardiac death has been evaluated in eight randomized trials. The largest of these trials, the Polish Amiodarone Study (PAS) compared the effects of amiodarone with placebo in 613 postinfarction patients who had contraindications to β-blocker therapy. Amiodarone therapy significantly reduced cardiac mortality and serious ventricular dysrhythmias and resulted in a trend toward less sudden death at 1-year follow-up. The BASIS trial, as previously described, revealed a reduction in mortality with amiodarone compared to control in 312 postinfarction patients. Teo et al.[4] performed a meta-analysis of all the reported trials evaluating the effect of amiodarone in 1,557 postinfarction patients. Treatment with amiodarone significantly reduced overall mortality by 23% (9.9% amiodarone vs. 12.9% control, P = 0.03) (Fig. 7-1).

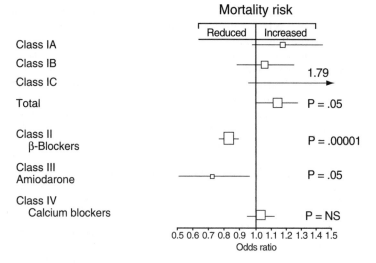

Figure 7-1. Effects of antiarrhythmic agents on mortality. (From Teo et al.,[4] with permission.)

Two large, recently completed trials—the European Myocardial Infarction Amiodarone Trial (EMIAT), which enrolled 1,486 patients, and the Canadian Amiodarone Myocardial Infarction Trial (CAMIAT), which enrolled 1,202 patients—will provide a more definitive answer regarding the role of prophylactic administration of amiodarone to patients after myocardial infarction.

AMIODARONE IN CONGESTIVE HEART FAILURE

Patients with severe congestive heart failure have a high frequency of complex ventricular ectopic activity and dysrhythmias. Sudden cardiac death, presumably caused by malignant dysrhythmias, accounts for over 40% of heart failure deaths. The effect of prophylactic amiodarone therapy in patients with congestive heart failure without symptomatic ventricular dysrhythmias has been evaluated in two clinical trials. The Groupa de Estudio de la Sobrevida en la Insuficiencia Cardiaca en Argentina (GESICA) trial randomized 516 patients with advanced congestive heart failure (New York Heart Association [NYHA] functional class III or IV) without symptomatic dysrhythmias to amiodarone therapy or control. This trial was terminated early after 13 months because of a significant 19% reduction in total mortality in the amiodarone group. Both subgroups of patients with and without nonsustained ventricular tachycardia on Holter monitor had reduced mortality with amiodarone.

The Survival Trial of Antiarrhythmic Therapy in Congestive Heart Failure (STAT-CHF) evaluated the effect of amiodarone compared with placebo on mortality in 674 patients with congestive heart failure and asymptomatic ventricular dysrhythmias (more than 10 PVCs per hour on Holter monitor). Although amiodarone therapy significantly suppressed ventricular dysrhythmias, there was no difference in overall mortality at 45-month follow-up. STAT-CHF may have failed to demonstrate an improvement in mortality with amiodarone therapy for two reasons. First, the patients enrolled in STAT-CHF (55% NYHA II, 43% NYHA III or IV) had less severe congestive heart failure compared to the patients enrolled in GESICA (100% NYHA III or IV). Amiodarone may provide a survival advantage only in patients with advanced congestive heart failure who are the patients with the highest mortality and incidence of ventricular dysrhythmias. Second, the proportion of patients with coronary artery disease in STAT-CHF (70%) was higher than in GESICA (39%). Amiodarone may provide more benefit among patients with nonischemic cardiomyopathy.

An interesting finding from both of these trials was that amiodarone meaningfully improved congestive symptoms and LVEF. Amiodarone therapy in the GESICA trial significantly reduced hospital admissions for congestive heart failure and improved the NYHA functional class. In the STAT-CHF trial, amiodarone therapy significantly improved the LVEF. The mechanism for improvement in congestive symptoms and ventricular function may be related to the β-adrenergic blocking effects or to the coronary and perhaps systemic vasodilatory effects of amiodarone. In a separate trial,[5] an improvement in exercise tolerance was observed in patients with congestive heart failure treated with low-dose amiodarone. Thus, prophylactic amiodarone therapy appears to reduce mortality and improve NYHA functional class and LVEF in at least some patients with advanced congestive heart failure.

β-Blocker Trials

The protective effect of β-adrenergic antagonists on overall survival after myocardial infarction is discussed in Chapter 4, "β-Blocker Trials." Long-term treatment with β-blockers is unequivocally associated with a reduction in the incidence of sudden cardiac death. The β-Blocker Heart Attack Trial (BHAT) demonstrated a 28% reduction in the incidence of sudden cardiac death (P < 0.05) among patients treated with propranolol after myocardial infarction over a 2-year follow-up period. The Goteborg Metoprolol Trial showed a reduction in the in-hospital incidence of ventricular fibrillation (P = 0.03) and the requirement for lidocaine (P < 0.01) among postinfarction patients treated with metoprolol compared to placebo. The Norwegian Propranolol Study demonstrated a 51% reduction in sudden cardiac death (P = 0.04) and a significant reduction in PVCs and nonsustained ventricular tachycardia among high-risk survivors of acute myocardial infarction treated with propranolol over a 1-year follow-up period. Finally, in the Norwegian Timolol Trial, sudden cardiac death was reduced by 45% (P = 0.0001) with timolol treatment for 3 years in patients surviving acute myocardial infarction. Thus, chronic administration of selected β-blockers to patients after myocardial infarction substantially decreases the incidence of sudden cardiac death.

Invasive Electrophysiologic Testing

The Electrophysiologic Study vs. Electrocardiographic Monitoring (ESVEM) trial was designed to determine which method, electrophysiologic (EP) testing or Holter monitoring with exercise testing, more accurately predicted the prevention of recurrence of ventricular dysrhythmias by antiarrhythmic therapy. A total of 486 patients with documented ventricular tachyarrhythmias that were inducible during EP study and who had more than 10 PVCs per hour during Holter monitoring were assigned to various drug therapies guided by EP study or Holter monitor. Patients assigned to EP testing had more predictions of drug efficacy compared to patients assigned to Holter monitor. Among patients with a prediction of drug efficacy, the mean actuarial recurrence rates of ventricular tachycardia were 64% for the EP study group compared with 67% for the Holter monitor group. In other words, both methods were equal in their ability to predict the success of a drug in preventing the recurrence of dysrhythmias.

Other trials have shown that patients who have a prediction of drug efficacy have a lower risk of arrhythmic death compared to patients who do not have a prediction of drug efficacy. In the ESVEM trial, the group of 190 patients in whom no drug was predicted to be efficacious were treated outside the protocol. This group had a risk of recurrence of dysrhythmia of 62%, which is similar to the recurrence rate found in patients with a prediction of drug efficacy by EP study (64%) and Holter monitor (67%). Thus, invasive EP testing and noninvasive Holter monitoring appear equal in their ability to predict the success of a drug in preventing dysrhythmias. Furthermore, the results of ESVEM suggest that the ability to predict the effectiveness of a drug has no significant effect on the rate of recurrence of dysrhythmia. Patients with a prediction of drug efficacy had an approximately 65% risk of recurrence of dysrhythmia compared to a 62% risk of recurrence of dysrhythmia in patients without a prediction of drug efficacy who were treated outside the study protocol.

Automatic Implantable Cardioverter/Defibrillator

Michel Mirowski designed the first AICD and had the first AICD implanted into a human patient at Johns Hopkins Hospital in 1980. These devices detect malignant ventricular dysrhythmias by continuously monitoring a patient's cardiac rhythm, and they then automatically cardiovert and terminate the dysrhythmia. The first-generation devices used epicardial patches and were bulky, requiring implantation in the abdomen. Newer devices are much smaller, allowing for subpectoral implantation, and use transvenous leads, obviating the need for thoracotomy. With more sophisticated detection algorithms and ease of implantation, these devices have the potential to significantly reduce mortality from ventricular tachyarrhythmias. The Amiodarone vs. Implantable Defibrillator (AVID) trial, the Cardiac Arrest Study in Hamburg (CASH), the Multicenter Unsustained Tachycardia Trial (MUSTT), the Multicenter Automatic Defibrillator (MADIT) trial, and the CABG PATCH trial are large ongoing clinical trials investigating the effects on survival of AICD therapy in various high-risk populations for sudden cardiac death.

Conclusions

Cardiac dysrhythmias account for a significant number of deaths from acute myocardial infarction and congestive heart failure. Antiarrhythmic drugs have enjoyed only limited success, which is due to frequent side effects, a lack of uniform effectiveness, and the potential for proarrhythmias. The use of encainide, flecainide, and moricizine increased mortality when administered to patients after myocardial infarction. Mexilitine was effective in reducing ventricular ectopy in patients after myocardial infarction but produced a trend toward increased mortality. Prophylactic lidocaine may increase mortality in the setting of acute myocardial infarction, as suggested by meta-analyses. Meta-analyses and retrospective studies have suggested that the chronic administration of quinidine to patients with atrial fibrillation increases mortality. Amiodarone appears to be more effective than conventional antiarrhythmic therapy and may improve survival when administered prophylactically to patients after myocardial infarction and to patients with advanced congestive heart failure. Long-term treatment with specific β-blockers, without the ability to stimulate β-receptors, unequivocally reduces the incidence of sudden cardiac death in postinfarction patients. Electrophysiologic testing and Holter monitoring appear to be equal in their ability to predict the success of a drug in preventing the recurrence of dysrhythmias. The AICD is undergoing intense clinical investigation, and it appears to have real potential for reducing mortality from ventricular dysrhythmias.

BASIS

Basel Antiarrhythmic Study of Infarct Survival

PURPOSE

Determine the effect of prophylactic antiarrhythmic treatment on mortality in patients with asymptomatic complex ventricular arrhythmias after myocardial infarction.

STUDY DESIGN

General

- 312 patients enrolled in this prospective, randomized, controlled trial.
- Eligible patients were randomized to one of three treatment groups:
  1. Individualized antiarrhythmic therapy: quinidine or mexilitine with dosage titration to suppress Lown class 4 arrhythmias, reduce premature ventricular contractions (PVCs) by ≥ 50%, eliminate runs of three-beat or more ventricular tachycardia, and reduce couplets by ≥ 90%. If both drugs failed, other antiarrhythmic drugs were used (ajmaline, disopyramide, flecainide, propafenone, sotalol). If none of these drugs were effective, amiodarone was used.
  2. Amiodarone therapy: 1,000 mg PO every day for 5 days, then 200 mg/day.
  3. Control group.

Inclusion. Patients included were < 71 years of age and were admitted with acute myocardial infarction. A Holter monitor, placed 1–3 days before hospital discharge, had to reveal frequent multiform PVC or repetitive ventricular arrhythmias (Lown class 3 or 4b) present in ≥ 2 of 24 hr.

Exclusion. The criteria for exclusion were symptomatic arrhythmias, cardiovascular surgery during hospitalization, or other life-threatening illness.

End Points. The criterion for end point was mortality, both sudden death and other cardiac death.

RESULTS

Cumulative mortality rates at 12 months were significantly reduced for amiodarone therapy compared to the control group (5% amiodarone vs. 13% control, $P = 0.048$). No significant difference in mortality was observed between the individual treatment group and control (10% individual treatment vs. 13% control). Amiodarone also significantly reduced sudden death and sustained ventricular tachycardia or ventricular fibrillation compared to control (5% amiodarone vs. 17% control, $P < 0.01$) (Fig. 7-2).

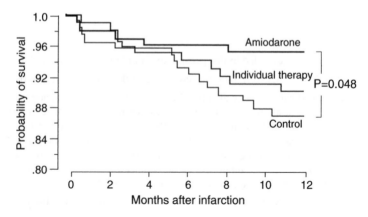

Figure 7-2. Probability of 12-month survival. (From Burkhart et al.,[6] with permission.)

CONCLUSIONS

Prophylactic amiodarone therapy significantly reduced 12-month mortality by 62% compared to control in a high-risk group of patients with asymptomatic persistent complex ventricular arrhythmias after myocardial infarction. Individualized treatment with a variety of antiarrhythmic drugs showed no benefit in survival compared to control.

(Data from Burkhart et al.[6]) ∎

CASCADE

Cardiac Arrest in Seattle: Conventional vs. Amiodarone Drug Evaluation

PURPOSE

Compare the effect of amiodarone vs. conventional drug therapy in survivors of out-of-hospital ventricular fibrillation not associated with a Q-wave myocardial infarction who were at especially high risk of recurrent ventricular fibrillation.

STUDY DESIGN

General

- 228 patients enrolled in this prospective, randomized trial.
- Eligible patients were randomized to one of two treatment groups:
  1. Amiodarone: the mean dose of amiodarone was 183 mg/day at 12 months, 158 mg/day at 24 months, and 185 mg/day at 36 months.
  2. Conventional therapy: procainamide (22%), quinidine (29%), disopyramide (3%), tocainide (4%), mexilitine (7%), flecainide (10%), propafenone (1%), moricizine (1%), or combination therapy (15%).
- Baseline radionuclide ventriculography and drug-free Holter monitor, electrophysiologic (EP) study, or both were performed.

Inclusion. Patients included were resuscitated from an episode of out-of-hospital ventricular fibrillation without a primary reversible cause or Q-wave myocardial infarction who were at risk of recurrent ventricular fibrillation estimated ≥ 20% at 1 year. These patients had > 10 PVCs per hour on Holter monitor or sustained ventricular tachycardia or fibrillation at EP study.

End Points. The criteria for end points were cardiac survival defined as survival free of cardiac mortality, resuscitated cardiac arrest that was due to documented ventricular fibrillation, and complete syncope followed by a shock from an automatic implantable cardioverter/defibrillator.

RESULTS

Early results at 2 years showed a favorable trend toward better cardiac survival for amiodarone, although the results were not statistically significant. At 6-year follow-up, amiodarone significantly improved cardiac survival by 33% compared to conventional therapy (53% amiodarone vs. 40% conventional, P = 0.007). The combined end point of cardiac survival and the absence of sustained ventricular arrhythmias at 6 years was also significantly better with amiodarone (41% amiodarone vs. 20% conventional, P < 0.001). Amiodarone was associated with a 10% incidence of pulmonary toxicity at 3 years and a significantly high rate of drug discontinuation at 1 year (Fig. 7-3).

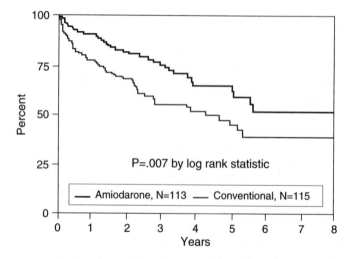

Figure 7-3. Cumulative cardiac survival for all patients. (From The CASCADE Investigators,[7] with permission.)

CONCLUSIONS

Treatment with amiodarone resulted in significantly better survival free of cardiac death and sustained ventricular arrhythmias compared to conventional therapy in patients surviving out-of-hospital ventricular fibrillation at 6-year follow-up. Amiodarone, however, also produced pulmonary toxicity in 10% of patients and resulted in more frequent discontinuation of therapy.

(Data from The CASCADE Investigators.[7]) ■

CASH

Cardiac Arrest Study Hamburg

PURPOSE

Compare the effects of metoprolol, amiodarone, propafenone, and an automatic implantable cardioverter/defibrillator (AICD) on mortality in patients surviving sudden cardiac death that was due to documented ventricular tachycardia or fibrillation.

STUDY DESIGN

General

- 230 patients enrolled to date in this prospective, randomized, multi-center trial.

- Eligible patients were randomized to one of four treatment groups:
  1. Metoprolol: initial dose of 12.5–25 mg/day titrated up to maximum of 200 mg/day as tolerated.
  2. Amiodarone: loading dose of 1,000 mg/day for 7 days, then 400–600 mg/day.
  3. Propafenone: initial dose of 450 mg/day titrated up to maximum of 900 mg/day as tolerated.
  4. AICD implantation: detection rate of 170–200 bpm with primary therapy given as electrical cardioversion. No subsequent antiarrhythmic medications were used.

- Echocardiography, Holter monitor, exercise testing, coronary and left ventricular angiography, and electrophysiologic (EP) study were performed in all patients.

- Patients with severe ischemia were revascularized.
- Patients assigned to medications had repeat EP study and Holter monitor performed after steady-state drug effect was obtained.

Inclusion. Patients included were survivors of sudden cardiac death that was due to documented ventricular tachycardia or fibrillation and were randomized within 3 months of the event.

End Points. The criteria for end points were total mortality, sudden cardiac death, and incidence of recurrent ventricular tachycardia or fibrillation.

RESULTS

After an average 11-month follow-up, the Safety Monitoring Board recommended early termination of the propafenone arm only. Compared to AICD treatment, the use of propafenone resulted in a significantly higher incidence of sudden death (12% propafenone vs. 0% AICD, $P < 0.05$) and sudden death or cardiac arrest (23% propafenone vs. 0% AICD, $P < 0.05$). The incidence of true-positive discharges during syncope in the AICD group (which represents the natural history of arrhythmia in medically untreated patients) was 23%, which is identical to that seen with propafenone treatment. No significant difference in the primary end points to date were observed between metoprolol, amiodarone, and AICD (Fig. 7-4).

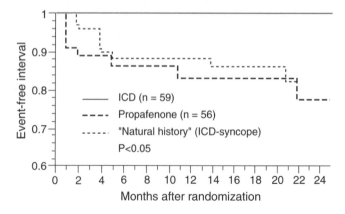

Figure 7-4. Sudden death survival and recurrence of cardiac arrest. (From Siebels et al.,[8] with permission.)

CONCLUSIONS
In this preliminary report at 11-month follow-up, propafenone resulted in a significantly increased incidence of sudden death and sudden death or cardiac arrest compared to patients treated with AICD. The propafenone arm was therefore terminated; the study continues with metoprolol, amiodarone, and AICD treatments.

(Data from Siebels et al.[8]) ■

CAST 1

Cardiac Arrhythmia Suppression Trial

PURPOSE
Determine if suppression of ventricular ectopy after myocardial infarction with encainide, flecainide, or moricizine reduces the incidence of sudden death.

STUDY DESIGN

General

- 1,498 patients enrolled in this prospective, randomized, double-blind, placebo-controlled trial.

- Patients first underwent an open-label titration phase using up to three drugs at two oral doses as follows:

  1. Encainide: 35 mg PO tid, then 50 mg PO tid

  2. Flecainide: 100 mg PO bid, then 150 mg PO bid

  3. Moricizine: 200 mg PO tid, then 250 mg PO tid

- This initial open-label titration period was used to determine which patients responded to drug therapy with at least 80% suppression of ventricular premature depolarizations and at least 90% suppression of runs of ventricular tachycardia on Holter monitor placed 4–10 days after each dose began. Patients who responded to drug therapy were then enrolled in the main study and randomly assigned to a titrated dose of drug or placebo. Flecainide was avoided in patients with left ventricular ejection fraction (LVEF) < 30%.

Inclusion. Patients included were 6 days to 2 years after myocardial infarction with an average of six or more PVCs per hour on ambulatory

Holter monitor of ≥ 18-hr duration. Patients were also required to have a LVEF ≤ 55% if the patient was recruited within 90 days of myocardial infarction or a LVEF was ≤ 40% if recruited after 90 days of myocardial infarction.

Exclusion. The criteria for exclusion were as follows: ventricular arrhythmias causing severe symptoms such as syncope or presyncope, nonsustained ventricular tachycardia with ≥ 15 successive beats at a rate ≥ 120 bpm, poor compliance, contraindications to the study drugs, other life-threatening illness, or electrocardiogram abnormalities that would make interpretation of the rhythm difficult.

End Points. The criteria for end points were death or cardiac arrest with resuscitation, either of which was due to arrhythmia.

RESULTS

The Data and Safety Monitoring Board recommended early termination of CAST 1. The use of encainide and flecainide resulted in a 2.64-fold increase in death or cardiac arrest compared to placebo during the average 10-month follow-up period (63 events flecainide/encainide vs. 26

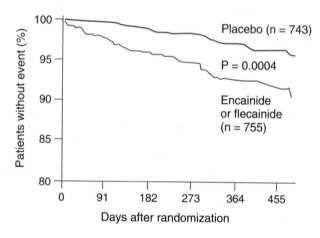

Figure 7-5. Actuarial probabilities of freedom from death or cardiac arrest due to arrhythmia. (From Echt et al.,[9] with permission.)

events placebo, P = 0.0004). The increased risk of death or cardiac arrest in patients receiving active drug was similar among the subgroups of patients with LVEF < 30% (risk ratio [RR] = 1.97) and patients with LVEF > 30% (RR = 3.38). In addition, more deaths and cardiac arrests that were not due to arrhythmia (acute myocardial infarction, congestive heart failure, after coronary artery bypass graft) occurred with encainide and flecainide compared to placebo (17 events flecainide/encainide vs. 5 deaths placebo, P = 0.01) (Fig. 7-5).

CONCLUSIONS
The use of encainide or flecainide in patients after myocardial infarction resulted in a significant 2.64-fold excess of death or cardiac arrest compared to placebo. The results of moricizine are reported in CAST 2.

(Data from Echt et al.[9]) ■

CAST 2

Cardiac Arrhythmia Suppression Trial

PURPOSE
Determine if suppression of ventricular ectopy after myocardial infarction with moricizine reduces the incidence of sudden death.

STUDY DESIGN

General

- CAST 2 was divided into two prospective, randomized, blinded, placebo-controlled trials as follows:

  1. Early, 14-day, low-dose exposure phase: 1,325 patients treated with moricizine 200 mg PO tid.

  2. Long-term phase: 1,155 patients underwent titration of moricizine starting with 200 mg PO tid, then 250 mg PO tid, and if necessary 300 mg PO tid until adequate suppression of ≥ 80% of premature ventricular contractions (PVCs) and ≥ 90% of runs of nonsustained ventricular tachycardia on ambulatory Holter monitor placed 4–10 days after each dose began. Patients who responded to drug therapy were then enrolled in the main study and randomly assigned to titrated dose of drug or placebo.

Inclusion. Patients included were within 90 days of a myocardial infarction with a Holter monitor demonstrating of an average of six or more PVCs per hour and a radionuclide left ventricular ejection fraction ≤ 40%.

Exclusion. The criteria for exclusion were as follows: ventricular arrhythmias causing severe symptoms such as syncope or presyncope, ventricular tachycardia lasting ≥ 30 sec at a rate ≥ 120 bpm, poor compliance, contraindications to the study drugs, other life-threatening illness, or electrocardiogram abnormalities that would make interpretation of the rhythm difficult. Patients with repetitive ventricular complexes ≥ 15 beats lasting up to 30 sec without symptoms were allowed to be enrolled.

End Points. The criteria for end points follow:

- Early low-dose phase: death or cardiac arrest
- Long-term phase: death or cardiac arrest with resuscitation, either of which was due to arrhythmia

RESULTS

The Data and Safety Monitoring Board recommended early termination of CAST 2. During the early, 2-week, low-dose phase, the use of moricizine

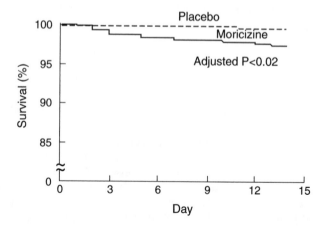

Figure 7-6. Survival of patients during the first 14 days of treatment. (From The Cardiac Arrhythmia Suppression Trial II Investigators,[10] with permission.)

resulted in a significant excess of death or cardiac arrest compared to placebo (17 events with moricizine vs. 3 events with placebo, P = 0.001). In addition, there was a trend toward more recurrent myocardial infarction, new or worsened congestive heart failure, and proarrhythmia with moricizine. In the long-term phase, at a mean follow-up of 18 months, there was no significant difference in the numbers of deaths or cardiac arrests due to arrhythmia between moricizine and placebo (49 events with moricizine vs. 42 events with placebo, P = 0.40) (Fig. 7-6).

CONCLUSIONS
The use of moricizine to reduce ventricular premature depolarizations after myocardial infarction significantly increased mortality compared to placebo during the initial 2 weeks of treatment with no benefit seen at 18-month follow-up.

––––––––––

(Data from The Cardiac Arrhythmia Suppression Trial II Investigators.[10]) ∎

ESVEM

Electrophysiologic Study vs. Electrocardiographic Monitoring Study

PURPOSE
Compare invasive electrophysiologic (EP) study with noninvasive Holter monitoring as predictors of drug efficacy in the treatment of ventricular tachyarrhythmias.

STUDY DESIGN

General

- 486 patients enrolled in this prospective, randomized, multicenter trial.

- Eligible patients were randomized to Holter monitor or EP testing group and then received up to seven antiarrhythmic drugs (imipramine, mexilitine, pirmenol, procainamide, propafenone, quinidine, and sotalol) in random order until one or more was predicted to be effective.

- Prediction of efficacy was defined as follows:

1. Holter monitor group: suppression of 100% of runs of ventricular tachycardia (VT) > 15 beats, 90% of shorter runs of VT, 80% of all couplets, 70% of all premature ventricular contractions (PVCs) as well as the absence of VT of ≥ 5 beats on exercise testing
2. Invasive EP testing: suppression of inducible VT lasting > 15 beats

Inclusion. Patients included met one or more of the following criteria:

1. Electrocardiographically documented sustained VT or ventricular fibrillation lasting ≥ 15 sec
2. Resuscitation from cardiac arrest
3. Syncope without electrocardiogram (ECG) documentation of the reproducible rhythm but with inducible VT by EP study

In addition, all patients had an average of 10 PVCs per hour during 48-hr Holter monitoring and reproducibly inducible sustained VT at EP study.

Exclusion. The criteria for exclusion were myocardial infarction within 3 weeks, a high likelihood of surgical revascularization within the next 2 months, Wolff-Parkinson-White syndrome, previous responsiveness to one of the study drugs, the presence of an automatic implantable cardioverter/defibrillator, or other serious illness.

End Points. The criteria for end points were recurrence of arrhythmia defined as ECG-documented VT of ≥ 15 beats; ventricular fibrillation; and death caused by arrhythmia, cardiac arrest, torsades de pointes, or unmonitored syncope.

RESULTS

An antiarrhythmic drug was predicted to be effective in 45% of patients in the EP study group compared to 77% of patients in the Holter monitor group. The mean actuarial recurrence rates of arrhythmia in patients with predictions for drug efficacy at 4 years was 64% for the EP study group vs. 67% for the Holter monitor group ($P = 0.69$). There was no significant difference between study groups in the type of recurrent arrhythmia ($P = 0.80$). The use of sotalol was an independent predictor of significant reduction in the recurrence of arrhythmia ($P = 0.01$) and a trend toward reduced mortality ($P = 0.07$).

The 190 patients in whom no drug was predicted to be effective were subsequently treated outside the study protocol. The risk of recurrence of arrhythmia was 62% in this group, which is similar to that among the 296 patients with predictions of drug efficacy.

CONCLUSIONS

In patients with ventricular tachyarrhythmias, there was no significant difference between invasive EP testing and Holter monitor regarding their ability to predict the success of drug therapy in preventing recurrence of arrhythmia. In addition, patients with predictions of drug efficacy by Holter monitor or EP study had rates of recurrence of arrhythmia similar to those of patients without predictions of drug efficacy who were treated empirically.

(Data from Mason.[11]) ■

GESICA

Grupo de Estudio de la Sobrevida en la Insuficiencia Cardiaca en Argentina

PURPOSE

Study the effect of amiodarone on mortality in patients with severe congestive heart failure without symptomatic ventricular arrhythmias.

STUDY DESIGN

General

- 516 patients enrolled in this prospective, randomized, multicenter trial.
- Eligible patients were randomized to one of two treatment groups:
  1. Amiodarone: loaded with 600 mg/day for 14 days, then 300 mg/day for 2 years
  2. Control
- All patients received diuretics, digitalis, and angiotensin-converting enzyme inhibitors.

- Patients were stratified according to the presence or absence of nonsustained ventricular tachycardia (NSVT) on admission 24-hr Holter monitor.

Inclusion. Patients included had advanced chronic congestive heart failure (New York Heart Association [NYHA] functional class advanced III or IV) adequately treated with salt restriction, diuretics, digoxin, and vasodilators. Patients were not receiving antiarrhythmic medications and had a marked reduction of left ventricular systolic function (defined as a cardiothoracic ratio > 0.55 on chest x-ray, left ventricular ejection fraction ≤ 35% by radionuclide ventriculography, and a left ventricular end-diastole diameter ≥ 3.2 cm/M^2).

Exclusion. The criteria for exclusion were symptomatic ventricular arrhythmias, amiodarone treatment during the previous 3 months, thyroid disease, severe respiratory failure, mitral or aortic stenosis, hypertrophic or restrictive cardiomyopathy, atrioventricular block, history of ventricular tachycardia or fibrillation, > 10-beat run of asymptomatic ventricular tachycardia with a rate > 100 bpm, angina pectoris, myocardial infarction, onset of congestive heart failure or syncope within the previous 3 months, or other serious illness.

End Point. The criterion for end point was total mortality.

RESULTS
On the recommendation of the steering committee, the trial was terminated early after an average of 13 months. The use of amiodarone significantly reduced total mortality by 19% compared to control (33.5% amiodarone vs. 41.4% control, P = 0.024). The benefit of amiodarone was due to a reduction of both sudden cardiac death and death that was due to progressive heart failure. Patients with and without NSVT on admission Holter monitor had reduced mortality with amiodarone. Amiodarone treatment resulted in fewer hospital admissions for congestive heart failure (45.8% amiodarone vs. 58.9% control, P = 0.0024). Amiodarone also resulted in a significantly higher proportion of patients who had improved functional class compared to control. Side effects were reported in 6.1% of patients taking amiodarone; however, pulmonary and thyroid status was followed clinically, not by serial thyroid and pulmonary function tests (Fig. 7-7).

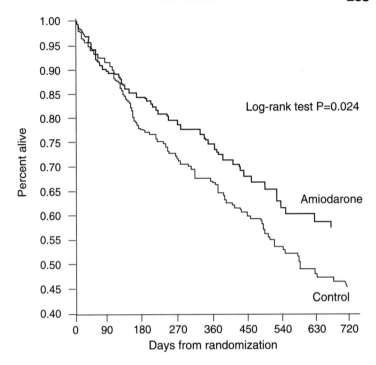

Figure 7-7. Total mortality. (From Doval et al.,[12] with permission.)

CONCLUSIONS

Amiodarone therapy significantly reduced total mortality by 19%, reduced hospital admissions for worsening congestive heart failure, and improved NYHA functional class compared to a control group in patients with severe congestive heart failure over a 13-month follow-up. This effect was independent of the presence of NSVT on admission Holter monitor.

(Data from Doval et al.[12])   ■

IMPACT

International Mexiletine and Placebo Antiarrhythmic Coronary Trial

PURPOSE

Determine the antiarrhythmic effect of mexiletine in patients with a recent myocardial infarction.

STUDY DESIGN

General

- 630 patients enrolled in this prospective, randomized, double-blind, placebo-controlled, multicenter trial.
- Eligible patients were randomized to one of two treatment groups:
  1. Mexiletine: 360-mg sustained release capsules PO bid
  2. Placebo
- Patients who required antianginal medication other than long-acting nitrates or antiarrhythmic medications other than β-blockers were withdrawn from the study.
- Clinical follow-up and serial Holter monitors continued to 12 months.

Inclusion. Patients included were men 30–74 years old and women 45–74 years old who were admitted to a hospital coronary care unit with evidence of a recent myocardial infarction. Patients were not required to have arrhythmias.

Exclusion. The criteria for exclusion were refractory congestive heart failure, cardiogenic shock, Wolff-Parkinson-White syndrome, left bundle branch block, second- or third-degree atrioventricular block, organic neurologic disorders, myocardial infarction secondary to a known cause other than atherosclerosis, the need for other antiarrhythmic drugs, contraindications to mexiletine, or other serious illness.

End Points. The criteria for end points were incidence of ≥ 30 single premature ventricular contractions (PVCs) in any two consecutive 30-min blocks or one or more run of two or more PVCs in 24 hr.

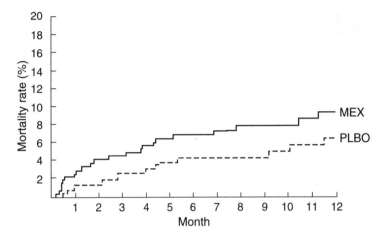

Figure 7-8. Life-table analysis for total mortality. MEX, mexiletine; PLBO, placebo. (From IMPACT Research Group,[13] with permission.)

RESULTS

A significant reduction in the occurrence of the primary end point was observed in the mexiletine group at 1 month (36.5% mexiletine vs. 58.0% placebo, Z value = -5.04) and at 4 months (41.7% mexiletine vs. 59.9% placebo, Z value = -3.98). At 1 year, however, the occurrence of primary end points was not statistically different (43.3% mexiletine vs. 53.6% placebo). The incidence of nonsustained ventricular tachycardia (NSVT) was also significantly reduced with mexilitine at 1 and 4 months only, but not at 12 months of follow-up. At an average of 9 months of follow-up, there was a trend toward higher mortality in the mexiletine group compared to placebo (7.6% mexiletine vs. 4.8% placebo, Z value = 1.45) (Fig. 7-8).

CONCLUSIONS

The use of sustained release mexiletine in patients with a recent myocardial infarction resulted in a significant reduction in the combined occurrence of frequent PVC, couplets, and NSVT at 1- and 4-month follow-up compared to placebo. However, there was a trend toward increased overall mortality at 9 months in the mexiletine group compared to placebo.

(Data from IMPACT Research Group.[13]) ■

PAS

Polish Amiodarone Study

PURPOSE

Determine the effect of amiodarone on mortality and ventricular arrhythmias in high-risk, postinfarction patients with contraindications to β-blocker therapy.

STUDY DESIGN

General

- 613 patients enrolled in this prospective, randomized, double-blind, placebo-controlled trial.
- Eligible patients were randomized to one of two treatment groups:
    1. Amiodarone: Initial dose of 800 mg/day for 7 days, then 400 mg PO 6 days a week for 12 months.

       Dose could be decreased to 200 mg or 100 mg per day if heart rate was < 55 bpm or Q-T interval corrected for heart rate (QTc) > 480 msec.
    2. Placebo.
- Serial 24-hr Holter monitors, echocardiograms, chest x-rays, and laboratory studies were obtained during the 12-month follow-up period.

Inclusion. Patients included were < 75 years old with a confirmed diagnosis of acute myocardial infarction and contraindication to β-blocker therapy.

Exclusion. The criteria for exclusion were hypotension, bradycardia, atrioventricular block, bundle branch blocks, prolonged QTc, a clear need for antiarrhythmic therapy, amiodarone use in the past 6 months, or other life-threatening illness.

End Points. The criteria for end points were cardiac mortality, total mortality, and serious (Lown grade 4) ventricular arrhythmias on Holter monitoring.

RESULTS

At 12-month follow-up, amiodarone therapy significantly reduced cardiac mortality compared to placebo (6.2% amiodarone vs. 10.7%

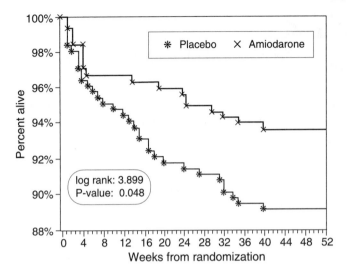

Figure 7-9. Survival curves for amiodarone and placebo groups. (From Ceremuzynski et al.,[14] with permission.)

placebo, P = 0.048). Amiodarone also produced a favorable trend toward less sudden death (3.3% amiodarone vs. 6.5% control, P = 0.07), although the results were not statistically significant. The incidence of serious ventricular arrhythmias (Lown grade 4) was significantly lower in the amiodarone group (7.5% amiodarone vs. 19.5% control, P < 0.001) (Fig. 7-9).

CONCLUSIONS

Amiodarone significantly reduced cardiac mortality and serious ventricular arrhythmias (Lown grade 4) and resulted in a trend toward less sudden death compared to placebo at 12-month follow-up in patients after acute myocardial infarction with contraindications to β-blocker therapy.

(Data from Ceremuzynski et al.[14]) ∎

Survival Trial of Antiarrhythmic Therapy in Congestive Heart Failure

PURPOSE

Determine the effect of amiodarone on mortality in patients with congestive heart failure and asymptomatic ventricular arrhythmias.

STUDY DESIGN

General

- 674 patients enrolled in this prospective, randomized, double-blind, placebo-controlled, multicenter trial.
- Eligible patients randomized to one of two treatment groups:
  1. Amiodarone: Initially, 800 mg/day for 14 days, then 400 mg/day for 50 weeks, then 300 mg/day until the end of the study
  2. Placebo
- All patients received vasodilatory therapy. Digoxin and diuretics were administered at the discretion of the local physician.
- Radionuclide ventriculography was performed at baseline, 6, 12, and 24 months.
- Echocardiograms were performed at baseline, 12, and 24 months.

Inclusion. Patients included had a documented history of congestive heart failure and ≥ 10 premature ventricular contractions (PVCs) per hour without symptoms on ambulatory Holter monitor. All patients had dyspnea on exertion or paroxysmal nocturnal dyspnea, an echocardiogram showing a left ventricular end-diastole diameter of ≥ 55 mm or chest x-ray with cardiothoracic ratio > 0.50, and a left ventricular ejection fraction (LVEF) ≤ 40% by radionuclide ventriculography.

Exclusion. The criteria for exclusion were women of childbearing age, myocardial infarction within the previous 3 months, symptomatic ventricular arrhythmias, history of aborted sudden cardiac death or sustained ventricular tachycardia, uncontrolled thyroid disease, clear need

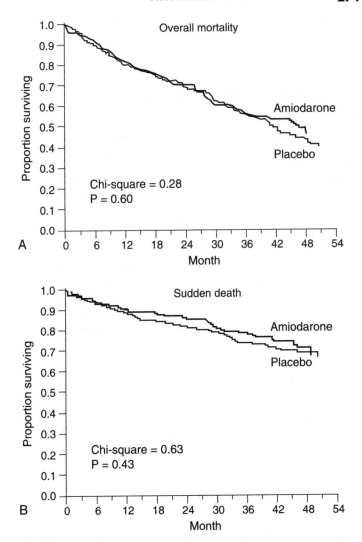

Figure 7-10. *(A & B)* Kaplan-Meier estimates of overall mortality and sudden death from cardiac causes. (From Singh et al.,[15] with permission)

for antiarrhythmic therapy, QRS interval ≥ 180 msec or Q-T interval corrected for heart rate ≥ 500 msec, symptomatic hypotension or systolic blood pressure < 90 mmHg, or other serious illness.

End Points. The criteria for end points were overall mortality, sudden cardiac death, and left ventricular ejection fraction.

RESULTS

During an average 45-month follow-up, there was no significant difference in overall mortality between amiodarone and placebo treatment (39% amiodarone vs. 42% placebo, P = 0.60). The incidence of sudden cardiac death was also similar between the two treatment groups (19% amiodarone vs. 22% placebo, P = 0.43). Amiodarone significantly reduced the frequency of PVC at 3 months (44 PVC per hour amiodarone vs. 266 PVC per hour placebo, P < 0.001) and the incidence of ventricular tachycardia at 2 weeks (33% amiodarone vs. 76% placebo, P < 0.001); however, neither of these subgroups with suppressed PVC or suppressed ventricular tachycardia on amiodarone had any survival benefit compared to placebo. The use of amiodarone did result in substantial improvements in LVEF at 2 years compared to placebo: LVEF with amiodarone was 24.9% baseline to 35.4% at 2 years (+42% improvement); LVEF with placebo was 25.7% baseline to 29.8% at 2 years (+16% improvement), P < 0.001. (Fig. 7-10).

CONCLUSIONS

The use of amiodarone in patients with congestive heart failure and asymptomatic arrhythmias had no effect on overall mortality or sudden cardiac death, despite significant suppression of ventricular arrhythmias and a substantial improvement in left ventricular ejection fraction compared to placebo over a 45-month follow-up period.

(Data from Singh et al.[15]) ■

References

1. MacMahon S, Collins R, Peto R et al: Effects of prophylactic lidocaine in suspected acute myocardial infarction: an overview of results from the randomized controlled trials. JAMA 260:1910, 1988

2. Coplen SE, Antmann EM, Berlin JA et al: Efficacy and safety of quinidine therapy for maintenance of sinus rhythm after cardioversion: a meta-analysis of randomized controlled trials. Circulation 82:1106, 1990

3. Flaker GC, Blackshear JL, McBride R et al: Antiarrhythmic drug therapy and cardiac mortality in atrial fibrillation. J Am Coll Cardiol 20:527, 1992

4. Teo KK, Yusuf S, Furberg CD: Effects of prophylactic antiarrhythmic drug therapy in acute myocardial infarction: an overview of results from randomized controlled trials. JAMA 270:1589, 1993

5. Hamer AW, Arkles LB, Johns JA: Beneficial effects of low dose amiodarone in patients with congestive heart failure: a placebo controlled trial. J Am Coll Cardiol 14:1768, 1989

6. Burkhart F, Pfisterer M, Kiowski W et al: Effect of antiarrhythmic therapy on mortality in survivors of myocardial infarction with asymptomatic complex ventricular arrhythmias: Basel Antiarrhythmic Study of Infarct Survival (BASIS). J Am Coll Cardiol 16:1711-8, 1990

7. The CASCADE Investigators: Randomized antiarrhythmic drug therapy in survivors of cardiac arrest (the CASCADE Study). Am J Cardiol 72:280-7, 1993

8. Siebels J, Cappato R, Rüppel R et al: Preliminary results of the Cardiac Arrest Study Hamburg (CASH). Am J Cardiol 72:109F-13F, 1993

9. Echt DS, Liebson PR, Mitchell LB et al: Mortality and morbidity in patients receiving encainide, flecainide, or placebo: the Cardiac Arrhythmia Suppression Trial. N Engl J Med 324:781-8, 1991

10. The Cardiac Arrhythmia Suppression Trial II Investigators: Effect of the antiarrhythmic agent moricizine on survival after myocardial infarction. N Engl J Med 327:227-33, 1992

11. Mason JW: A comparison of electrophysiologic testing with Holter monitoring to predict antiarrhythmic-drug efficacy for ventricular tachyarrhythmias. N Engl J Med 329:445-51, 1993

12. Doval HC, Nul DR, Grancelli HO et al: Randomised trial of low-dose amiodarone in severe congestive heart failure. Lancet 344:493-8, 1994

13. IMPACT Research Group: International Mexiletine and Placebo Antiarrhythmic Coronary Trial: I. Report on arrhythmia and other findings. J Am Coll Cardiol 4:1148-63, 1984

14. Ceremuzynski L, Kleczar E, Krzeminska-Pakula M et al: Effect of amiodarone on mortality after myocardial infarction: a double-blind, placebo-controlled, pilot study. J Am Coll Cardiol 20:1056-62, 1992

15. Singh SN, Fletcher RD, Fisher SG et al: Amiodarone in patients with congestive heart failure and asymptomatic venticular arrhythmia. N Engl J Med 333:77-82, 1995

CHAPTER 8

Atrial Fibrillation Trials

OVERVIEW

Atrial fibrillation is the most common form of cardiac dysrhythmia, affecting 0.4% of the adult population. Among patients over the age of 69 years, the incidence of atrial fibrillation is more than 5%. Hypertensive heart disease is the most common cause of atrial fibrillation, but other causes include coronary artery disease, dilated and restrictive cardiomyopathies, tachycardia-bradycardia syndrome, valvular heart disease, hyperthyroidism, pericarditis, Wolff-Parkinson-White syndrome, alcohol, and pulmonary emboli; commonly, it is idiopathic. The development of atrial fibrillation is associated with a twofold increase in mortality and a fivefold increase in morbidity. The major morbidity associated with atrial fibrillation consists of embolic disorders, particularly embolic stroke, presumably arising from thrombus residing in the left atrial appendage. Among patients with valvular heart disease, especially rheumatic mitral stenosis, the yearly incidence of embolic stroke is nearly 15%, which represents a 17-fold increase compared to the 0.9% yearly incidence of stroke in the general population. Patients without valvular heart disease have a more modestly increased yearly incidence of stroke of 3% to 5%. When atrial fibrillation occurs without detectable structural heart disease, known as idiopathic or "lone" atrial fibrillation, the incidence of embolic stroke is low and approaches that found in the general population, according to the Mayo Clinic experience.

In the presence of mitral stenosis, the risk of stroke in patients with atrial fibrillation is sufficiently high that chronic anticoagulation is usually recommended, even though little evidence from randomized trials supports this treatment. However, among patients with nonrheumatic atrial fibrillation with a more modest risk of embolic stroke, the benefit of chronic oral anticoagulation has been less clear. This subgroup of patients, with nonrheumatic atrial fibrillation, has provided the arena for most of the anticoagulation trials in atrial fibrillation.

Warfarin and Aspirin in Stroke Prevention in Nonrheumatic Atrial Fibrillation

The Copenhagen AFASAK trial was the first to examine the role of aspirin and warfarin in patients with chronic nonrheumatic atrial fibrillation. This trial randomized over 1,000 patients to warfarin titrated to keep the international normalized ratio (INR) 2.4 to 4.2, aspirin 75 mg/day, or placebo and found a significant 63% reduction in the incidence of thromboembolic events with use of warfarin only compared to placebo. Treatment with low-dose aspirin produced no benefit. The use of warfarin, however, also resulted in significantly more bleeding complications compared to placebo. These findings raised the question of whether a lower target level of anticoagulation would still protect against embolic events without conferring an increase in the risk of bleeding.

The Boston Area Anticoagulation Trial for Atrial Fibrillation (BAATAF) was designed to address this question by randomizing 420 patients to warfarin, titrated to keep the INR 1.5 to 2.7, or control. This trial was terminated early by the Data Monitoring Committee because of a significant, 86%, reduction in the risk of ischemic stroke with warfarin treatment compared to control at 2.3-year follow-up. In addition, this lower level of anticoagulation did not confer a significant increase in the incidence of major bleeds. The Veterans Affairs Stroke Prevention in Nonrheumatic Atrial Fibrillation (SPINAF) study used a dose of warfarin (INR 1.4 to 2.8) similar to that used in BAATAF and reconfirmed a significant, 80%, reduction in the incidence of ischemic stroke without an increase in the incidence of major hemorrhage at 1.7-year follow-up.

The Stroke Prevention in Atrial Fibrillation (SPAF 1) trial was designed to re-examine the role of aspirin, at a higher dose than used in AFASAK, as primary treatment for stroke prevention. Approximately 1,300 patients were randomized to warfarin titrated to keep the INR 2.0 to 3.5, aspirin 325 mg/day, or placebo. A significant reduction in the incidence of ischemic stroke or systemic embolization was observed with warfarin, by 67%, and aspirin, by 42%, compared to control. No direct comparison between warfarin and aspirin could be made in this trial, since the exclusion criteria were different for the aspirin and warfarin treatment groups (i.e., warfarin-ineligible patients were included in the aspirin group).

SPAF 2 was designed to directly compare aspirin with warfarin by randomizing approximately 1,100 patients with nonrheumatic atrial fibrillation to warfarin (INR 2.0 to 4.5) or aspirin (325 mg/day). Patients were separated according to age above or below 75 years and according to the presence of risk factors for thromboembolism (history of hypertension, previous thromboembolism, or recent heart failure). Among all patients, there was only a modest statistically insignificant reduction in ischemic stroke with warfarin over aspirin. Patients over 75 years of age with clinical risk factors for thromboembolism had a nonsignificant reduction in the risk of ischemic stroke with use of warfarin (4.2%/year) compared to aspirin (7.2%/year); however, the use of warfarin in this group was associated with more "major" hemorrhages. A combined end point of all strokes with residual deficits (hemorrhagic and ischemic) revealed no meaningful difference between aspirin and warfarin treatment. Patients less than 75 years of age without clinical risk factors for thromboembolism had a low incidence of ischemic stroke (0.5%/year) with the use of aspirin alone.

Secondary Prevention Trials

Patients who have already succumbed to an embolic stroke represent a subgroup of patients at increased risk for future embolic events. The role of aspirin or warfarin in this population was studied in The European Atrial Fibrillation Trial (EAFT), which randomized approximately 1,000 patients with recent transient ischemic attack or minor stroke to warfarin (INR 2.5 to 4.0), aspirin (325 mg/day), or placebo. Patients receiving placebo had a 12% yearly incidence of stroke. Treatment with warfarin produced a significant 66% reduction in the incidence of ischemic stroke over a 2.3-year follow-up. Treatment with aspirin provided no meaningful protection against stroke. Warfarin did, however, substantially increase "major" bleeding episodes compared to placebo, which is perhaps due to the high utilized INR of 2.5 to 4.0.

Optimal Dose of Warfarin

The level of anticoagulation, assessed by the INR range, appears to play a key role in determining the risk of bleeding. Anticoagulation with warfarin substantially reduced the incidence of ischemic stroke in all of the trials. The administration of warfarin, however, was also associated with an increase in the risk of bleeding complications in some studies. When the dose of warfarin was adjusted to keep the INR above 2.5, significant bleeding complications were observed. However, lower doses of warfarin titrated to keep the INR 1.5 to 2.5, which were used in the BAATAF and SPINAF trials, produced significant reductions in stroke without a concomitant increased risk of bleeding. Therefore, the optimal level of anticoagulation appears to be an INR from 1.5 to 2.5, which provides protection against ischemic strokes equivalent to that of higher levels of anticoagulation without an associated increase in bleeding events. The optimal level of anticoagulation is currently being investigated in two dose-ranging trials of warfarin, PATAF and AFASAK 2 (Table 8-1).

Antiarrhythmic Therapy for Atrial Fibrillation

Antiarrhythmic agents are frequently administered to patients with atrial fibrillation acutely to attempt cardioversion to sinus rhythm and chronically to prevent recurrence of atrial fibrillation. The most widely used agent, quinidine, has been studied in several small randomized trials to determine its effectiveness in maintaining sinus rhythm after electrical cardioversion. The proportion of patients remaining in sinus rhythm after 1 year is 50% with chronic quinidine therapy compared to 25% with no antiarrhythmic therapy. Because of the small numbers of patients enrolled in each of these trials, no conclusions could be made regarding the effect of chronic quinidine therapy on long-term mortality. Coplen et al.[1] performed a meta-analysis of six small randomized trials evaluating chronic quinidine therapy and found a significant 3.6-fold excess in mortality with use of quinidine compared to no antiarrhyth-

Table 8-1. Comparison of the Level of International Normalized Ratio, Efficacy of Stroke Prevention, and Risk of Bleeding Events Among Randomized Trials of Warfarin in Nonrheumatic Atrial Fibrillation

CLINICAL TRIAL	INR	STROKE PREVENTION	INCREASED BLEEDING RISK
SPAF 2	2.0–4.5	+	+
AFASAK	2.8–4.2	+	+
EAFT	2.5–4.0	+	+
SPAF 1	2.0–3.5	+	–
CAFA	2.0–3.0	+	+
BAATAF	1.5–2.7	+	–
SPINAF	1.4–2.8	+	–

mic therapy (2.9% mortality rate with quinidine vs. 0.8% mortality rate with control, P < 0.05). In addition, a retrospective analysis of the 1,330 patients enrolled in SPAF 1[3] was performed to examine the effect of antiarrhythmic therapy on mortality. Among patients with a history of congestive heart failure, those given antiarrhythmic medications, most commonly quinidine, had a relative risk of cardiac death of 4.7 (P < 0.001) and a relative risk of arrhythmic death of 3.7 (P = 0.01) compared to patients not treated with antiarrhythmic medications. Patients without a history of congestive heart failure had no increase in mortality during antiarrhythmic drug therapy. These findings raise concerns over the safety of chronic quinidine therapy. To date, no large randomized prospective trial has examined the effect of antiarrhythmic therapy used to treat atrial fibrillation on long-term mortality or the incidence of embolic stroke.

Conclusions

Atrial fibrillation is a common disorder that confers considerable morbidity and mortality. Patients with lone atrial fibrillation not treated with aspirin or warfarin appear to have a very low incidence of stroke. When atrial fibrillation is associated with valvular heart disease, particularly rheumatic mitral stenosis, the risk of embolic stroke is high, and chronic anticoagulation is usually indicated.

Among patients with nonrheumatic atrial fibrillation, the use of warfarin significantly reduces the incidence of embolic stroke at a potential expense of increased risk of bleeding. The risk of bleeding with warfarin therapy appears directly related to the level of anticoagulation. Titrating the dose of warfarin to keep the INR from 1.5 to 2.5 provides significant protection from ischemic strokes without producing an increase in bleeding complications. However, maintaining an INR above 2.5 results in substantially increased bleeding events. Aspirin given as 325 mg/day also protects against embolic stroke, but aspirin therapy is not as effective as warfarin.

The risk of thromboembolic stroke appears to increase with older age and the presence of risk factors for thromboembolism (history of hypertension, previous thromboembolism, or recent heart failure). Young patients less than 75 years of age without risk factors for thromboembolism have a low, 0.5%, annual incidence of embolic stoke with aspirin therapy alone. Among patients with a previous stoke or transient ischemic attack, who represent a high-risk group for future thromboembolic events, only warfarin provides protection against future embolic events, whereas aspirin therapy provides no benefit. Older patients with risk factors for thromboembolism have the highest incidence of embolic stoke and therefore benefit the most from warfarin therapy; however, this subgroup also has the highest incidence of bleeding complications associated with chronic anticoagulation with INRs of 2.0 to 4.5. The best treatment plan in this high-risk group of older patients with risk factors for thromboembolism may be a lower dose of warfarin titrated to keep the INRs from 1.5 to 2.5. The combination of aspirin and a fixed low dose of warfarin (i.e., 1 or 2 mg/day) is currently being investigated in clinical trials.

From meta-analyses and retrospective analyses, the use of chronic antiarrhythmic therapy to treat atrial fibrillation appears to be associated with significantly increased mortality and arrhythmic deaths, particularly in patients with congestive heart failure. Prospective randomized trials examining the effect of antiarrhythmic therapy on mortality in patients with atrial fibrillation are needed to clarify this issue.

AFASAK

PURPOSE
Determine the effect of warfarin and aspirin on the incidence of thromboembolic events in patients with chronic nonrheumatic atrial fibrillation.

STUDY DESIGN

General
- 1,007 patients enrolled in this prospective, randomized, placebo-controlled trial.
- Eligible patients were randomized to one of three treatment groups:
  1. Warfarin: dose titrated to keep the international normalized ratio (INR) 2.8–4.2, with protime monitored at least every month
  2. Aspirin: 75 mg PO every day
  3. Placebo

Inclusion. Patients included were at least 18 years of age with electrocardiogram-verified chronic atrial fibrillation.

Exclusion. Criteria for exclusion were previous anticoagulation for more than 6 months, a cerebrovascular event within the past month, a contraindication for aspirin or warfarin, current treatment with aspirin or warfarin, pregnancy or breastfeeding, blood pressure > 180/100 mmHg, psychiatric illness, prosthetic heart valve, or rheumatic heart disease.

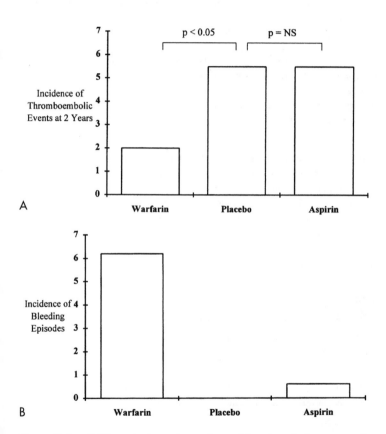

Figure 8-1. *(A)* The reduction in the incidence of thromboembolic events and *(B)* increased incidence of bleeding episodes with warfarin therapy compared to placebo. Aspirin therapy was not different from placebo.

End Points. The criteria for end points were mortality and thromboembolic events (transient ischemic attack, minor stroke, nondisabling stroke, disabling stroke, fatal stroke, peripheral embolism).

RESULTS

At 2-year follow-up, warfarin produced a significant reduction in the yearly incidence of thromboembolic events by 63% compared to placebo (2.0% warfarin vs. 5.5% placebo, P < 0.05). Aspirin resulted in no significant change in the yearly incidence of thromboembolic events compared to placebo (5.5% aspirin vs. 5.5% placebo). Only three vascular deaths (cerebrovascular and cardiovascular) occurred in the warfarin group compared to 12 in the aspirin group and 15 in the placebo group (P < 0.02). No significant difference in total mortality was observed. Bleeding episodes occurred much more commonly with warfarin (6.2%) compared to aspirin (0.6%) and placebo (0.0%) (Fig. 8-1).

CONCLUSIONS

Warfarin significantly reduced the incidence of thromboembolic events by 63% in patients with chronic nonrheumatic atrial fibrillation compared to placebo. Warfarin, at the dose used in this study (INR of 2.8–4.2) was also associated with higher bleeding complications. Aspirin, at a dose of 75 mg/day did not reduce the incidence of thromboembolic events compared to placebo.

(Data from Petersen et al.[3]) ∎

BAATAF

Boston Area Anticoagulation Trial for Atrial Fibrillation

PURPOSE

Determine the effect of low-dose warfarin on the incidence of ischemic stroke in patients with nonrheumatic atrial fibrillation.

STUDY DESIGN

General

- 420 patients enrolled in this prospective, randomized, unblinded, multicenter trial.

- Eligible patients were randomized to one of two treatment groups:
    1. Warfarin: dose adjusted to maintain prothrombin time 1.2–1.5 × control (international normalized ratio [INR] 1.5–2.7) with prothrombin time monitored every 3 weeks. Patients were not allowed to take aspirin.
    2. Control: not placebo controlled. Patients were allowed to take aspirin at their discretion.
- Normal thyroid function tests were required.

Inclusion. Patients included were adults with chronic sustained or intermittent atrial fibrillation with no echocardiographic evidence of rheumatic heart disease and two separate electrocardiograms documenting atrial fibrillation.

Exclusion. Criteria for exclusion were as follows: transient atrial fibrillation during an acute illness, echocardiographic evidence of intracardiac thrombus, left ventricular aneurysm, severe congestive heart failure, prosthetic heart valves, stroke within the previous 6 months, transient ischemic attack for which the patient was being treated, predisposition for intracranial hemorrhage, or clear clinical indication or contraindication to warfarin or aspirin.

End Points. The criteria for end points were ischemic stroke—defined as the sudden onset of neurologic deficit lasting $\geq$ 24 hr with no hemorrhage on computed tomography scan—and major bleeding—defined as intracranial hemorrhage, fatal bleeding, or requirement of $\geq$ 4-U blood transfusion within 48 hr.

RESULTS

The Data Monitoring Committee recommended early termination of the study. The use of warfarin resulted in a significant reduction in the incidence of ischemic stroke by 86% compared to placebo during the average 2.3 years of follow-up (0.41%/year warfarin vs. 3.0%/year control, P = 0.002). Patients with intermittent atrial fibrillation and those with sustained atrial fibrillation had similar rates of stroke. Older age and mitral annular calcification were clearly associated with increased risk of stroke. Overall mortality was significantly lower in the warfarin group compared to the control group (2.3% warfarin vs. 6.0% control, P = 0.005) (Fig. 8-2).

The number of major bleeds was low in both warfarin and control groups (two major bleeds with warfarin vs. one major bleed with con-

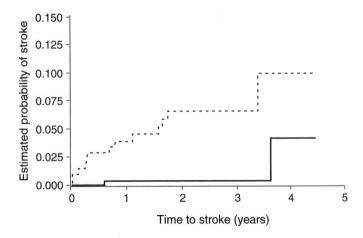

Figure 8-2. Cumulative probability of stroke. - - -,control; —, warfarin. (From The Boston Area Anticoagulation Trial for Atrial Fibrillation Investigators,[4] with permission.)

trol). Minor bleeding was more common with warfarin (38 minor bleeds with warfarin vs. 21 minor bleeds with control).

CONCLUSIONS

The use of low-dose warfarin (INR 1.5–2.7) in patients with chronic intermittent or sustained nonrheumatic atrial fibrillation significantly reduced the incidence of ischemic stroke by 86% compared to control with no increase in the incidence of major bleeds.

(Data from The Boston Area Anticoagulation Trial for Atrial Fibrillation Investigators.[4]) ■

CAFA

Canadian Atrial Fibrillation Anticoagulation Study

PURPOSE
Determine the effect of warfarin in preventing thromboembolic events in patients with chronic or paroxysmal nonrheumatic atrial fibrillation.

STUDY DESIGN

General

- 378 patients enrolled in this prospective, randomized, double-blind, placebo-controlled, multicenter trial.
- Eligible patients were randomized to one of two treatment groups:
  1. Warfarin: dose adjusted to maintain INR 2.0–3.0 with prothrombin time monitored every 3 weeks
  2. Placebo
- Study medications were stopped 6 days before any surgery and restarted on hospital discharge.
- Patients were advised not to take aspirin or other antiplatelet therapy.

Inclusion. Patients included were ≥ 19 years old with chronic atrial fibrillation documented to be present for ≥ 1 month or with paroxysmal atrial fibrillation occurring at least three times in the previous 3 months. The patients had no mitral valve prosthesis, mechanical aortic valve prosthesis, or mitral stenosis on echocardiogram.

Exclusion. Criteria for exclusion were a clear indication for or contraindication to anticoagulation, stroke or transient ischemic attack (TIA) within 1 year, requirement for antiplatelet drug therapy, hyperthyroidism, uncontrolled hypertension, or myocardial infarction within 1 month.

End Points. The criteria for end points were ischemic stroke, other systemic embolism, and intracranial or fatal hemorrhage.

RESULTS
Part way through recruitment, the results of AFASAK and SPAF became available to the Steering Committee. They believed that the cumulative

evidence favoring the benefit of warfarin was significantly persuasive to warrant early termination of the study because it would be unethical to continue to withhold warfarin from the enrolled patients. At 15.2-month follow-up, use of warfarin resulted in a 37% risk reduction in the annual rate of primary outcome events (3.5% warfarin vs. 5.2% control, P = 0.17) (Fig. 8-3).

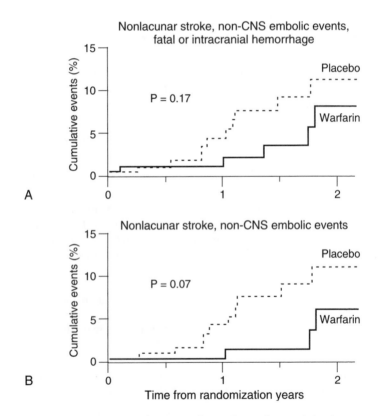

Figure 8-3. *(A & B)* Cumulative rate of events for warfarin and placebo groups. (From Connolly et al.,[5] with permission.)

CONCLUSIONS

This study was terminated early due to available results from AFASAK and SPAF that demonstrated clear benefit of warfarin in preventing ischemic stroke. Warfarin reduced the annual rate of primary outcome by 37% compared to placebo at 15.2-month follow-up in this truncated study.

(Data from Connolly et al.[5]) ■

EAFT

European Atrial Fibrillation Trial—Secondary Prevention of Thromboembolic Events

PURPOSE

Determine the effect of oral anticoagulants and aspirin on the incidence of thromboembolic events in patients with nonrheumatic atrial fibrillation and a recent transient ischemic attack (TIA) or minor ischemic stroke.

STUDY DESIGN

General

- 1,007 patients enrolled in this prospective, randomized, placebo-controlled, multicenter trial.
- Eligible patients were randomized to one of three treatment groups:
    1. Oral anticoagulants: free choice of oral anticoagulants. Most used coumarin derivatives with a target international normalized ratio (INR) of 2.5–4.0.
    2. Aspirin: 300 mg/day.
    3. Placebo.
- Prerandomization computed tomography brain scans, echocardiograms, and Holter monitor were obtained.
- Other medications were left to the discretion of each physician.

Inclusion. Patients included were > 25 years old with a TIA or minor ischemic stroke within the previous 3 months and nonrheumatic chronic or paroxysmal atrial fibrillation.

Exclusion. Criteria for exclusion were as follows: hyperthyroidism; the use of a nonsteroidal anti-inflammatory drug, other antiplatelet drugs, or oral anticoagulants; prosthetic heart valves; cardiac aneurysm; atrial myxoma; cardiothoracic ratio > 0.65; myocardial infarction within the previous 3 months; a scheduled carotid endarterectomy within the next 3 months; other serious illness; or clear indication or contraindication to the study drugs.

End Points. The criteria for end points were composite end point of mortality, nonfatal strokes, nonfatal myocardial infarction, and systemic embolization.

RESULTS

Anticoagulation vs. Control. During an average 2.3-year follow-up, the use of oral anticoagulants significantly reduced the composite end point by 53% compared to control (8%/year anticoagulants vs. 17%/year control, P = 0.001). Specifically, oral anticoagulants substantially reduced the risk of stroke by 66% (4%/year anticoagulants vs. 12% control) with no significant benefit on mortality.

Aspirin vs. Placebo. Treatment with aspirin produced a trend toward a reduction in the composite end point compared to placebo, but the

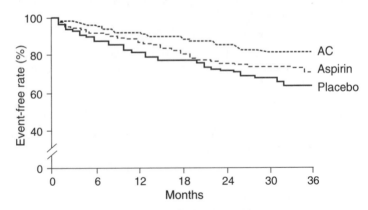

Figure 8-4. Survival analysis for primary outcome of death, nonfatal stroke, nonfatal myocardial infarction, or nonfatal systemic embolism. AC, anticoagulation. (From EAFT [European Atrial Fibrillation Trial] Study Group,[6] with permission.)

results were not statistically significant (15%/year aspirin vs. 19%/year placebo, P = 0.12).

Oral anticoagulants were significantly more effective at preventing the occurrence of primary events compared to aspirin (8%/year anticoagulants vs. 15%/year aspirin, P = 0.008). Oral anticoagulants also resulted in a significantly higher yearly incidence of major and minor bleeding (11.8%/year) compared to aspirin (4.2%/year, P < 0.001) and placebo (3.5%/year, P < 0.001). The incidence of cerebral hemorrhage was very low: one in the placebo group and two in the aspirin group only (Fig. 8-4).

CONCLUSIONS

In patients with nonrheumatic atrial fibrillation and a recent TIA or minor ischemic stroke, oral anticoagulation significantly reduced the risk of recurrent stroke by 66%, whereas aspirin had no significant benefit at 2.3-year follow-up. Oral anticoagulation was also associated with a substantial excess of major and minor bleeding episodes.

(Data from EAFT [European Atrial Fibrillation Trial] Study Group.[6]) ∎

SPAF 1

Stroke Prevention in Atrial Fibrillation

PURPOSE

Determine the benefit of warfarin and aspirin in preventing ischemic stroke and systemic thromboembolism in patients with sustained or intermittent nonrheumatic atrial fibrillation.

STUDY DESIGN

General

- 1,330 patients enrolled in this prospective, randomized, double-blind, placebo-controlled, multicenter trial.
- Eligible patients were randomized to one of three treatment groups:
  1. Warfarin: dose adjusted to maintain an international normalized ratio (INR) of 2.0–3.5 (prothrombin time 1.3–1.8 × control)
  2. Aspirin: enteric-coated aspirin 325 mg PO every day
  3. Placebo
- Other medications were left to the discretion of each physician.

Inclusion. Patients included were adults with electrocardiographic documentation of constant or intermittent atrial fibrillation in the preceding 12 months, with no prosthetic heart valve, and with no echocardiographic evidence of rheumatic mitral stenosis.

Exclusion. Criteria for exclusion were as follows: cerebral ischemic syndromes in the previous 2 years, previous thromboembolism, congestive heart failure that was due to severe mitral regurgitation or idiopathic dilated cardiomyopathy, myocardial infarction or percutaneous transluminal coronary angioplasty within the previous 3 months, coronary artery bypass graft within the previous 1 year, or contraindications to or clear indications for warfarin or aspirin.

End Points. The criteria for end points were ischemic stroke or systemic embolism.

RESULTS

The rate of ischemic stroke or systemic embolism was substantially reduced by 67% in those assigned to warfarin compared to placebo

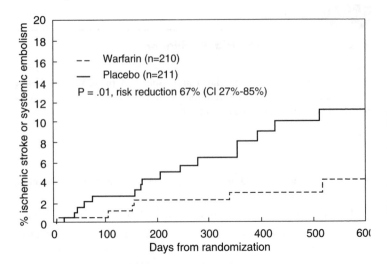

Figure 8-5. Cumulative rate of primary events for warfarin and placebo groups. CI, confidence intervals. (From Stroke Prevention in Atrial Fibrillation Investigators,[7] with permission.)

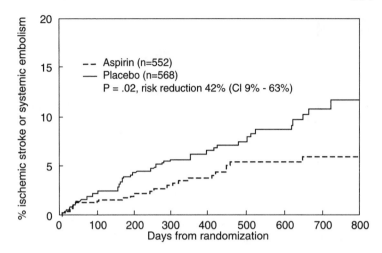

Figure 8-6. Cumulative rate of primary events for aspirin and placebo groups. CI, confidence intervals. (From Stroke Prevention in Atrial Fibrillation Investigators,[7] with permission.)

(2.3%/year warfarin vs. 7.4%/year placebo, P = 0.01). The risk of a primary event or death was significantly reduced by 58% in those taking warfarin (P = 0.01).

The rate of ischemic stroke or systemic embolism in patients taking aspirin was significantly reduced by 42% compared with placebo (3.6%/year aspirin vs. 6.3% placebo, P = 0.02). Primary events and death were also substantially reduced by 32% with aspirin (P = 0.02) (Figs. 8-5 and 8-6).

The risk of significant bleeding per year in patients receiving warfarin, aspirin and placebo was 1.5%, 1.4%, and 1.6%, respectively.

CONCLUSIONS
Warfarin and aspirin significantly reduced the rate of ischemic stroke and systemic embolism by 67% and 42%, respectively, compared to placebo in patients with sustained or intermittent nonrheumatic atrial fibrillation. No significant difference in bleeding complications was observed between the three groups.

(Data from Stroke Prevention in Atrial Fibrillation Investigators.[7]) ■

SPAF 2

Stroke Prevention in Atrial Fibrillation

PURPOSE

Compare warfarin with aspirin for preventing ischemic stroke and systemic embolism in patients with sustained or intermittent nonrheumatic atrial fibrillation.

STUDY DESIGN

General

- 1,100 patients enrolled in this prospective, randomized, multicenter trial.
- Two parallel clinical trials separated by patients aged ≤ 75 years (715 patients) and > 75 years (385 patients).
- Eligible patients were randomized to one of two treatment groups:
  1. Warfarin: dose adjusted to maintain an international normalized ratio (INR) of 2.0–4.5
  2. Aspirin: enteric-coated aspirin 325 mg PO every day
- Other medications were left to the discretion of each physician.

Inclusion. Patients included were adults with atrial fibrillation in the previous 12 months without prosthetic heart valves, mitral stenosis, or requirements for or contraindications to warfarin or aspirin.

Exclusion. Criteria for exclusion were ischemic stroke or transient ischemic attack within the previous 2 years and patients < 60 years old without overt cardiovascular disease (lone atrial fibrillation).

End Points. The criteria for end points were primary events defined as ischemic stroke and systemic embolism.

RESULTS

Patients ≤ 75 Years of Age at Entry. After a mean of 2.3 years of follow-up, the rate of primary events in patients assigned to aspirin was 1.9%/year compared to 1.3%/year for patients taking warfarin (P = 0.24). The incidence of major hemorrhage was 0.9%/year for aspirin vs.

1.7%/year for warfarin (P = 0.17).

Patients > 75 Years of Age at Entry. Patients taking aspirin had a 4.8%/year rate of primary events compared to 3.6%/year for warfarin (P = 0.39). The incidence of major hemorrhage was significantly higher for warfarin (4.2%/year) than for aspirin (1.6%/year, P = 0.04). The rate of all strokes with residual deficits (hemorrhagic and ischemic) was not statistically different between warfarin and aspirin (4.6% warfarin vs. 4.3% aspirin, P = NS).

Older patients assigned to warfarin had substantially higher rates of intracranial hemorrhage than younger patients taking warfarin (1.8%/year age > 75 vs. 0.5%/year age ≤ 75, P = 0.05). Patients assigned to aspirin with clinical risk factors for thromboembolism (history of hypertension, previous thromboembolism, or recent heart failure) had higher rates of thromboembolism than those without clinical risk factors (P < 0.001). In patients ≤ 75 years of age without clinical risk factors for thromboembolism, the use of aspirin resulted in a very low incidence of primary events (0.5%/year) (Table 8-2 and Fig. 8-7).

CONCLUSIONS
In patients of any age with sustained or intermittent nonrheumatic atrial fibrillation, there was only a modest benefit in the reduction of ischemic strokes by warfarin over aspirin; the results were not statistically significant. Patients > 75 years of age taking warfarin (INR 2.0–4.5) had signifi-

Table 8-2. Antithrombotic Efficacy in Patients With Risk Factors for Thromboembolism[a]

| | CLINICAL RISK FACTORS FOR THROMBOEMBOLISM | |
AGE GROUP	YES	NO
< 75 years old		
% of cohort	57%	43%
Aspirin event rate (95% CI)	2.9% (1.9–4.6)	0.5% (0.1–1.9)
Warfarin event rate (95% CI)	1.5% (0.8–2.9)	1.0% (0.4–2.4)
> 75 years old		
% of cohort	61%	39%
Aspirin event rate (95% CI)	7.2% (4.3–11.9)	1.8 (0.6–5.5)
Warfarin event rate (95% CI)	4.2% (2.3–7.9)	2.5 (1.0–6.8)

[a]Includes all primary events. No statistically significant difference between aspirin and warfarin in any subset.
(From Stroke Prevention in Atrial Fibrillation Investigators,[8] with permission.)

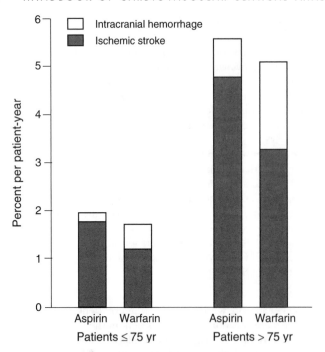

Figure 8-7.   Combined rate of ischemic stroke and intracranial hemorrhage according to antithrombotic therapy and age group. (From Stroke Prevention in Atrial Fibrillation Investigators,[8] with permission.)

cantly higher rates of major hemorrhage compared to aspirin and significantly higher rates of intracranial hemorrhage compared to patients < 75 years of age taking warfarin.

In patients < 75 years of age with no clinical risk factors for thromboembolism (history of hypertension, previous thromboembolism, or recent heart failure), the risk of ischemic stroke with aspirin was so low (0.5%/year) that use of warfarin in this population may not be advantageous.

(Data from Stroke Prevention in Atrial Fibrillation Investigators.[8])   ■

SPINAF

Veterans Affairs Stroke Prevention in Nonrheumatic Atrial Fibrillation

PURPOSE

Determine if low-intensity anticoagulation with warfarin would reduce the risk of stroke in patients with chronic nonrheumatic atrial fibrillation.

STUDY DESIGN

General

- 525 patients enrolled in this prospective, randomized, double-blind, placebo-controlled trial.
- Eligible patients were randomized to one of two treatment groups:
  1. Warfarin: initially 4 mg PO every day, with prothrombin time (PT) monitored weekly. The dose of warfarin was adjusted in 1-mg increments to maintain the patients' PT at 1.2-1.5 × control (corresponding to an international normalized ratio [INR] of 1.4-2.8)
  2. Placebo
- Aspirin and other nonsteroidal anti-inflammatory drugs (NSAIDs) were withdrawn if both the patient and physician agreed.
- Sporadic use of aspirin or an NSAID was discouraged.

Inclusion. Patients included were male veterans of any age without echocardiographic evidence of rheumatic heart disease and with atrial fibrillation documented by two electrocardiograms at least four weeks apart. These patients had a normal baseline PT and no baseline anticoagulation for 6 months preceding randomization.

Exclusion. Criteria for exclusion were intermittent atrial fibrillation, clear indication for or contraindication to anticoagulation or antiplatelet therapy, or an uninterpretable echocardiogram.

End Points. The criteria for end points were clinically evident cerebral infarction, cerebral hemorrhage, and death.

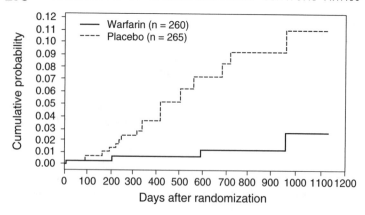

Figure 8-8. Cumulative probability of cerebral infarction. (From Ezekowitz et al.,[9] with permission.)

RESULTS

The Data Monitoring Board recommended early termination of the study. At an average follow-up of 1.75 years, treatment with low-intensity warfarin significantly reduced the incidence of cerebral infarction by 80% (1.5% warfarin vs. 7.2% placebo, P = 0.001). The benefit of warfarin was also observed among the subgroup of patients > 70 years of age (annualized stroke rate: 0.9%/year warfarin vs. 4.8%/ year placebo, P = 0.02). No significant difference was found in overall mortality (5.7% warfarin vs. 8.3% placebo, P = 0.19). The incidence of major hemorrhage (admission to an intensive care unit, transfusion of blood, or emergency procedure to terminate bleeding) was not significantly different between warfarin and placebo (2.3% warfarin vs. 1.5% placebo, P = 0.54) (Fig. 8-8).

CONCLUSIONS

Low-intensity anticoagulation with warfarin (INR 1.4–2.8) significantly reduced cerebral infarction by 80% compared to placebo in patients with chronic nonrheumatic atrial fibrillation without producing an excess risk of major hemorrhage.

(Data from Ezekowitz et al.[9]) ■

References

1. Coplen SE, Antmann EM, Berlin JA et al: Efficacy and safety of quinidine therapy for maintenance of sinus rhythm after cardioversion: a meta-analysis of randomized controlled trials. Circulation 82:1106, 1990

2. Flaker GC, Blackshear JL, McBride R et al: Antiarrhythmic drug therapy and cardiac mortality in atrial fibrillation. J Am Coll Cardiol 20:527, 1992

3. Petersen P, Boysen G, Godtfredsen J et al: Placebo-controlled, randomised trial of warfarin and aspirin for prevention of thromboembolic complications in chronic atrial fibrillation: the Copenhagen AFASAK Study. Lancet 1:175-9, 1989

4. The Boston Area Anticoagulation Trial for Atrial Fibrillation Investigators: The effect of low-dose warfarin on the risk of stroke in patients with non-rheumatic atrial fibrillation. N Engl J Med 323:1505-11, 1990

5. Connolly SJ, Laupacis A, Gent M et al: Canadian Atrial Fibrillation Anticoagulation (CAFA) study. J Am Coll Cardiol 18:349-55, 1991

6. EAFT (European Atrial Fibrillation Trial) Study Group: Secondary prevention in non-rheumatic atrial fibrillation after transient ischaemic attack or minor stroke. Lancet 342:1255-62, 1993

7. Stroke Prevention in Atrial Fibrillation Investigators: Stroke Prevention in Atrial Fibrillation study: final results. Circulation 84:527-39, 1991

8. Stroke Prevention in Atrial Fibrillation Investigators: Warfarin versus aspirin for prevention of thromboemblism in atrial fibrillation: Stroke Prevention in Atrial Fibrillation II study. Lancet 343:687-91, 1994

9. Ezekowitz MD, Bridgers SL, James KE et al: Warfarin in the prevention of stroke associated with nonrheumatic atrial fibrillation. N Engl J Med 327:1406-12, 1992

CHAPTER 9

Lipid-Lowering/Primary Prevention Trials

OVERVIEW

Epidemiologic evidence exists demonstrating a strong correlation and possibly a causal relationship between serum cholesterol level and the risk of coronary heart disease (CHD). Data from the Seven Countries Study[1] and the Multiple Risk Factor Intervention Trial (MRFIT)[2] clearly show a positive relationship between total serum cholesterol and CHD mortality. Furthermore, the Framingham Heart Study[3] revealed that serum low-density lipoprotein (LDL) cholesterol level is more predictive of CHD likelihood than total serum cholesterol (Fig. 9-1).

It is also clear from many clinical trials that reducing serum cholesterol decreases CHD events. A reduction in serum cholesterol of 1% typically confers a reduction in the risk of myocardial infarction of 2% and a reduction in CHD mortality of 1.4%. However, there have been concerns about the overall benefit of cholesterol lowering because of the lack of a reduction in all-cause mortality. A few trials have, in fact, suggested increased mortality from cholesterol reducing agents. The lack of a uniform benefit in overall mortality may be due to inadequately short follow-up periods, to an insufficient size and power in many trials to reveal mortality reductions, and to differences in the various agents used to lower cholesterol. Gould et al.[4] performed a meta-analysis of 35 randomized cholesterol-lowering trials and found that a 10% reduction in serum cholesterol was associated with reduced CHD mortality by 13% (P < 0.002) and reduced overall mortality by 10% (P < 0.05). This meta-analysis, however, raised concerns about the safety of specific types of lipid-lowering agents, since some regimens

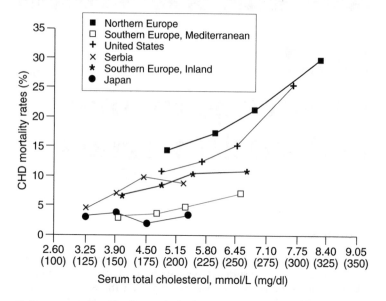

Figure 9-1. Effect of serum total cholesterol on 25-year coronary heart disease mortality rates adjusted for age, cigarette smoking, and systolic blood pressure. (From Verschuren et al.,[1] with permission.)

appeared to increase CHD and overall mortality. Specifically, the use of fibrates (clofibrate and gemfibrozil) and the use of hormones in men (estrogen and dextrothyroxine) resulted in significantly increased non-CHD mortality, despite effective reductions in serum cholesterol. The 3-hydroxy-3-methylglutaryl coenzyme A (HMG CoA) reductase inhibitors have recently accrued considerable evidence demonstrating reduced CHD events and overall mortality. Bile acid sequestrants and niacin have also been proven to reduce CHD events. Therefore, in addition to the degree of cholesterol lowering, the specific agent used to lower cholesterol appears to determine overall clinical benefit.

Bile Acid Sequestrant Trials

The two most commonly used bile acid sequestrants are cholestyramine and colestipol. These agents act solely in the gastrointestinal tract by binding and inhibiting the reabsorption of bile acids. The resulting reduction in hepatic bile acids stimulates conversion of cholesterol to bile acids in the liver. The expression of hepatic LDL receptors is subsequently increased, which mediates the decrease in serum LDL cholesterol. The major limitation to bile acid sequestrants is the high incidence of bothersome gastrointestinal side effects resulting in poor compliance.

The Lipid Research Clinics—Coronary Primary Prevention Trial (LRC-CPPT) examined the effect of cholestyramine as primary prevention of CHD in middle-aged men with primary hypercholesterolemia. A total of 3,806 men with a mean total cholesterol of 291 mg/dl and LDL cholesterol of 215 mg/dl were randomized to cholestyramine or placebo. Treatment with cholestyramine significantly reduced the incidence of CHD (death and nonfatal myocardial infarction) by 19% over the 7.4-year follow-up period. In addition, cholestyramine therapy reduced the incidence of angina by 20%, the development of a new positive exercise stress test by 25%, and the incidence of coronary artery bypass graft (CABG) by 21%. Overall mortality was not meaningfully different between the two treatment groups. A dose–response effect was observed between the amount of cholestyramine ingested and the degree of reduction in LDL cholesterol. The amount of LDL reduction strongly correlated with the degree of reduction in CHD events.

The Cholesterol Lowering Atherosclerosis Study (CLAS) examined the effect of combination colestipol-niacin therapy in reducing angiographically documented atherosclerosis in 162 men with previous CABG. Treatment with colestipol-niacin produced dramatic changes in total cholesterol, LDL cholesterol, high-density lipoprotein (HDL) cholesterol, and triglycerides of -25%, -40%, +37%, and -18%, respectively. Angiographic outcomes revealed significantly more nonprogression and regression in native coronary arteries and fewer new lesions in both native coronary arteries and saphenous vein grafts with colestipol-niacin therapy over a 4-year follow-up period. No analysis of clinical end points was attempted in this trial. Two other trials demonstrating improved angiographic end points with bile acid sequestrants are the Familial Atherosclerosis Treatment Study (FATS)[5] and the National Heart, Lung, and Blood Institute (NHLBI)—Type II Coronary Intervention Study.[6] The FATS trial demonstrated that patients with established coronary artery disease treated with combination lovastatin-colestipol or niacin-colestipol therapy had substantially less progression and more regression of coronary artery lesions and a reduced incidence of cardiovascular events over a 32-month follow-up period. In the NHLBI trial, patients with hypercholesterolemia treated with cholestyramine had significantly less progression of atherosclerotic lesions. Collectively, these trials provide evidence that bile acid sequestrants are relatively safe and effective in reducing serum cholesterol, improving angiographic outcomes, and reducing CHD events.

Nicotinic Acid Trials

Niacin is a B vitamin that has potent cholesterol-lowering effects at high doses. The mechanism of action appears to be decreasing the production of very-low-density lipoprotein (VLDL) particles by the liver and inhibiting the release of free fatty acids from adipose tissue. The specific effect of niacin on serum cholesterol is to decrease VLDL triglycerides and raise HDL cholesterol. Major side effects include flushing, which can usually be controlled with concomitant daily aspirin therapy, and gastrointestinal discomfort.

The major trial to demonstrate a clinical benefit of niacin is the Coronary Drug Project (CDP), which randomized 8,341 men with previous myocardial infarction to two doses of estrogen, dextrothyroxine, clofibrate, niacin, or placebo. Both estrogen arms and the dextrothyroxine arm were terminated early because of unfavorable trends in mortality with these treatments. At 5-year follow-up, treatment with niacin significantly reduced the incidence of nonfatal myocardial infarction by 27%. No effect on overall mortality was observed until the 15-year follow-up analysis, which revealed a significant 11% reduction in overall mortality with niacin treatment.

Trials combining niacin with another lipid-lowering agent, including FATS,[5] CLAS, and the Stockholm Ischemic Heart Disease Study,[7] have demonstrated substantial reductions in total cholesterol and LDL cholesterol, improved angiographic outcomes, and reduced CHD mortality.

Fibric Acid Trials

The two most commonly used fibrates are gemfibrozil and clofibrate. Fibric acids have a variety of actions, including increasing the activity of LDL receptors, inhibiting the synthesis of triglycerides in the liver, and interfering with the release of free fatty acids from adipose tissue. The main mechanism of action remains unknown. Fibric acids are most effective in lowering triglycerides and raising HDL cholesterol and are usually well tolerated.

The Helsinki Heart Study evaluated the effect of gemfibrozil in preventing CHD events among 4,081 asymptomatic men with primary hypercholesterolemia. After 5 years of follow-up, treatment with gemfibrozil significantly reduced a combined end point of cardiac death and nonfatal myocardial infarction. Despite a 26% lower mortality from CHD, there were slightly more overall deaths in the gemfibrozil group; the deaths were mainly due to accidents or violence and intracranial hemorrhage. These differences in overall mortality were not statistically significant.

The World Health Organization (WHO) Cooperative study evaluated the effect of clofibrate in preventing CHD in men with hypercholesterolemia. During a treatment period of 5.3 years, clofibrate administration significantly reduced the incidence of nonfatal myocardial infarction by 25%. However, there was a 47% increase in overall mortality (P < 0.05) and an increase in non-CHD mortality in the clofibrate-treated group. This excess in mortality could not be accounted for by any particular disease process (cancer, violence, etc.). During the 7.9 years after completion of the trial, there was no meaningful difference in mortality between patients who had received clofibrate or placebo during the trial period. Therefore, the excess in mortality was observed only during active treatment with clofibrate, which raises the concern that clofibrate therapy was, in some way, causally related to the excess deaths. The Coronary Drug Project revealed no difference in overall mortality between clofibrate therapy and placebo over a 5-year treatment period in men with previous myocardial infarction.

HMG CoA Reductase Inhibitor Trials

HMG CoA reductase inhibitors, the newest class of lipid-lowering drugs, inhibits the rate-limiting step of cholesterol synthesis in the liver. Decreased hepatic cholesterol synthesis stimulates the expression of LDL receptors, which subsequently produces reductions in serum LDL cholesterol and triglycerides. These agents are generally well tolerated and have a low incidence of side effects, the most common being myopathy and hepatotoxicity. Numerous clinical trials have documented the efficacy of these agent in improving angiographic outcomes. However, because of the relatively small numbers of patients in these trials, definitive conclusions regarding CHD and total mortality could not be made. Two landmark trials, the Scandinavian Simvastatin Survival Study (4S) and the West of Scotland Coronary Prevention Study (WOSCOPS), have recently reported the effects of certain HMG CoA reductase inhibitors on CHD events and overall mortality.

The 4S trial examined the effects of simvastatin in reducing mortality and CHD events in 4,444 patients with a history of coronary artery disease and elevated total serum cholesterol. Treatment with simvastatin produced changes in total cholesterol, LDL cholesterol, HDL cholesterol, and triglycerides of -25%, -35%, +8%, and -10%, respectively, during the 5.4-year follow-up period. Simvastatin therapy reduced overall mortality by 29% (P = 0.0003) and CHD mortality by 42% (P < 0.05) compared to placebo. In addition, significantly fewer "major" coronary events, a reduced need for CABG or percutaneous transluminal coronary angioplasty (PTCA), and fewer fatal and nonfatal cerebrovascular events were observed with simvastatin therapy. Patients tolerated simvastatin well and had a low incidence of discontinuation of drug therapy.

The WOSCOPS was a primary prevention trial examining the effect of pravastatin on mortality and CHD events in 6,595 men with hypercholesterolemia and no previous myocardial infarction. Only 5% of patients had a history of angina pectoris. Pravastatin produced changes in total cholesterol, LDL cholesterol, HDL cholesterol, and triglycerides of -20%, -26%, +5%, and -12%, respectively. During an average 4.9-year follow-up, the use of pravastatin reduced the incidence of nonfatal myocardial infarction by 29% (P < 0.001) and death from all cardiovascular causes by 30% (P = 0.03) compared to placebo. Pravastatin therapy produced a trend toward reduced overall and CHD mortality, but the results were not statistically significant. There was a reduced need for subsequent revascularization with PTCA or CABG in patients receiving pravastatin.

The recently reported Cholesterol and Recurrent Events (CARE) trial examined the effect of pravastatin in patients after a recent myocardial infarction with normal or mildly elevated total serum cholesterol (< 240 mg/dl). During a mean follow-up of 5 years, the use of pravastatin significantly reduced a combined end point of fatal coronary heart disease or nonfatal myocardial infarction, the overall incidence of myocardial infarction, and the requirement for revascularization procedures. There was a trend toward lower mortality with pravastatin treatment, although the results were not statistically significant. Thus, HMG CoA reductase inhibitors significantly reduce the development of ischemic heart disease events when used as primary prevention in patients with elevated cholesterol and when used as secondary prevention in patients with normal or elevated cholesterol.

Primary Prevention Trials

Most clinical and epidemiologic evidence of primary prevention therapies comes from meta-analyses and observational studies. The reliability of data from such methods is not ideal, and conclusions made may be misleading. Evidence from observational studies[8] is accruing that all of the following produce reductions in the risk of myocardial infarction: cessation of smoking by approximately 50%, treatment of hypertension by 2%–3% for each decline of 1 mmHg in the diastolic blood pressure, maintaining an active lifestyle and ideal body weight by 40% each, consuming mild amounts of alcohol by approximately 30%, and replacement of estrogen in postmenopausal women by 40%.

Randomized, prospective trials have examined the effects of lipid-lowering and aspirin therapy in the primary prevention of CHD. The primary prevention lipid-lowering trials—the Helsinki Heart Study using gemfibrozil, the WHO Cooperative using clofibrate, the LRC-CPPT using cholestyramine, and the WOSCOPS using pravastatin—have all demonstrated a significant reduction in the incidence of nonfatal myocardial infarction in men with hypercholesterolemia. Overall mortality was meaningfully increased in the WHO Cooperative trial but not significantly affected in the other trials. The role of aspirin in the primary prevention of CHD was examined in the Physician Health Study, a prospective, randomized trial of 22,071 male physicians. A significant, 44%, reduction in the incidence of myocardial infarction was observed in physicians taking aspirin over the 5-year follow-up period. This benefit was limited to physicians aged 50 years and older. Cardiovascular and overall mortality were not significantly reduced with aspirin therapy; this was perhaps due to the markedly low mortality rate observed in this physician population. The use of aspirin produced significantly more bleeding ulcers, "minor" bleeding, and blood transfusions.

Conclusions

The risk of CHD is strongly correlated to total serum cholesterol level, particularly serum LDL cholesterol. Reducing serum cholesterol clearly decreases CHD events; however, the effect on overall mortality has been controversial. For every 1% reduction in total cholesterol, the risk of myocardial infarction decreases by 2% and the risk of CHD mortality decreases by 1.4%. Table 9-1 summarizes the important findings from the major cholesterol-lowering clinical trials.

Table 9-1. Summary of Findings From the Major Cholesterol-Lowering Clinical Trials

TRIAL	DRUG	PRIMARY/ SECONDARY PREVENTION	NONFATAL MYOCARDIAL INFARCTION	CHD MORTALITY	OVERALL MORTALITY
LRC-CPPT	Cholestyramine	Primary	↓	↓	No change
HHS	Gemfibrozil	Primary	↓	↓	No change
WHO	Clofibrate	Primary	↓	No change	↑
WOSCOPS	Pravastatin	Primary	↓	↓	No change
4S	Simvastatin	Secondary	↓	↓	↓
CARE	Pravastatin	Secondary	↓	No change	No change
CDP	Niacin	Secondary	↓	↓	↓
CDP	Clofibrate	Secondary	No change	No change	No change

Thus, overall mortality was reduced by lipid-lowering therapy only in certain secondary prevention trials. The primary prevention trials failed to demonstrate a significant reduction in overall mortality. Aspirin therapy was effective in the primary prevention of myocardial infarction in men over the age of 50 years at a cost of increased bleeding complications. Aspirin therapy did not significantly reduce overall mortality.

ACAPS

Asymptomatic Carotid Artery Progression Study

PURPOSE

Determine the effect of lovastatin and low-dose warfarin on the progression of carotid atherosclerosis and clinical outcome in asymptomatic patients with early carotid atherosclerosis and moderately elevated low-density lipoprotein (LDL) cholesterol.

STUDY DESIGN

General

- 919 patients enrolled in this prospective, randomized, double-blind, placebo-controlled, multicenter trial.

- Over 15,000 asymptomatic patients were screened for inclusion criteria; eligible patients were randomized to one of four treatment groups:

1. Active lovastatin/active warfarin
2. Active lovastatin/warfarin placebo
3. Lovastatin placebo/active warfarin
4. Lovastatin placebo/warfarin placebo

- Lovastatin: initial dose of 20 mg/day taken with the evening meal; after 4 months, the dose was titrated between 10 and 40 mg/day to keep LDL between 90 and 110 mg/dl.
- Warfarin: fixed low dose of 1 mg/day.
- All patients were encouraged to take one aspirin 81 mg/day with the other study medications.
- B-mode ultrasound examinations were used to assess for carotid atherosclerosis at baseline and every 6 months.

Inclusion. Patients included were 40–79 years old with serum LDL 130–159 mg/dl with any number of coronary risk factors, serum LDL 160–189 mg/dl with one or more coronary risk factor, triglycerides ≤ 400 mg/dl, and at least one B-mode image measurement reflecting an intimal medial wall thickness (IMT) ≥ 1.5 mm (common or internal carotid) or 1.6 mm (bifurcation) and < 3.5 mm.

Exclusion. The criteria for exclusion were as follows: history of myocardial infarction, stroke, or angina; serum triglycerides > 400 mg/dl or alanine aminotransferase (ALT) > 20% the upper limits of normal; uncontrolled hypertension (diastolic blood pressure > 94 mmHg or systolic blood pressure > 180 mmHg); the use of lipid-lowering agents within the past 1 year; the regular use of anticoagulants; bleeding disorders; alcohol abuse; prothrombin time > 16.8 sec during 1-mg warfarin test dosing, or other serious illness.

End Points. The criteria for end points were change in mean maximum IMT over the study period and major clinical events.

RESULTS

This report was limited to the lovastatin component of the trial. During a mean follow-up of 34 months, the use of lovastatin significantly reduced the mean maximum IMT compared to placebo (–0.009 mm/year lovastatin vs. +0.006 mm/year placebo, P = 0.001). 1.1% of patients in the

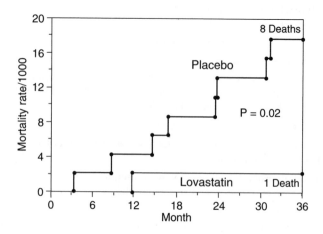

Figure 9-2. All-cause mortality rates. (From Furberg et al.,[9] with permission.)

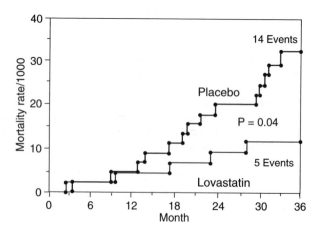

Figure 9-3. Incidence of fatal or nonfatal cardiovascular disease. (From Furberg et al.,[9] with permission.)

lovastatin group had a major cardiovascular event (all nonfatal myocardial infarction) compared with 3.1% of patients in the placebo group (4 ischemic deaths, 5 strokes, 5 nonfatal myocardial infarction, P = 0.04). Significantly fewer deaths occurred with the use of lovastatin (0.22% lovastatin vs. 1.74% placebo, P = 0.02). Lovastatin produced changes in LDL and high-density lipoprotein cholesterol of –28% and +5%, respectively (Figs. 9-2 and 9-3).

CONCLUSIONS

In patients with asymptomatic carotid atherosclerosis and moderately elevated LDL cholesterol, the use of lovastatin significantly reduced the mean intimal medial thickness in the carotid arteries and reduced the risk of cardiovascular events and mortality compared to placebo over a 3-year follow-up period. The results of low-dose warfarin therapy will be reported separately.

(Data from Furberg et al.[9]) ■

CARE

Cholesterol and Recurrent Events

PURPOSE

Determine the effects of pravastatin on mortality and cardiac events in survivors of recent myocardial infarction with normal or mildly elevated serum cholesterol.

STUDY DESIGN

General

- 4,159 patients enrolled in this prospective, randomized, double-blind, placebo-controlled, multicenter trial.
- Eligible patients were randomized to one of two treatment groups:
  1. Pravastatin: 40 mg PO daily
  2. Placebo
- Study medications were added to optimal medical therapy as defined by the treating physician.
- All patients were advised to follow an American Heart Association step 1 cholesterol-lowering diet.

Inclusion. Patients included were 21–75 years old, surviving a myocardial infarction during the previous 3–20 months. Patients had a total cholesterol < 240 mg/dl, low-density lipoprotein (LDL) cholesterol between 115 and 174 mg/dl, and serum triglycerides < 350 mg/dl.

Exclusion. The criteria for exclusion were as follows: the need for lipid-lowering therapy, left ventricular ejection fraction (LVEF) < 25%, overt congestive heart failure, hepatic or renal disease, or other serious illness.

End Points. The criteria for end points were combined end point of fatal coronary heart disease or nonfatal myocardial infarction.

RESULTS

Baseline characteristics revealed a mean age of 59 years, with 14% women and 14% diabetic patients. The mean LVEF was 53%. Concomitant therapy consisted of aspirin in 83%, β-blockers in 40%, calcium channel blockers in 39%, and angiotensin-converting enzyme inhibitors in 14% of patients. The mean baseline total cholesterol, LDL, high-density lipoprotein (HDL), and triglyceride levels were 209, 139, 39, and 155 mg/dl, respectively. During a mean follow-up of 5 years, treatment with pravastatin significantly reduced the primary end point of fatal coronary heart disease or nonfatal myocardial infarction by 24% compared to placebo (9.9% pravastatin vs. 12.9% placebo, $P = 0.002$). Treatment with pravastatin also substantially reduced the incidences of revascularization with coronary artery bypass graft (CABG) or percutaneous transluminal coronary angioplasty (PTCA) by 27% (14.0% pravastatin vs. 18.6% placebo, $P = 0.0001$) and of total myocardial infarction by 25% (7.1% pravastatin vs. 9.4% placebo, $P = 0.007$). There was a trend toward lower total mortality (8.6% pravastatin vs. 9.4% placebo, $P = NS$) and coronary heart disease mortality (4.6% pravastatin vs. 5.7% placebo, $P = NS$) in patients receiving pravastatin, although the results were not statistically significant. A higher incidence of breast cancer was found in women receiving pravastatin (0.57% pravastatin vs. 0.04% placebo, $P = 0.002$). Pravastatin produced changes in total cholesterol, LDL, HDL, and triglycerides of –20%, –28%, +5%, and –14%, respectively (Fig. 9-4).

CONCLUSIONS

Treatment with pravastatin in patients surviving a recent myocardial infarction with normal or mildly elevated serum cholesterol significantly reduced a combined end point of fatal coronary heart disease or nonfatal

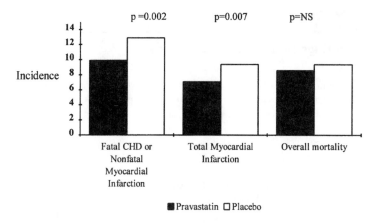

Figure 9-4. Significant reductions in the primary combined end point and the incidence of total myocardial infarctions and a trend toward reduced overall mortality with pravastatin therapy.

myocardial infarction, the incidence of total myocardial infarctions, and the requirement for revascularization with PTCA or CABG compared to placebo during a 5-year follow-up period.

(Data presented at the annual meeting of the American College of Cardiology, Orlando, FL, 1996.) ∎

CHAOS

Cambridge Heart Antioxidant Study

PURPOSE
Determine the effect of vitamin E therapy in preventing nonfatal myocardial infarction and cardiovascular death among patients with angiographically established coronary artery disease.

STUDY DESIGN

General

- 2,002 patients enrolled in this prospective, randomized, double-blind, placebo-controlled trial.
- Eligible patients were randomized to one of two treatment groups:
  1. Vitamin E: the first 546 patients received 800 IU daily; the dose was subsequently reduced to 400 IU daily.
  2. Placebo.
- Patients were followed with serial questionnaires.
- Serum α-tocopherol concentrations were measured at baseline and in patients who were readmitted.

Inclusion. Patients included were with angiographically proven coronary atherosclerosis.

Exclusion. The criteria for exclusion was prior use of vitamin supplements containing vitamin E.

End Points. The criteria for end points were combined end point of cardiovascular death and nonfatal myocardial infarction.

RESULTS
The baseline serum α-tocopherol concentration was 34.2 μmol/L and did not change with placebo treatment, but increased to 51.1 μmol/L on 400 IU vitamin E daily and 64.5 μmol/L on 800 IU vitamin E daily. Mean serum cholesterol was 5.77 mmol/L and did not significantly change with vitamin E supplementation. More than 90% of patients had angina, evidence of reversible ischemia, or both. During a median follow-up of 510 days, ther-

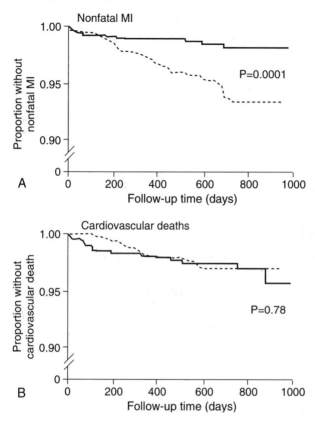

Figure 9-5. Kaplan-Meier survival curves for (A) nonfatal myocardial infarction and (B) cardiovascular deaths. —, vitamin E; - - -, placebo. (From Stephens et al.,[10] with permission.)

apy with vitamin E significantly reduced the incidence of the combined end point of cardiovascular deaths and nonfatal myocardial infarction by 47% (4.0% vitamin E vs. 6.6% placebo, P = 0.015) and the incidence of non-fatal myocardial infarction by 77% (1.4% vitamin E vs. 4.2% placebo, P = 0.0001). This beneficial treatment effect became apparent after approxi-mately 200 days. However, there was a nonsignificant excess of cardiovascular deaths (2.6% vitamin E vs. 2.4% placebo, P = 0.61) and total mortality (3.5% vitamin E vs. 2.8% placebo, P = 0.31). Treatment with vitamin E was well tolerated with few side effects (Fig. 9-5)

CONCLUSIONS
Therapy with vitamin E (400–800 IU daily) in patients with angiographically proven symptomatic coronary artery disease significantly reduced the incidence of nonfatal myocardial infarction without meaningfully affecting cardiovascular mortality compared to placebo during a median follow-up of 510 days.

(Data from Stephens et al.[10])   ∎

CLAS

Cholesterol-Lowering Atherosclerosis Study

PURPOSE
Determine the effect of combined colestipol-niacin therapy on angiographically evaluated atherosclerosis in men with previous coronary artery bypass grafting and hypercholesterolemia.

STUDY DESIGN

General

- 162 men enrolled in this prospective, randomized, double-blind, placebo-controlled, multicenter trial.
- Eligible patients were randomized to one of two treatment groups:
  1. Colestipol-niacin: colestipol 30 g PO daily and niacin 3–12 g PO daily
  2. Placebo
- All patients were nonsmokers and were treated with concomitant dietary therapy.
- Angiography was performed at randomization, 2 and 4 years.

Figure 9-6.   Increased incidence of *(A)* nonprogression, *(B)* regression, and *(C)* fewer new lesions with colestipol-niacin therapy compared to placebo.

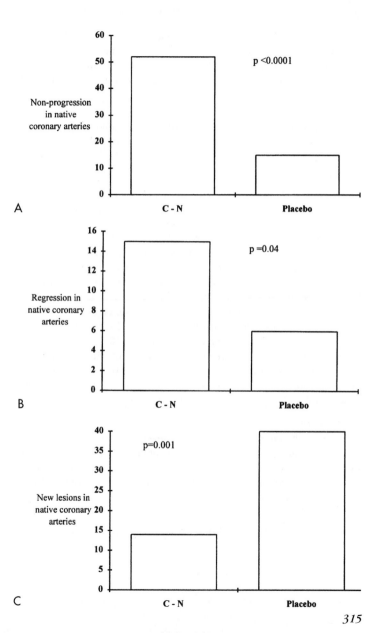

Inclusion. Patients included were nonsmoking men 40–59 years old who had undergone previous CABG at least 3 months before enrollment with a total cholesterol between 185 and 350 mg/dl. All patients had to have a confirmed lipid-lowering response to the study medications before randomization.

End Points. The criteria for end points were angiographically documented nonprogression or regression of coronary atherosclerosis at 4 years.

RESULTS
The average daily dose of colestipol was 30.1 g, and niacin was 4.2 g. The mean changes in lipid profiles in patients treated with colestipol-niacin for total cholesterol, low-density lipoprotein, high-density lipoproteins, and triglycerides were –25%, –40%, +37%, and –18%, respectively. Significantly more patients treated with colestipol-niacin demonstrated nonprogression (52% colestipol-niacin vs. 15% placebo, P < 0.0001) and regression (18% colestipol-niacin vs. 6% placebo, P = 0.04) of native coronary atherosclerosis compared to placebo at 4-year follow-up. Treatment with colestipol-niacin, compared to placebo, resulted in substantially less progressing lesions (45% colestipol-niacin vs. 74% placebo, P = 0.001) and fewer new lesions (14% colestipol-niacin vs. 40% placebo, P = 0.001) in native coronary arteries. In vein grafts, treatment with colestipol-niacin also produced significantly fewer new lesions (16% colestipol-niacin vs. 38% placebo, P = 0.006). The small patient size of this trial precluded meaningful analysis of clinical outcomes (Fig. 9-6).

CONCLUSIONS
Treatment with combination colestipol-niacin therapy in men with previous CABG and hypercholesterolemia resulted in significantly more nonprogression and regression of native coronary atherosclerosis and substantially fewer new lesions in native coronary arteries and bypass vein grafts compared to placebo at 4-year follow-up.

(2-year follow-up data from Blankenhorn et al.[11]; 4-year follow-up data from Cashin-Hemphill et al.[12]) ■

CORONARY DRUG PROJECT

PURPOSE

Determine the effects of niacin and clofibrate on mortality and cardiac events in men with previous myocardial infarction.

STUDY DESIGN

General

- 8,341 men enrolled in this prospective, randomized, placebo-controlled, multicenter trial.
- Eligible patients were randomly assigned to one of the following six treatment groups:
    1. Estrogen 2.5 mg/day
    2. Estrogen 5 mg/day
    3. Dextrothyroxine 6.0 mg/day
    4. Clofibrate 1.8 g/day
    5. Niacin 3.0 g/day
    6. Placebo
- Drug treatment was continued to the scheduled end of the 5-year trial.
- A 15-year follow-up was reported; however, drug treatment was not controlled after 5 years.

Inclusion. Patients included were men 30–64 years old with verified evidence of previous myocardial infarction, at least 3 months prior, with stable New York Heart Association functional class I or II.

End Points. The criterion for end point was total mortality.

RESULTS

Five-Year Follow-up. Both estrogen groups and the dextrothyroxine group were discontinued early because of unfavorable trends in mortality. Total cholesterol and triglycerides were reduced by 6.5% and 22.3%, respectively, for clofibrate therapy and by 9.9% and 26.1%, respectively, for niacin therapy. Treatment with clofibrate resulted in no significant

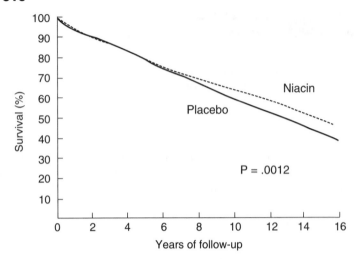

Figure 9-7. Survival curves for niacin and placebo groups. (From Canner et al.,[14] with permission.)

reduction in total mortality (20.0% clofibrate vs. 20.9% placebo, P = NS) or the incidence of nonfatal myocardial infarction (11.6% clofibrate vs. 12.2% placebo, P = NS). Treatment with niacin significantly reduced the incidence of nonfatal myocardial infarction by 27% compared to placebo (8.9% niacin vs. 12.2% placebo, Z = –2.88). No significant reduction in total mortality was observed with niacin treatment (21.2% niacin vs. 20.9% placebo, P = NS).

Fifteen-Year Follow-up. A mean follow-up of 15 years was performed, nearly 9 years after termination of the trial and its study medications. Treatment with niacin resulted in a statistically significant 11% reduction in total mortality (52.0% niacin vs. 58.2% placebo, P = 0.0004). Treatment with clofibrate did not meaningfully decrease mortality compared to placebo (57.8% clofibrate vs. 58.2% placebo, P = NS). The late benefit of niacin was postulated to be due to the early effect of niacin in reducing nonfatal myocardial infarction or as a result of the cholesterol-lowering effect of niacin, or both (Fig. 9-7).

CONCLUSIONS

Treatment with niacin in men with hypercholesterolemia and previous myocardial infarction reduced the incidence of nonfatal myocardial infarction at 5-year follow-up and total mortality at 15-year follow-up compared to placebo. Clofibrate therapy provided no beneficial effect. Estrogen and dextrothyroxine therapy produced an unfavorable trend in total mortality.

(5-year follow-up data from The Coronary Drug Project Research Group[13]; 15-year follow-up data from Canner et al.[14]) ∎

HELSINKI HEART STUDY

PURPOSE

Determine the effect of gemfibrozil therapy for primary prevention of coronary heart disease among asymptomatic men with primary dyslipidemia.

STUDY DESIGN

General

- 4,081 men enrolled in this prospective, randomized, double-blind, placebo-controlled, multicenter trial.
- Eligible patients were randomized to one of two treatment groups:
  1. Gemfibrozil: 600 mg PO bid
  2. Placebo
- In addition to drug therapy, all patients were recommended to adhere to a cholesterol-lowering diet, increased physical activity, weight reduction, and smoking cessation.
- Clinical follow-up was performed every 3 months.

Inclusion. Patients were men aged 40–55 years who were asymptomatic with non-high-density lipoprotein cholesterol (low-density lipoproteins [LDLs] plus very-low-density lipoproteins [VLDL]) ≥ 200 mg/dl on two successive measurements. Patients with hypertension and mild non-insulin-dependent diabetes were accepted.

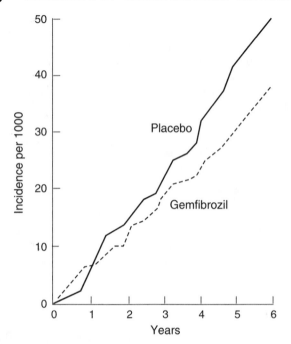

Figure 9-8. Kaplan-Meier cumulative incidence of cardiac end points. (From Frick et al.,[15] with permission.)

Exclusion. The criteria for exclusion were clinical manifestations of coronary heart disease, electrocardiographic abnormalities, congestive heart failure, or other serious illness.

End Points. The criteria for end points were combined end point of fatal and nonfatal myocardial infarction and cardiac death at 5 years.

RESULTS

At the time of enrollment, the mean total cholesterol was 289 mg/dl, with an HDL of 47 mg/dl, non-HDL of 242 mg/dl, and triglycerides of 176 mg/dl. Gemfibrozil therapy produced changes in total cholesterol, LDL, HDL, and triglycerides of -7%, -9%, +9%, and -35%, respectively. After 5 years of follow-up, treatment with gemfibrozil significantly reduced combined cardiac end points by 34% compared to placebo (2.7% gemfibrozil vs. 4.1% placebo, P < 0.002). Analysis of individual end points revealed a substantial reduction in nonfatal myocardial infarction with gemfibrozil treatment (2.2% gemfibrozil vs. 3.5% placebo, P < 0.02). Total mortality, however, was not significantly different between the two groups (2.2% gemfibrozil vs. 2.1% placebo, P = not significant) (Fig. 9-8).

CONCLUSIONS

Among middle-aged asymptomatic men with primary dyslipidemia, defined as a non-HDL cholesterol ≥ 200 mg/dl, the use of gemfibrozil significantly reduced the incidence of combined cardiac end points (cardiac death and nonfatal myocardial infarction) by 34% and the incidence of nonfatal myocardial infarction by 37% compared to placebo over a 5-year follow-up period. Total mortality was not meaningfully reduced by treatment with gemfibrozil.

(Data from Frick et al.[15]) ■

LRC-CPPT

Lipid Research Clinics—Coronary Primary Prevention Trial

PURPOSE

Determine the effect of cholestyramine on reducing mortality in asymptomatic middle-aged men with primary hypercholesterolemia.

STUDY DESIGN

General

- 3,806 men enrolled in this prospective, randomized, double-blind, placebo-controlled, multicenter trial.
- Eligible patients were randomized to one of two treatment groups:
  1. Cholestyramine: goal of 24 g/day divided into two to four doses
  2. Placebo
- All patients followed a moderate cholesterol-lowering diet.

Inclusion. Patients included were men 35–59 years old with a total cholesterol ≥ 265 mg/dl and a low-density lipoprotein (LDL) cholesterol ≥ 190 mg/dl without symptomatic coronary artery disease.

Exclusion. The criteria for exclusion were as follows: a history of definite or suspected myocardial infarction; angina pectoris; electrocardiogram abnormalities such as left bundle branch block, heart block, left ventricular hypertrophy, or atrial fibrillation; congestive heart failure; secondary hypercholesterolemia (diabetes mellitus, hypothyroidism, obesity, etc.); history of hypertension, serum triglycerides $\geq$ 300 mg/dl; or other serious illness.

End Points. The criteria for end points were coronary heart disease (CHD) mortality and nonfatal myocardial infarction.

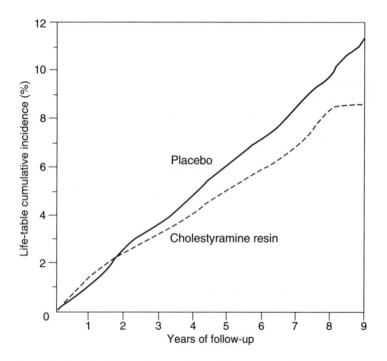

Figure 9-9. Life-table cumulative incidence of the primary end point. (From Lipid Research Clinics Program,[16] with permission.)

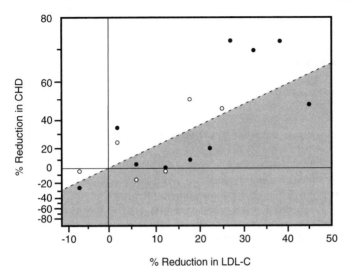

Figure 9-10. Relationship of reduction in low-density lipoprotein cholesterol (LDL-C) to reduction in coronary heart disease (CHD). (From Lipid Research Clinics Program,[16] with permission.)

RESULTS

During an average of 7.4 years of follow-up, treatment with cholestyramine resulted in a decrease in total cholesterol of 8% and LDL cholesterol of 12% compared to the placebo diet-only group. The incidence of coronary heart disease (deaths and nonfatal myocardial infarction) was significantly lower by 19% in patients treated with cholestyramine (8.1% cholestyramine vs. 9.8% placebo, P < 0.05). The individual end point of CHD mortality was reduced by 24% and of nonfatal myocardial infarction by 19%; however, the statistical significance of these results was not reported. All-cause mortality was not meaningfully different between cholestyramine therapy and placebo (3.6% cholestyramine vs. 3.7% placebo, P = NS). Cholestyramine also reduced the incidence of angina by 20% (P < 0.01), the development of a new positive exercise test by 25% (P < 0.001), and the incidence of coronary bypass surgery by 21% P = 0.06).

Analysis of the effect of cholesterol lowering on the risk of CHD was also performed for patients assigned to cholestyramine therapy. A 19%

reduction in CHD risk was associated with each decrement of 8% in total cholesterol or 11% in LDL cholesterol. Among men with a 25% reduction in total cholesterol, which is the typical response to 24 mg/day of cholestyramine, there was a 50% reduction in the risk of CHD. The number of packets taken per day correlated with the percentage decrease in cholesterol. When five or more packets were taken per day, total cholesterol and LDL cholesterol were reduced by 20% and 28%, respectively. A correlation also existed between the percentage reduction in LDL and the percentage reduction in CHD risk (Figs. 9-9 and 9-10).

CONCLUSIONS

Treatment with cholestyramine in asymptomatic middle-aged men with primary hypercholesterolemia significantly reduced the incidence of CHD (death and nonfatal myocardial infarction), angina, positive exercise treadmill test, and coronary bypass surgery compared to placebo over 7.4 years of follow-up. The reduction in CHD events was directly related to the degree of reduction in total and LDL cholesterol.

(Data from Lipid Research Clinics Program.[16]) ■

PHYSICIANS HEALTH STUDY: ASPIRIN IN PRIMARY PREVENTION

PURPOSE

Determine the effects of aspirin on cardiovascular mortality and the incidence of myocardial infarction in healthy male physicians.

STUDY DESIGN

General

- 22,071 male physicians enrolled in this prospective, randomized, double-blind, placebo-controlled, multicenter trial.
- Eligible physicians were randomized to one of four treatment groups:
    1. Active aspirin/active β-carotene
    2. Active aspirin/β-carotene placebo
    3. Aspirin placebo/active β-carotene
    4. Aspirin placebo/β-carotene placebo

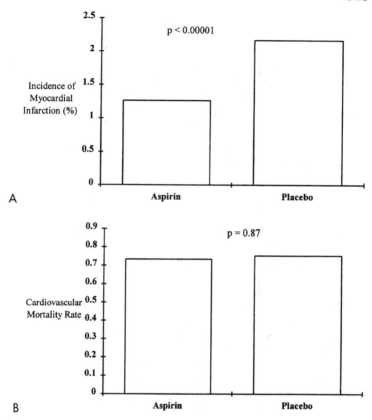

Figure 9-11. *(A)* A reduced incidence of myocardial infarction with *(B)* no effect on cardiovascular mortality for aspirin therapy compared to placebo.

- Aspirin: buffered aspirin 325 mg PO taken every other day.
- β-Carotene: 50 mg PO taken every other day.
- Yearly questionnaires were obtained to evaluate for relevant outcome events. When an event was reported by the physician, all medical records were reviewed by the End Points Committee to confirm the event.

Inclusion. Patients included were male physicians 40–84 years old residing in the United States.

Exclusion. The criteria for exclusion were as follows: history of myocardial infarction, stroke, or transient ischemic attack; cancer (except nonmelanoma skin cancer); current liver or renal disease, peptic ulcer disease, or gout; current use of aspirin, other platelet active drugs, a nonsteroidal anti-inflammatory drug, or vitamin A supplement; or contraindications to aspirin.

End Points. The criteria for end points were cardiovascular mortality and myocardial infarction or stroke.

RESULTS

During an average 5-year follow-up period, there was a significant 44% reduction in the incidence of myocardial infarction (fatal and nonfatal) in physicians taking aspirin compared to placebo (1.26% aspirin vs. 2.17% placebo, $P < 0.00001$). This reduced incidence of myocardial infarction was limited to physicians aged 50 years and older. No significant difference in the incidence of total stroke was observed. Aspirin use, however, was associated with an increased risk of borderline significance of hemorrhagic stroke compared to placebo (23 hemorrhagic strokes with aspirin vs. 12 hemorrhagic strokes with placebo, $P = 0.06$). Total cardiovascular mortality and overall mortality were not substantially different between the two treatment groups (81 cardiovascular deaths with aspirin vs. 83 cardiovascular deaths with placebo, $P = 0.87$). However, the total cardiovascular mortality rate in this physician population was exceptionally low (only 15% of that expected in a matched group of white males in the general population), which may have made if difficult to demonstrate a statistically significant difference in mortality. Aspirin use was associated with a higher incidence of bleeding ulcers (64 patients aspirin vs. 30 patients placebo, $P = 0.04$), minor bleeding (2,979 aspirin vs. 2,248 placebo, $P < 0.00001$), and transfusions (48 aspirin vs. 28 placebo, $P = 0.02$). A combined end point of nonfatal myocardial infarction, nonfatal stroke, and cardiovascular death was significantly reduced with the use of aspirin compared to placebo (307 events with aspirin vs. 370 events with placebo, $P = 0.01$) (Fig. 9-11).

CONCLUSIONS

The use of aspirin in healthy male physicians for the primary prevention of cardiovascular disease resulted in a significant 44% reduction in the risk of myocardial infarction but did not reveal a substantial reduction in stroke rate or cardiovascular mortality, perhaps because of the inadequate numbers of physicians with these later two end points.

(Data from Steering Committee of the Physicians' Health Study Research Group.[17]) ∎

REGRESS

Regression Growth Evaluation Statin Study

PURPOSE

Determine the effect of pravastatin on progression and regression of coronary atherosclerosis in patients with symptomatic coronary artery disease and normal to moderately elevated serum cholesterol.

STUDY DESIGN

General

- 885 men enrolled in this prospective, randomized, double-blind, placebo-controlled, multicenter trial.
- Eligible patients were randomized to one of two treatment groups:
   1. Pravastatin: initial dose of 40 mg/day was administered at bedtime. If the total cholesterol decreased to < 2.0 mmol/l, the dose was reduced to 20 mg/day. If the total cholesterol rose above 8.0 mmol/l, open-label cholestyramine was added. Pravastatin was continued for 1 year.
   2. Placebo.
- Patients were requested to remain on a stable diet of calories derived from protein, 10%–15%; lipid, 30%–35%; and carbohydrate, 50% 55%.
- Potential candidates receiving therapy with lipid-lowering agents or drugs that could significantly affect serum lipids had their drugs withdrawn before randomization.
- Patients with a recent myocardial infarction had their total cholesterol obtained at least 8 weeks after the myocardial infarction.
- Repeat quantitative coronary angiography was performed at 2-year follow-up.

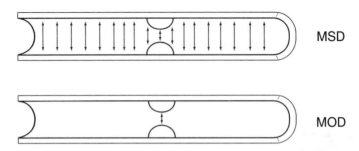

Figure 9-12. Mean segment diameter (MSD) and minimum obstruction diameter (MOD). (From Jukema et al.,[18] with permission.)

Inclusion. Patients included were men < 70 years old undergoing coronary angiography for symptomatic coronary artery disease with at least one coronary stenosis ≥ 50% in a major coronary artery with a baseline total cholesterol between 4 and 8 mmol/L after ≥ 4 weeks of dietary advice.

Exclusion. The criteria for exclusion were as follows: fasting cholesterol < 4.0 or ≥ 8.0 mmol/L or triglycerides ≥ 4.0 mmol/L, requirement for valve replacement, cardiomyopathy, previous coronary artery bypass graft (CABG), percutaneous transluminal coronary angioplasty (PTCA) within 1 year, cardiac pacemaker, clinical congestive heart failure requiring diuretics or left ventricular ejection fraction < 30%, complete atrioventricular block, left bundle branch block, Wolff-Parkinson-White syndrome, ethanol abuse, or other serious illness.

End Points. The criteria for end points were as follows: the change in average mean segment diameter (MSD) per patient, the change in average minimum obstruction diameter (MOD) per patient, cardiovascular clinical events (nonfatal and fatal myocardial infarction, ischemic death, nonscheduled PTCA or CABG, stroke, or transient ischemic attack) (Fig. 9-12).

RESULTS

At 2-year follow-up, the MSD decreased 0.06 mm in the pravastatin group compared to 0.10 mm in the placebo group (P = 0.019). The median MOD decreased 0.03 mm in the pravastatin group compared to 0.09 mm in the

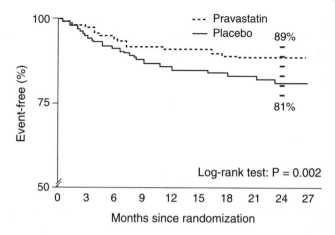

Figure 9-13. Kaplan-Meier curves for time to first event. (From Jukema et al.,[18] with permission.)

placebo group (P = 0.001). Significantly more patients treated with pravastatin remained free of new cardiovascular events (89% pravastatin vs. 81% placebo, P = 0.002). Pravastatin produced changes in total cholesterol, LDL cholesterol, HDL cholesterol, and triglycerides by −20%, −29%, +10%, and −7%, respectively, during the study period. Maximum lipid reduction was achieved within 2 months of initiation of pravastatin (Fig. 9-13).

CONCLUSIONS

In men with symptomatic coronary artery disease and normal to moderately elevated serum cholesterol, the use of pravastatin resulted in significantly less angiographic progression of coronary atherosclerosis and fewer new cardiovascular events compared to placebo over a 2-year follow-up period.

(Data from Jukema et al.[18]) ■

Scandinavian Simvastatin Survival Study

PURPOSE

Determine the effect of simvastatin on morbidity and mortality in patients with coronary artery disease and elevated total serum cholesterol.

STUDY DESIGN

General
- 4,444 patients enrolled in this prospective, randomized, double-blind, placebo-controlled, multicenter trial.
- Eligible patients were randomly assigned to one of two treatment groups:
  1. Simvastatin: initial dose of 20 mg/day taken before the evening meal with titration of the dose between 10 and 40 mg/day to maintain total serum cholesterol between 116 and 200 mg/dl.
  2. Placebo.
- Therapy with other medications was left to the discretion of the local physician.
- Clinical follow-up was every 6 months with monitoring of liver function tests and creatine kinase.

Inclusion. Patients were 35–70 years old with a history of angina pectoris or acute myocardial infarction and total serum cholesterol of 213–310 mg/dl and serum triglyceride ≤ 230 mg/dl after 8 weeks of dietary therapy.

Exclusion. The criteria for exclusion were as follows: women of child-bearing potential; secondary hypercholesterolemia; unstable or Prinzmetal angina; tendon xanthoma; planned coronary artery bypass graft (CABG) or percutaneous transluminal coronary angioplasty (PTCA); myocardial infarction within the previous 6 months; antiarrhythmic therapy; congestive heart failure requiring digitalis, diuretics, or vasodilators; persistent atrial fibrillation; cardiomegaly; significant valvular disease; history of stroke; impaired hepatic function; partial ileal bypass; history of drug or alcohol abuse; contraindication to 3-hydroxy-3-methylglutaryl coenzyme A reductase inhibitors; or other serious illness.

End Points. The criteria for end points were total mortality and major coronary events defined as coronary deaths, nonfatal acute myocardial infarction, resuscitated cardiac arrest, and definite silent myocardial infarction.

RESULTS

During an average 5.4-year follow-up, the use of simvastatin significantly reduced total mortality by 29% (8.2% simvastatin vs. 11.5% placebo, P = 0.0003) and cardiac mortality by 42% (5.0% simvastatin vs.

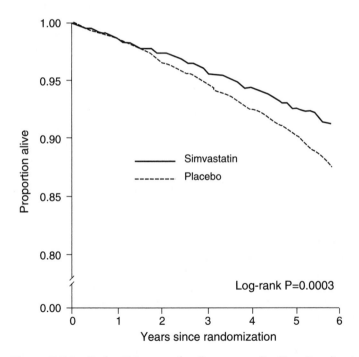

Figure 9-14. Kaplan-Meier curves for all-cause mortality. (From Scandinavian Simvastatin Survival Study Group,[19] with permission.)

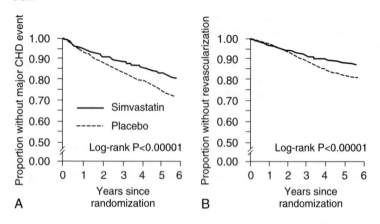

Figure 9-15. *(A & B)* Kaplan-Meier curves for secondary and tertiary end points. (From Scandinavian Simvastatin Survival Study Group,[19] with permission.)

8.5% placebo, P < 0.05) compared to placebo. Substantially fewer major coronary events occurred in patients receiving simvastatin (19% simvastatin vs. 28% placebo, P < 0.00001). Simvastatin also significantly reduced the risk of undergoing CABG or PTCA (11.3% simvastatin vs. 17.2% placebo, P < 0.00001) and significantly reduced the incidence of fatal and nonfatal cerebrovascular events (2.7% simvastatin vs. 4.3% placebo, P = 0.024). Simvastatin produced changes in total cholesterol, low-density lipoproteins, high-density lipoproteins, and triglycerides of −25%, −35%, +8%, and −10%, respectively, with few adverse effects (Figs. 9-14 and 9-15).

CONCLUSIONS
The use of simvastatin in patients with coronary artery disease and elevated total serum cholesterol significantly reduced total mortality by 29%, cardiac mortality by 42%, major coronary events by 32%, the need for revascularization by 34%, and cerebrovascular events by 37% compared to placebo over a 5.4-year follow-up period.

(Data from Scandinavian Simvastatin Survival Study Group.[19]) ■

West of Scotland Coronary Prevention Study

PURPOSE

Determine the effect of pravastatin on the incidence of nonfatal myocardial infarction and coronary mortality in men with moderate hypercholesterolemia and no previous myocardial infarction.

STUDY DESIGN

General

- 6,595 men enrolled in this prospective, randomized, double-blind, placebo-controlled, multicenter trial.
- Eligible patients were randomized to one of two treatment groups:
  1. Pravastatin: 40 mg PO in the evening
  2. Placebo
- All patients had 8 weeks of lipid-lowering dietary therapy before randomization and smoking cessation counseling during the trial.
- Clinical follow-up was performed every 3 months.

Inclusion. Patients included were men 45–64 years old with a fasting low-density lipoprotein (LDL) cholesterol of 155–232 mg/dl without serious electrocardiographic (ECG) abnormalities or arrhythmias such as atrial fibrillation and with no history of previous myocardial infarction. Patients with stable angina pectoris who had not been hospitalized within the previous 12 months were eligible.

Exclusion. The criteria for exclusion were as follows: previous myocardial infarction, angina pectoris requiring hospitalization for treatment or investigation within the past 12 months, serious ECG abnormalities, uncontrolled hypertension, rheumatic or congenital heart disease, congestive heart failure, significant valvular heart disease, current lipid-lowering therapy, or other serious illness.

End Points. The criteria for end points were nonfatal myocardial infarction and mortality from coronary heart disease.

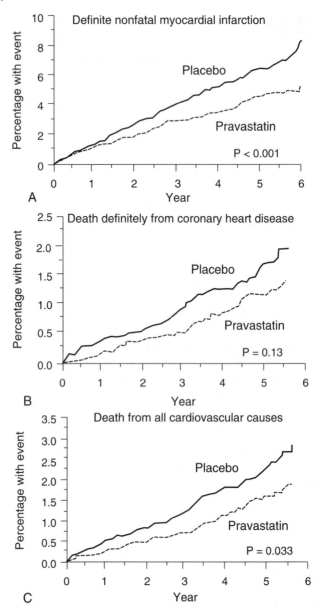

Figure 9-16. *(A–C)* Kaplan-Meier curves for primary end points. (From Shepherd et al.,[20] with permission.)

RESULTS

During an average follow-up of 4.9 years, the use of pravastatin significantly reduced the incidence of nonfatal myocardial infarction by 29% (4.6% pravastatin vs. 6.5% placebo, P < 0.001) and death from all cardiovascular causes by 30% (1.6% pravastatin vs. 2.3% placebo, P = 0.033) compared to placebo. Pravastatin produced a trend toward fewer definite deaths from coronary heart disease compared to placebo, but the results were not statistically significant (1.2% pravastatin vs. 1.7% placebo, P = 0.13). Similarly, a nonsignificant trend toward reduced overall mortality was observed in the pravastatin group (3.2% pravastatin vs. 4.1% placebo, P = 0.051). Patients receiving pravastatin underwent significantly less coronary angiography (2.8% pravastatin vs. 4.2% placebo, P = 0.007) and revascularization with percutaneous transluminal coronary angioplasty or coronary artery bypass graft (1.7% pravastatin vs. 2.5% placebo, P = 0.009). The beneficial effects of pravastatin were evident in all of the predefined subgroups including age, current smoking status, presence of multiple risk factors for coronary artery disease, cholesterol levels, and prior vascular disease. Pravastatin produced changes in total cholesterol, LDL, triglycerides, and high-density lipoproteins of –20%, –26%, –12% and +5%, respectively (Fig. 9-16).

CONCLUSIONS

The use of pravastatin in middle-aged men with moderate hypercholesterolemia and no history of previous myocardial infarction significantly reduced the incidence of nonfatal myocardial infarction by 29%, death from all cardiovascular causes by 30%, and the need for revascularization, while producing a trend toward fewer deaths from coronary heart disease compared to placebo over a 4.9-year follow-up period.

(Data from Shepherd et al.[20])   ■

References

1. Verschuren WM, Jacobs DR, Bloemberg BP et al: Serum total cholesterol and long-term coronary heart disease mortality in different cultures. JAMA 274:131, 1995

2. Multiple risk factor intervention trial research group: Multiple risk factor intervention trial: risk factor changes and mortality results. JAMA 248:1465, 1982

3. Anderson KM, Castelli WP, Levy D: Cholesterol and mortality: 30 years of follow-up from the Framingham study. JAMA 257:2176, 1987

4. Gould AL, Rossouw JE, Santanello NC: Cholesterol reduction yields clinical benefit: a new look at old data. Circulation 91:2274, 1995

5. Brown G, Albers JJ, Fisher LD et al: Regression of coronary artery disease as a result of intensive lipid-lowering therapy in men with high levels of apolipoprotein B. N Engl J Med 323:1289, 1990

6. Levy RI, Brensike JF, Epstein SE et al: The influence of changes in lipid values induced by cholestyramine and diet on progression of coronary artery disease: results of the NHLBI type II coronary intervention study. Circulation 69:325, 1984

7. Carlson LA, Rosenhamer G: Reduction of mortality in the Stockholm ischemic heart disease secondary prevention study by combined treatment with clofibrate and nicotinic acid. Acta Med Scand 223:405, 1988

8. Mandon JE, Tosleson H, Ridker PM et al: The primary prevention of myocardial infarction (review). N Engl J Med 326:1406, 1992

9. Furberg CD, Adams HP, Applegate WB et al: Effect of lovastatin on early carotid atherosclerosis and cardiovascular events. Circulation 90:1679-87, 1994

10. Stephens NG, Parsons A, Schofield PM et al: Randomised controlled trial of vitamin E in patients with coronary disease: Cambridge Heart Antioxidant Study (CHAOS). Lancet 347:781-6, 1996

11. Blankenhorn DH, Nessim SA, Johnson RL et al: Beneficial effects of combined colestipol-niacin therapy on coronary atherosclerosis and coronary venous bypass grafts. JAMA 257:3233-40, 1987

12. Cashin-Hemphill L, Mack WJ, Pogoda JM et al: Beneficial effects of colestipol-niacin on coronary atherosclerosis: a 4-year follow-up. JAMA 264:3013-7, 1990

13. The Coronary Drug Project Research Group: Clofibrate and niacin in coronary heart disease. JAMA 231:360-81, 1975

14. Canner PL, Berge KG, Wenger NK et al: Fifteen year mortality in coronary drug project patients: long-term benefit with niacin. J Am Coll Cardiol 8:1245-55, 1986

15. Frick MH, Elo O, Haapa K et al: Helsinki Heart Study: primary-prevention trial with gemfibrozil in middle-aged men with dyslipidemia. N Engl J Med 317:1237-45, 1987

16. Lipid Research Clinics Program: The Lipid Research Clinics coronary primary prevention trial results: I. Reduction in incidence of coronary heart disease. JAMA 251:351-74, 1984

17. Steering Committee of the Physicians' Health Study Research Group: Final report on the aspirin component of the ongoing Physician's Health Study. N Engl J Med 321:129–35, 1989

18. Jukema JW, Bruschke AVG, van Boven AJ et al: Effects of lipid lowering by pravastatin on progression and regression of coronary artery disease in symptomatic men with normal to moderately elevated serum cholesterol levels: the Regression Growth Evaluation Statin Study (REGRESS). Circulation 91: 2529–40, 1995

19. Scandinavian Simvastatin Survival Study Group: Randomised trial of cholesterol lowering in 4444 patients with coronary heart disease: the Scandinavian Simvastatin Survival Study (4S). Lancet 344:1383–9, 1994

20. Shepherd J, Cobbe SM, Ford I et al: Prevention of coronary heart disease with pravastatin in men with hypercholesterolemia. N Engl J Med 333:1301–7, 1995

CHAPTER 10

Revascularization Versus Medical Therapy Trials

OVERVIEW

Postmortem observations at the end of the eighteenth century suggested that cardiac muscle death was due to narrowing in the coronary arteries, resulting in decreased myocardial blood flow. This led several investigators in the mid-1900s to experiment with the concept of myocardial revascularization. Initial clinical success was obtained by implanting the bleeding end of an internal mammary pedicle directly into the myocardium with the hope of supplying collateral blood flow and relieving angina. In 1962, the first coronary artery bypass graft (CABG) procedure was performed using a reversed saphenous vein graft to the right coronary artery. Refinement of this technique led to widespread use of CABG to relieve angina over the ensuing 20 years. Although CABG clearly was effective in relieving angina, concerns were raised over the influence of CABG on mortality and prevention of myocardial infarction. In the early 1970s, three large randomized clinical trials were begun to examine the effect of surgical revascularization compared with medical therapy on long-term survival (Table 10-1).

CABG vs. Medical Therapy Trials

The Veterans Affairs (VA) Coronary Artery Bypass Surgery Cooperative Study randomized 686 men with stable angina pectoris and more than 50% stenosis in at least one major coronary artery to CABG or medical

Table 10-1. The Three Major Surgery Trials

	VA	CASS	ECSS
n	686	780	768
Date	1972–1974	1974–1979	1973–1976
Angina (%)			
Asymptomatic	0	26%	0
Mild to moderate	42%	74%	57%
Lesion requirement	$\geq 50\%$	$\geq 70\%$	$\geq 50\%$
Ejection fraction	$> 35\%$	$> 35\%$	$> 50\%$
Operative mortality	5.8%	1.4%	3.3%

(Adapted from Ferguson and Wilson,[1] with permission.)

therapy. Two subgroups were defined as high angiographic risk (three-vessel disease with a left ventricular ejection fraction [LVEF] less than 50%) and high clinical risk (two or more of the following: ST-segment depression on resting electrocardiogram, history of myocardial infarction, history of hypertension). For the entire study population over an 18-year follow-up period, surgical therapy significantly improved survival compared to medical therapy only at the 7-year follow-up review. No significant difference in mortality was observed at 5, 11, 15, or 18 years. The subgroup of patients with left main disease had significantly better survival with CABG up to 7 years only; however, after 7 years, the mortality rate for the surgically treated patients increased, presumably as the result of progression of the coronary artery disease or occlusion of the saphenous vein graft. For all patients without left main disease, no significant difference in mortality was observed up to 11-year follow-up. After excluding patients with left main disease, the subgroups of patients with high angiographic or clinical risk had better survival with CABG for 11 years. After 11 years, survival was the same for both treatment groups. Relief of angina among all patients was significantly better with surgical therapy at 5 years. Graft closure rates at 1, 5, and 10 years were 29%, 36%, and 50%, respectively. Thus, the VA trial revealed that only patients with left main disease or high angiographic or clinical risk had improved survival with surgical therapy up to a maximum of 11 years. After 11 years, there was no difference in survival among any subgroups, which was perhaps due to vein graft closure or progression of the coronary vascular disease by 10 years.

The Coronary Artery Surgery Study (CASS) randomized 780 patients with mild stable angina pectoris to medical therapy or CABG. Patients

Table 10-2. Subgroups of Patients With Significantly Improved Survival From Surgical Therapy Compared to Medical Therapy

VA	CASS	ECSS[a]
1. Left main disease up to 11 years only	1. LVEF < 50%, especially when associated with triple-vessel at 10 years	1. Significant triple-vessel disease at 12 years
2. High angiographic risk up to 11 years only		2. Significant two-vessel disease with > 50% proximal stenosis of the LAD coronary artery at 12 years
3. High clinical risk up to 11 years only		

[a]All patients had LVEF > 50%.

with left main disease and patients with LVEF less than 35% were excluded. Among all patients, there was no significant difference in mortality or the incidence of myocardial infarction at both 5- and 10-year follow-up. Subgroup analyses according to the number of diseased vessels showed no significant difference in survival. Only the subgroup with LVEF less than 50%, particularly if associated with significant triple-vessel disease, had significantly better 10-year survival with CABG treatment. Patients with LVEF greater than 50% had no survival benefit from surgical treatment. Thus, the CASS trial showed that only the subgroup of patients with impaired LVEF, especially when associated with triple-vessel disease, had significantly better survival with surgical therapy at 10-year follow-up.

The European Coronary Surgery Study (ECSS) randomized 768 men with two- or three-vessel coronary artery disease and preserved left ventricular function (LVEF greater than 50%) to medical or surgical therapy. Among all patients, treatment with CABG significantly improved survival at 5-, 10-, and 12-year follow-up compared to medical therapy. Subgroup analysis of all patients with two-vessel disease revealed no significant difference in survival between surgical and medical therapy. The subgroup of patients with significant triple-vessel disease and patients with more than 50% proximal stenosis of the left anterior descending coronary artery as a component of two-vessel disease had increased survival from CABG. Table 10-2 summarizes the subgroups of patients in each study that had significantly improved survival with surgical treatment.

Limitations to CABG Trials

There are several limitations to these trials that raise concern over the applicability of their results to current practice. First, the medical therapy groups in all of the trials had no specified protocol for treatment but instead consisted of individual treatment plans according to each local physician. Only a small percentage of patients received aspirin, β-blockers or lipid-lowering therapy, which are three medications proven to prolong survival in patients with coronary artery disease. In fact, in the VA trial at 5-year follow-up, 12% of patients assigned to medical treatment were not taking any medications. The routine use of aspirin, β-blockers, and cholesterol-lowering agents like 3-hydroxy-3-methylglutaryl coenzyme A reductase inhibitors will significantly improve survival in medically treated patients. Second, since the major limitation of CABG appears to be vein graft closure by 10 years, the increased use of arterial conduits, especially the internal thoracic artery, which is now commonly used for left anterior descending coronary artery revascularization, may significantly improve survival with CABG. Finally, all analyses were performed by intention-to-treat analysis. This means that patients initially assigned to medical therapy were always analyzed with the medical cohort even if they subsequently underwent surgical revascularization. In the VA, CASS, and ECSS trials, the percentages of the medical cohort who subsequently underwent surgical treatment were 62% at 18 years, 37% at 10 years, and 36% at 12 years, respectively. Using intention-to-treat analysis with this high incidence of crossover from medical to surgical treatment has the effect of diluting the benefit of surgical therapy.

PTCA vs. Medical Therapy Trials

The Angioplasty Compared to Medicine (ACME) trial randomized 212 patients with stable single-vessel coronary artery disease to angioplasty or medical therapy consisting of a combination of aspirin, calcium channel blockers, β-blockers, and nitrates. Patients treated with percutaneous transluminal coronary angioplasty (PTCA) had significant improvements in total exercise duration, incidence of clinical angina, and residual stenosis at 6-month follow-up. Mortality was not a specified end point because of the small number of patients analyzed.

The Medicine Angioplasty Surgery Study (MASS)[2] randomized 214 patients with stable angina, normal left ventricular function, and a single stenosis greater than 80% of the proximal left anterior descending coronary artery to internal mammary artery bypass surgery, PTCA, or medical therapy. At 3-year follow-up, overall mortality and infarction rates were not significantly different between the three groups. Both revascularization techniques resulted in a significant reduction in angina compared to medical therapy.

Conclusions

Three large clinical trials, the VA, CASS, and ECSS, have evaluated the effect of medical vs. surgical treatment in patients with coronary artery disease. Patients with more severe ischemic heart disease—that is, those with significant triple-vessel disease and depressed LVEF, significant left main coronary artery disease and more recently identified, those with significant two-vessel disease where the very proximal left anterior descending (LAD) artery has a stenosis $\geq 90\%$—appear to gain the most survival benefit from surgical revascularization. Patients with one- or two-vessel disease, especially when the proximal LAD artery is not involved, and normal LVEF derived no survival benefit from surgical therapy in any of the above-mentioned trials. Several limitations to these surgical trials raise concern over applying the results to current clinical practice. The development of interventional cardiology techniques, like PTCA and stenting, appears to be more effective than medical therapy at relieving symptoms, improving exercise tolerance, and reducing residual stenosis in patients with single-vessel coronary artery disease. The effect of these interventional procedures on long-term survival in patients with multivessel coronary artery disease remains to be shown, but these new options coupled with appropriate medical therapy, especially marked reduction of cholesterol and LDL, may have their own favorable impacts on both symptoms and survival in subsets of patients with coronary heart disease in the future.

ACME

Angioplasty Compared to Medicine

PURPOSE
Compare the effect of percutaneous transluminal coronary angioplasty (PTCA) to medical therapy on the incidence of angina and exercise tolerance in patients with stable, single vessel coronary artery disease.

STUDY DESIGN

General

- 212 patients enrolled in this prospective, randomized, multicenter trial.
- Eligible patients with a positive baseline exercise thallium test were randomized to one of two treatment groups:
    1. PTCA: standard angioplasty was performed within 3 days of randomization. Treatment with aspirin 325 mg/day, calcium channel blockers for 1 month, and intravenous heparin and nitroglycerin during the procedure was used. Patients who developed restenosis were encouraged to undergo repeat angioplasty.
    2. Medical therapy: aspirin 325 mg/day, calcium channel blockers, β-blockers, oral nitrates, or a combination of these drugs was used.
- After 6 months, all patients had repeat cardiac catheterization and exercise testing (those in the PTCA group had antianginal medications discontinued for 24 hr before exercise testing, while those in

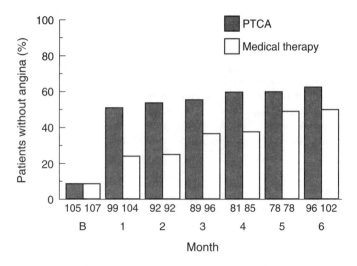

Figure 10-1. Percent of patients who were free of angina each month after revascularization. (From Parisi et al.,[3] with permission.)

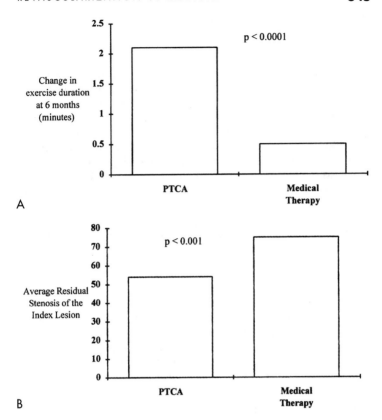

Figure 10-2. (A) Increased exercise duration and (B) reduced 6-month residual stenosis in patients treated with PTCA compared to medical therapy.

the medical therapy group were continued on medications during the exercise test).

Inclusion. Patients included had stable angina, a strikingly positive exercise tolerance test, or myocardial infarction within the past 3 months and had a 70%–99% diameter stenosis of one major epicardial coronary artery associated with a positive exercise thallium test.

End Points. The criteria for end points were changes in exercise tolerance and frequency of anginal attacks.

RESULTS

At 6-month follow-up, treatment with PTCA resulted in a 2.1-min increase in total exercise duration, which was significantly better than the 0.5-min increase in exercise duration observed with medical treatment (P < 0.0001). The change in heart rate × blood pressure double product was significantly improved with PTCA therapy as well (increase by 1,800 U with PTCA vs. decrease by 2,800 U with medical therapy, P < 0.0001). A greater proportion of the PTCA group was free of angina at 6 months (64% PTCA vs. 46% medical therapy, P = 0.01) and exercised longer before the development of angina (8.2-min exercise with PTCA vs. 6.5-min exercise with medical therapy, P < 0.01). The average residual stenosis of the index lesion at 6 months was significantly better with PTCA (54% stenosis with PTCA vs. 75% stenosis with medical therapy, P < 0.001). Significantly more patients treated with PTCA underwent CABG, with two bypass procedures performed emergently (7% PTCA vs. 0% medical, P < 0.01) (Figs. 10-1 and 10-2).

CONCLUSIONS

The use of PTCA in patients with single-vessel coronary artery disease resulted in significant improvements in total exercise duration, maximal heart rate × systolic blood pressure double product, angina-free exercise duration, incidence of clinical angina, and residual stenosis of the index lesions compared to medical therapy at 6-month follow-up.

(Data from Parisi et al.[3])   ■

CASS

Coronary Artery Surgery Study

PURPOSE
Determine the long-term effects of coronary artery bypass graft (CABG) on mortality and the incidence of myocardial infarction in patients with mild stable angina pectoris and angiographically documented coronary artery disease.

STUDY DESIGN

General

- 780 patients enrolled in this prospective, randomized trial.
- Eligible patients were randomized to medical or surgical therapy.
- Three subgroups of patients were defined as follows:

    Group A: Canadian Cardiovascular Society (CCS) angina class I or II with normal left ventricular function (left ventricular ejection fraction [LVEF] ≥ 50%)

    Group B: CCS angina class I or II with mild-to-moderate left ventricular dysfunction (LVEF 35%–50%)

    Group C: no angina after myocardial infarction

Inclusion. Patients included had mild stable angina or were free of angina after myocardial infarction with operable coronary artery disease defined as ≥ 70% stenosis of the right, left anterior descending, or left circumflex coronary arteries or with 50%–70% stenosis of the left main coronary artery.

Exclusion. The criteria for exclusion were ≥ 70% left main coronary artery stenosis, confirmed LVEF < 35%, CCS angina class III or IV, previous CABG, or other serious cardiac diseases requiring other procedures like valve replacement or resection of a ventricular aneurysm.

End Points. The criteria for end points were total mortality and the incidence of myocardial infarction.

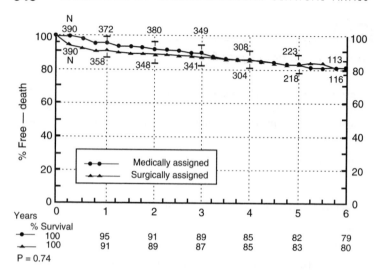

Figure 10-3. Probability of remaining alive and free of myocardial infarction for medical and surgical groups. (From Coronary Artery Surgery Study [CASS] Principal Investigators and Associates,[4] with permission.)

RESULTS

Five-Year Follow-up. The likelihood of death in the 5-year follow-up period was 8% in the medical cohort compared to 5% in the surgical cohort (P = NS). The cumulative incidence of Q-wave myocardial infarction over 5 years was not significantly different between medical and surgical treatment (11% medical vs. 14% surgical, P = not significant [NS]). There were also no statistically significant differences in the survival rate or in the infarction rate between subgroups A, B, or C or between subgroups of patients divided by number of diseased vessels or ejection fraction at 5-year follow-up. The subgroup of patients with LVEF < 50% and triple-vessel disease had significantly higher 5-year survival and freedom from nonfatal myocardial infarction with surgical treatment (86% surgical vs. 68% medical, P = 0.029), whereas patients with LVEF > 50% and two-vessel disease had significantly better 5-year survival and freedom from nonfatal myocardial infarction with medical therapy (89% surgical vs. 95% medical, P = 0.038).

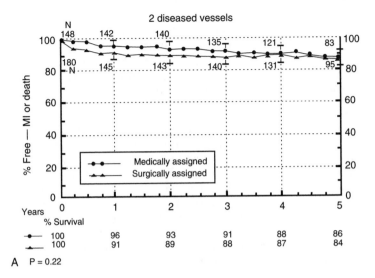

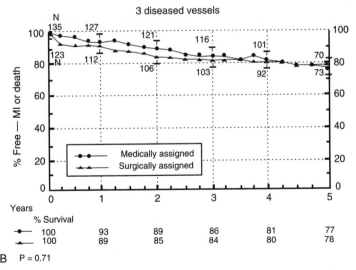

Figure 10-4. Survival and absence of myocardial infarction in patients with (A) two- or (B) three-vessel disease. (From Coronary Artery Surgery Study [CASS] Principal Investigators and Associates,[4] with permission.)

Ten-Year Follow-up. At 10 years, mortality was 21.8% in the medical group compared to 19.2% in the surgical group (P = NS). The survival rates for the subgroups of patients with LVEF < 50% (79% surgical vs. 61% medical, P = 0.01) and patients with both LVEF < 50% and triple-vessel disease (75% surgical vs. 58% medical, P = 0.08) were significantly better with surgical therapy (Figs. 10-3 and 10-4).

CONCLUSIONS

Coronary artery bypass surgery, compared to medical therapy, did not significantly prolong survival or prevent myocardial infarction overall in patients who have mild stable angina pectoris or patients who are asymptomatic after myocardial infarction during the 10-year follow-up. Subgroup analysis according to the number of diseased vessels also revealed no significant difference in mortality or the incidence of myocardial infarction. However, the subgroup of patients with LVEF < 50%, and particularly those with both LVEF < 50% and triple-vessel disease, had significantly higher 10-year survival and freedom from myocardial infarction with surgical treatment.

(5-year follow-up data from Coronary Artery Surgery Study [CASS] Principal Investigators and Associates[4]; 10-year follow-up data from Rogers et al.[5]) ∎

EUROPEAN CABG

European Coronary Artery Bypass Graft Surgery Study

PURPOSE

Compare the effect of coronary artery bypass graft (CABG) to medical therapy in patients with angina pectoris with at least two-vessel coronary artery disease and preserved left ventricular function.

STUDY DESIGN

General

- 768 patients enrolled in this prospective, randomized trial.
- Eligible patients underwent coronary angiography and left ventriculography.
- Patients with ≥ 50% stenosis in at least two major coronary arteries with left ventricular ejection fraction (LVEF) ≥ 50% were randomized to medical or surgical therapy.
- Medical care was not standardized in detail.
- Patients in the medical group who had unacceptable symptoms despite adequate medical treatment were eligible for surgical revascularization.

Inclusion. Patients included were men < 65 years old with angina pectoris of > 3-month duration and normal left ventricular function (LVEF > 50%).

Exclusion. The criteria for exclusion were severe anginal pain refractory to medical therapy, poor surgical candidates, LVEF ≤ 50%, or other serious illness.

End Points. The criterion for end point was mortality.

RESULTS

Cumulative survival rates were significantly higher among all patients receiving surgical treatment compared to medical therapy throughout the 12-year follow-up period (5 years: 83% medical vs. 92% surgical, P = 0.0001;

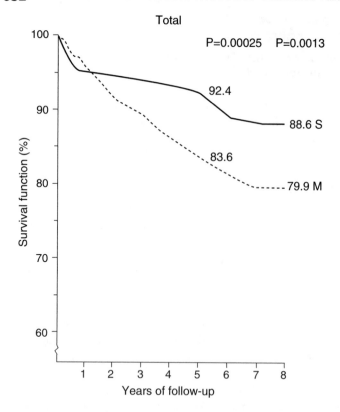

Figure 10-5. Survival curves in the total population. M, medical groups; S, surgical groups. (From European Coronary Surgery Study Group,[6] with permission.)

10 years: 70% medical vs. 76% surgical, P = 0.02; 12 years: 67% medical vs. 71% surgical, P = 0.04). At 8-year follow-up, treatment with CABG resulted in significantly higher survival rates among the subset of patients with triple-vessel disease (91.8% surgical vs. 76.7% medical, P = 0.0001) and ≥

Figure 10-6. Survival curves in patients with *(A)* three-vessel (3VD) or *(B)* two-vessel disease (2VD). (From European Coronary Surgery Study Group,[6] with permission.)

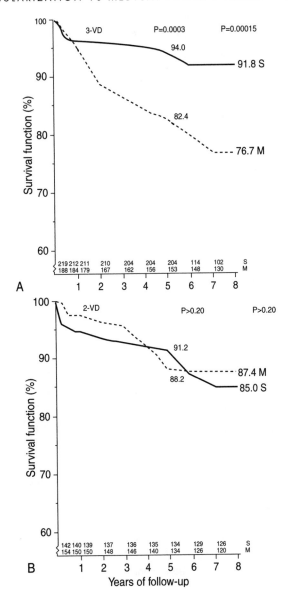

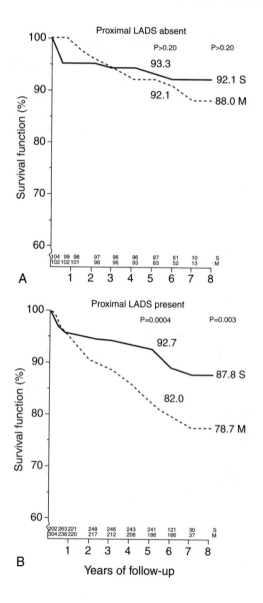

50% proximal stenosis of the left anterior descending coronary artery as a component of two- or three-vessel disease (87.8% surgical vs. 78.7% medical, P = 0.003). However, all patients with two-vessel disease treated with CABG had no significant survival benefit over medical therapy. Subgroup analysis revealed that the benefit of surgery tended to be greater, but not significantly so, in patients with left main disease, age > 53 years, with an abnormal resting electrocardiogram, a markedly positive exercise treadmill test, and peripheral vascular disease (Figs. 10-5 to 10-7).

CONCLUSIONS

A significant overall improvement in survival after CABG, compared with medical therapy, was observed in patients with stable angina pectoris and multivessel coronary artery disease with preserved left ventricular function over a 12-year follow-up period. The survival advantage of CABG was especially prominent among the subgroup of patients with triple-vessel disease and patients with proximal stenosis of the left anterior descending coronary artery as a component of two-vessel disease.

(5-year follow-up data from European Coronary Surgery Study Group[6]; 12-year follow-up data from Varnauskas E and European Coronary Surgery Study Group.[7]) ■

Figure 10-7. (A & B) Survival curves for the subgroups of patients with and without stenosis in the proximal segment of the left anterior descending coronary artery (LADS) as a component of two- or three-vessel disease. M, medical groups; S, surgical groups. (From European Coronary Surgery Study Group,[6] with permission.)

Veterans Affairs Coronary Artery Bypass Surgery Cooperative Study

PURPOSE

Compare the long-term survival after coronary artery bypass graft surgery (CABG) to medical therapy in patients with stable angina pectoris and angiographically confirmed coronary artery disease.

STUDY DESIGN

General

- 686 patients enrolled in this prospective, randomized trial.
- All eligible patients underwent coronary arteriography and left ventriculography.
- Patients with $\geq$ 50% stenosis in at least one major coronary artery with a graftable distal segment without ventricular aneurysm and with sufficient ventricular function to permit CABG at a reasonable surgical risk were randomized to medical or surgical treatments.
- High angiographic risk was defined as three-vessel disease and impaired left ventricular function (left ventricular ejection fraction < 50%).
- High clinical risk was defined as two or more of the following: ST-segment depression on resting electrocardiogram (ECG), history of myocardial infarction, or history of hypertension.

Inclusion. Patients included were men with stable angina pectoris of > 6-month duration receiving medical therapy for $\geq$ 3 months with resting or exercise ECG evidence of myocardial ischemia or previous myocardial infarction.

Exclusion. The criteria for exclusion were as follows: myocardial infarction within 6 months; persistent diastolic hypertension > 100 mmHg; marked cardiac enlargement; the presence of ventricular aneurysm or other serious cardiac disease such as valvular heart disease, unstable angina, uncompensated congestive heart failure, previous CABG; or other serious illness.

End Points. The criteria for end points were total mortality, myocardial infarction, and the severity of angina pectoris.

RESULTS

The primary treatment comparisons were made according to intent to treat; however, 44% of the medical cohort underwent CABG during a mean 16.8-year follow-up. Cumulative survival for all patients was significantly higher in the surgical group only at 7 years (70% medical vs. 77% surgical, P = 0.043) but not substantially different at 5 years (78% medical vs. 83% surgical, P = 0.12), at 11 years (57% medical vs. 58% surgical, P = 0.45), or at 18 years (33% medical vs. 30% surgical, P = 0.60). The subgroup of patients with left main disease had significantly better survival with CABG up to 7 years only, with no significant difference between medical and surgical groups after 7-year follow-up. For all patients without left main disease, no significant difference in cumulative survival was observed at 5 years (80% medical vs. 82% surgical, P = 0.53) or at 11 years (58% medical vs. 58% surgical, P = 0.81).

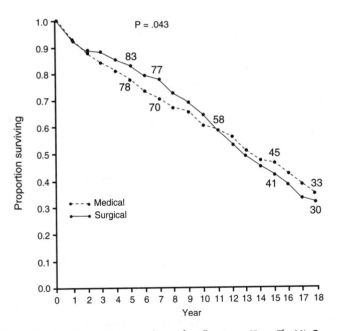

Figure 10-8. Cumulative survival rates for all patients. (From The VA Coronary Artery Bypass Surgery Cooperative Study Group,[9] with permission.)

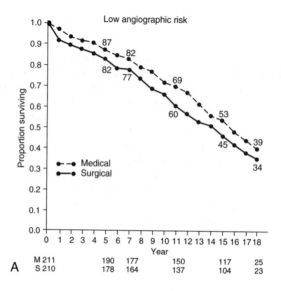

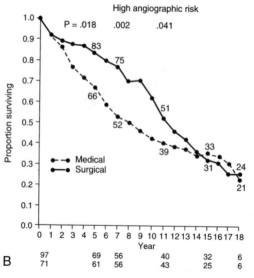

Figure 10-9. *(A & B)* Cumulative survival rates for patients without left main coronary artery disease according to angiographic risk. (From The VA Coronary Artery Bypass Surgery Cooperative Study Group,[9] with permission.)

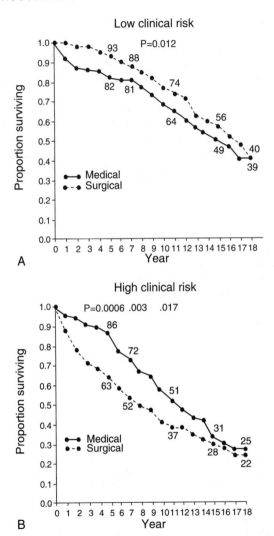

Figure 10-10. *(A & B)* Cumulative survival rates for patients without left main coronary artery disease according to clinical risk. (From The VA Coronary Artery Bypass Surgery Cooperative Study Group,[9] with permission.)

Subgroup analysis of patients without left main coronary disease showed a significant survival advantage for surgical therapy with impaired left ventricular function at 7 years only, with high angiographic risk at 5, 7, and 11 years only, and with high clinical risk at 5, 7, and 11 years only. A significant survival advantage for medical therapy was observed in the low clinical risk subgroup at 5 years and in patients with two-vessel disease at 11 years (Figs. 10-8 to 10-10).

Cumulative 18-year rates of myocardial infarction were not significantly different between medical therapy (41%) and surgical therapy (49% with 13% perioperative infarction rate, P = 0.15). Significantly more surgical patients were free of angina at 5 years only with no significant difference at 10 or 15 years. Graft closure rates at 1, 5, and 10 years were 29%, 36%, and 50%, respectively.

CONCLUSIONS

Surgical therapy significantly improved survival compared to medical therapy only in patients with left main stenosis, high angiographic risk, and high clinical risk, but the benefits began to diminish after 5 years and lasted < 11 years. No significant survival difference was observed in any group at 18-year follow-up. Patients with low clinical risk or low angiographic risk did not have a survival benefit from surgical therapy at any time over the 18-year follow-up period.

_____

(11-year follow-up data from The Veterans Administration Coronary Artery Bypass Surgery Cooperative Study Group[8]; 18-year follow-up data from The VA Coronary Artery Bypass Surgery Cooperative Study Group.[9])   ∎

References

1. Ferguson JJ, Wilson JM: Coronary artery bypass surgery and percutaneous transluminal coronary angioplasty. pp. 670–701. In Willerson JT, Cohn JN (eds): Cardiovascular Medicine. Churchill Livingstone, New York, 1995

2. Hueb WA, Bellotti G, Almeida de Oliveira S et al: The medicine, angioplasty, or surgery study (MASS): a prospective randomized trial of medical therapy, balloon angioplasty, or bypass surgery for single proximal left anterior descending coronary artery stenosis. J Am Coll Cardiol 26:1600, 1995

3. Parisi AF, Folland ED, Hartigan P et al: A comparison of angioplasty with medical therapy in the treatment of single-vessel coronary artery disease. N Engl J Med 326:10–16, 1992

4. Coronary Artery Surgery Study (CASS) Principal Investigators and Associates: Myocardial infarction and mortality in the Coronary Artery Surgery Study (CASS) randomized trial. N Engl J Med 310:750–8, 1984

5. Rogers WJ, Coggin J, Gersh BJ et al: Ten-yar follow-up of quality of life in patients randomzied to receive medical therapy or coronary artery bypass graft surgery: the Coronary aRtery Surgery Study (CASS). Circulation 82: 1629-58, 1990

6. European Coronary Surgery Study Group: Coronary-artery bypass surgery in stagle angina pectoris: survival at two years. Lancet 2:1173-80, 1982

7. Varnauskas E, European Coronary Surgery Study Group: Twelve-year follow-up of survival in the randomized European Coronary Surgery Study. N Engl J Med 319:332-7, 1988

8. The Veterans Administration Coronary Artery Bypass Surgery Cooperative Study Group: Eleven-year survival in the Veterans Administration Randomized Trial of Coronary Bypass Surgery for Stagle Angina. N Engl J Med 311:1333-9, 1984

9. The VA Coronary Artery Bypass Surgery Cooperative Study Group: Eighteen-year follow-up in the Veterans Affairs Cooperative Study of Coronary Artery Bypass Surgery for Stable Angina. Circulation 86:121-30, 1992

CHAPTER 11

Angioplasty Versus Coronary Artery Bypass Graft Trials

OVERVIEW

In the mid-1980s, Dotter and Judkins originated the idea of endovascular revascularization in which catheter interventions were used to reduce flow-limiting stenosis in atherosclerotic plaques. Their concept, which gradually became known as the *Dotter technique,* used progressively larger rigid dilators, which were advanced over a guidewire to sequentially compress the atherosclerotic plaque against the vessel wall, resulting in a larger luminal diameter. Andrea Gruentzig further developed this concept by designing a noncompliant balloon-tipped catheter, which was introduced percutaneously and positioned at a stenotic lesion. The balloon was then inflated to a high pressure, deflated, and removed, leaving a larger endovascular lumen. After refining this technique in peripheral and renal arteries, he performed the first percutaneous transluminal coronary angioplasty (PTCA) in September of 1977, a procedure that eventually revolutionized the field of myocardial revascularization. The development of smaller profile balloons, over-the-wire catheters, and high-pressure inflation balloons along with increasing skills of angioplasty operators have made coronary angioplasty an accepted, widely used procedure with a high success rate and low complication rate. In fact, today many more angioplasty procedures are performed than coronary artery bypass grafting (CABG) procedures.

Recent clinical investigations have focused on defining which revascularization technique, PTCA or CABG, provides better clinical outcomes in patients eligible for either therapy. Eight prospective, randomized clinical trials have directly compared PTCA with CABG with respect to the end points of mortality, nonfatal myocardial infarction, angina, and need for repeat revascularization procedures. These trials have included patients with single-, double-, and triple-vessel coronary artery disease with normal and impaired left ventricular function. A ninth trial, the unpublished Bypass Angioplasty Revascularization Investigation (BARI), will be reported after 5-year follow-up is complete.

Clinical Trials

The Randomized Intervention Treatment of Angina (RITA) trial was the first study to report outcomes among patients randomized to PTCA or

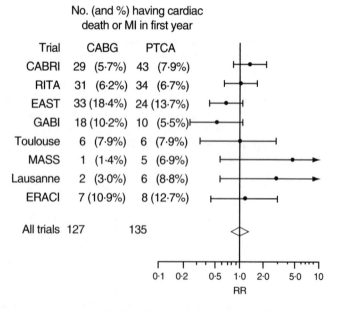

Figure 11-1. Cardiac death and myocardial infarction (MI) for the PTCA group compared with the CABG group in the first year since randomization. (From Pocock et al.,[1] with permission.)

CABG with one-, two-, or three-vessel coronary artery disease at 2.5-year follow-up. Overall, no significant difference was observed between PTCA and CABG regarding total mortality or the combined end point of mortality and nonfatal infarction. In addition, the risk of death or nonfatal infarction was not related to the number of treatment vessels present at the time of randomization. Patients treated with PTCA had a significant increase in the need for repeat revascularization with PTCA or CABG and also required more antianginal therapy. Patients treated with CABG had significantly longer hospitalizations. Left ventricular ejection fraction was not changed in either group at 6-month follow-up.

The Argentine Randomized Trial of PTCA vs. CABG in Multivessel Disease (ERACI) randomized 127 patients with multivessel coronary artery disease to PTCA or CABG and found similar results. No significant difference in mortality or the incidence of acute myocardial infarction was detected between PTCA and CABG treatment groups. Treatment with PTCA substantially increased the incidence of angina and the need for a repeat revascularization procedure, which was mostly due to restenosis by 6 months. Interestingly, after 6-month follow-up, when repeat revascularizations were completed and further restenosis was less likely, the incidence of angina was similar in both groups. Treatment with PTCA resulted in significantly lower costs even when repeat revascularization procedures were included in the analysis.

The Emory Angioplasty vs. Surgery Trial (EAST) and Coronary Angioplasty vs. Bypass Revascularization Investigation (CABRI) trials, which both randomized patients with symptomatic multivessel coronary artery disease, produced similar results. No significant difference was found in mortality or the incidence of myocardial infarction between PTCA and CABG groups; however, treatment with PTCA resulted in an increased need for antianginal medications and repeat revascularizations. The German Angioplasty Bypass Surgery Investigation (GABI) trial surprisingly reported a high incidence of procedure-related Q-wave myocardial infarctions after CABG (8.1%), which consequently resulted in a significant increase in the cumulative risk of death or myocardial infarction with CABG treatment compared to PTCA at 1-year follow-up. A meta-analysis of all the published randomized trials including 3,371 patients, recently performed by Pocock et al.,[1] revealed no significant difference in the combined incidence of death or myocardial infarction between PTCA and CABG treatment groups in the first year of follow-up (Fig. 11-1).

Limitations

Before generalizing the results of these trials to all patients with coronary artery disease, several limitations must be taken into account. First, a minority of screened patients met eligibility criteria, and only a small percentage of these eligible patients were actually randomized to the studies. Thus, enrolled patients represented only a fraction of the general population encountered with coronary artery disease. The requirement that a cardiologist and cardiovascular surgeon judge a patient to be eligible for either procedure may have introduced some selection bias against patients with more severe ischemic heart disease. It may have been perceived that this group of patients, with triple-vessel disease and impaired left ventricular function, would benefit more from surgical treatment than angioplasty. The small number of patients studied, even in the meta-analysis of 3,371 patients, makes it difficult to detect small but meaningful differences in the primary end points. Furthermore, subgroup analysis according to age, the presence of diabetes mellitus, or other potentially predictive variables becomes difficult to perform because of the limited number of enrolled patients. The relatively short follow-up periods (maximum of 3 years) do not permit conclusions regarding the long-term success of these procedures. Finally, the field of angioplasty has advanced considerably during the past 5 years, particularly with the advent of coronary stents. Coronary stenting reduces the incidence of restenosis from approximately 32% with standard angioplasty to 22% (BENESTENT 1 study), and possibly even lower with heparin-coated stents (BENESTENT 2 study) (see Ch. 12). This reduction in restenosis may confer an advantage to angioplasty/stent procedures over CABG, because the major limitation of PTCA appears to be restenosis and the concomitant need for repeat revascularizations.

Conclusions

Revascularization with PTCA compared with CABG in selected patients with coronary artery disease produces no significant difference in overall mortality or the incidence of myocardial infarction up to 3-year follow-up. Treatment with PTCA is associated with a significant increase in the need for antianginal medications and repeat revascularization procedures, likely as a result of both incomplete initial revascularization and restenosis. CABG requires longer hospitalizations and rehabilitation. The use of coronary stents and other techniques to reduce the incidence of restenosis after angioplasty should enhance the effectiveness of interventional procedures further. In the patients with extensive three-vessel coronary artery disease with and without reduced LVEF, CABG appears to be the preferred modality.

CABRI

Coronary Angioplasty vs. Bypass Revascularization Investigation

PURPOSE

Compare the effects of percutaneous transluminal coronary angioplasty (PTCA) with coronary artery bypass graft (CABG) on clinical outcome in patients with symptomatic multivessel coronary artery disease.

STUDY DESIGN

General

- 1,054 patients enrolled in this prospective, randomized multicenter trial.
- Eligible patients were randomized to one of two treatment groups:
    1. PTCA: in addition to standard angioplasty, newer techniques, including stents and atherectomy, were included. Aspirin was the only required medication.
    2. CABG.
- The protocol permitted incomplete revascularization and patients with totally occluded vessels.
- Operators had to have performed > 500 procedures.
- The cardiologist and cardiovascular surgeon had to agree that the patient was a suitable candidate for either PTCA or CABG.

Inclusion. Patients included were ≤ 75 years old who had typical angina pectoris, unstable angina, or unequivocal evidence of myocardial ischemia with angiographically documented > 50% stenosis in two or more major epicardial coronary arteries.

Exclusion. The criteria for exclusion were single-vessel or left main disease, myocardial infarction within the previous 10 days, overt congestive

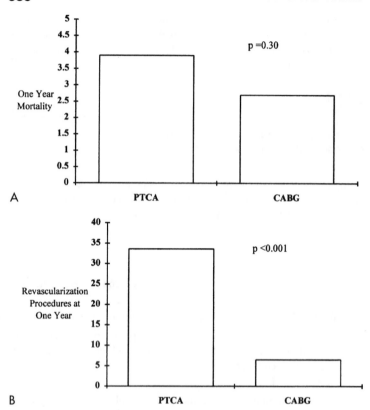

Figure 11-2. *(A)* Similar mortality rates at 1 year between PTCA and CABG. *(B)* The need for revascularization procedures was higher with PTCA.

heart failure, previous CABG or PTCA, other serious cardiac diseases, recent stroke, or other serious illness.

End Points. The criteria for end points were mortality and symptom status.

RESULTS

Left ventricular ejection fraction was normal, mildly impaired, moderately impaired, and severely impaired in 65%, 23%, 7%, and 1% of patients, respectively. Two-vessel disease was present in 57% of patients and three-vessel disease in 42%. No significant difference in total mortality was observed between treatment with PTCA or CABG at 1 year (3.9% PTCA vs. 2.7% CABG, P = 0.30), 28 months (P = 0.083) or 65 months (P = 0.068). The risk of nonfatal myocardial infarction was also not significantly different between the two treatment groups (P = 0.23). Treatment with PTCA resulted in a substantially increased need for repeat revascularization (33.6% PTCA vs. 6.5% CABG, P < 0.001) and increased use of antianginal medications (P < 0.001) during the first year of follow-up. More patients treated with PTCA had clinically significant angina at 1-year follow-up (Fig. 11-2).

CONCLUSIONS
In symptomatic patients with multivessel coronary artery disease, treatment with PTCA compared with CABG resulted in similar mortality and incidence of nonfatal myocardial infarction during the first year of follow-up. However, treatment with PTCA significantly increased the need for repeat revascularizations and the use of antianginal medications.

(Data from CABRI Trial Participants.[2]) ■

EAST

Emory Angioplasty vs. Surgery Trial

PURPOSE
Compare the effect of percutaneous transluminal coronary angioplasty (PTCA) with coronary artery bypass graft (CABG) in reducing mortality and the incidence of Q-wave myocardial infarction at 3-year follow-up in patients with multivessel coronary artery disease.

STUDY DESIGN

General

- 392 patients enrolled in this prospective, randomized trial.

- Patients with arteriographically proven coronary artery disease were considered for enrollment if myocardial revascularization was thought necessary on clinical grounds.

- Patients were stratified according to the number of diseased vessels (two or three) and the severity of the lesions.

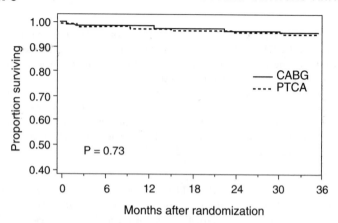

Figure 11-3. Survival of patients with multivessel coronary artery disease for CABG and PTCA treatments. (From King et al.,[3] with permission.)

- PTCA was performed by standard methods with the aim to open lesions thought to be contributing to ischemia. In 40% of the PTCA group, the procedure was staged.
- CABG was performed to provide complete revascularization.

Inclusion. Patients included had multivessel coronary artery disease and had not previously undergone PTCA or CABG.

Exclusion. The criteria for exclusion were old (> 8-week duration) chronic occlusions of bypassable vessels serving viable myocardium, left main stenosis of $\geq 30\%$, left ventricular ejection fraction (LVEF) $\leq 25\%$, insufficient symptoms or ischemia to warrant surgery, myocardial infarction within the previous 5 days, other serious illness, or procedures thought to be unsafe by cardiologist or surgeon.

End Points. The criteria for the composite end point were death, Q-wave myocardial infarction within 3 years, or large ischemic burden detected by thallium scanning.

RESULTS

No significant difference in the composite primary end point was observed between CABG and PTCA (27.3% CABG vs. 28.8% PTCA, P =

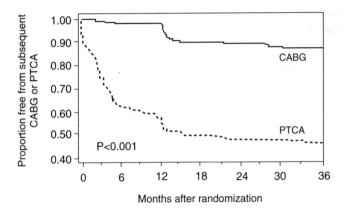

Figure 11-4. Proportion of patients remaining free from CABG or PTCA after the initial revascularization procedure. (From King et al.,[3] with permission.)

0.81). Overall mortality during the 3-year follow-up occurred in 6.2% of patients randomized to CABG compared to 7.1% of patients randomized to PTCA (P = 0.73). In addition, no significant difference was observed between the two groups regarding incidence of Q-wave myocardial infarction (19.6% CABG vs. 14.6% PTCA, P = 0.21) or incidence of large ischemic deficits by thallium scanning (5.7% CABG vs. 9.6% PTCA, P = 0.17). Subsequent revascularization with either PTCA or CABG was required in 13% of the CABG group compared to 54% of the PTCA group (P < 0.001). LVEF at 3 years was similar in both groups (mean of 69% by contrast ventriculography) (Figs. 11-3 and 11-4).

CONCLUSIONS
No significant difference between revascularization with PTCA or CABG was found with regard to total mortality, composite primary end point (death, Q-wave myocardial infarction, or large ischemic burden), or LVEF at 3-year follow-up in patients with multivessel coronary artery disease. Patients initially treated with PTCA required significantly more subsequent revascularization with either repeat PTCA or CABG.

_____

(Data from King et al.[3]) ∎

Argentine Randomized Trial of PTCA vs. CABG in Multivessel Disease

PURPOSE

Compare the effect of percutaneous transluminal coronary angioplasty (PTCA) with coronary artery bypass graft (CABG) on mortality and cardiac events in patients with multivessel coronary artery disease.

STUDY DESIGN

General

- 127 patients enrolled in this prospective, randomized, multicenter trial.

- Eligible patients were randomized to one of two treatment groups:

  1. PTCA: standard angioplasty of significant lesions with > 70% stenosis and evidence of ischemia by noninvasive testing was performed in staged procedures if needed. Pretreatment with aspirin 325 mg/day and calcium channel blocker was started 24 hr before the procedure and intravenous heparin for 24 hr after the procedure.

  2. CABG: performed using the left internal mammary artery (76.5% of patients) and saphenous vein grafts.

- Successful angioplasty was defined as a gain in lumen diameter of ≥ 20% and a final residual stenosis of < 50%.

Inclusion. Patients included had > 70% stenosis in more than one major epicardial coronary artery and were amenable to both PTCA and CABG. They had severely limiting stable angina or unstable angina refractory to medical therapy or minimal symptoms but with a large area of myocardium at risk assessed by exercise testing.

Exclusion. The criteria for exclusion were dilated ischemic cardiomyopathy, left main disease, severe triple-vessel disease with a left ventricular ejection fraction ≤ 35%, associated valvular heart disease or hypertrophic cardiomyopathy, evolving acute myocardial infarction, or other serious illness.

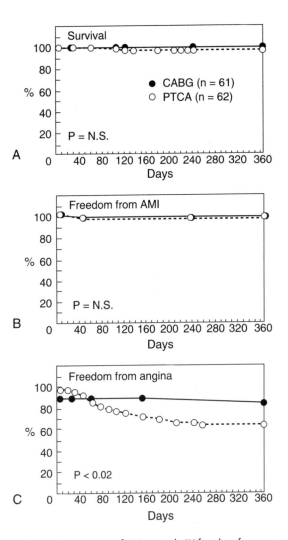

Figure 11-5. Comparison of *(A)* survival, *(B)* freedom from acute myocardial infarction (AMI), and *(C)* freedom from angina. (From Rodriguez et al.,[4] with permission.)

End Points. The criteria for end points were freedom from combined cardiac events (death, myocardial infarction, repeat revascularization procedures, and angina) and mortality.

RESULTS

In-Hospital Outcomes. No significant difference was found between PTCA and CABG with respect to in-hospital mortality (1.5% PTCA vs. 4.6% CABG, P = NS), incidence of Q-wave myocardial infarction (6.3% PTCA vs. 6.2% CABG, P = NS), incidence of revascularization procedures (1.5% both, P = NS), and incidence of stroke (1.5% PTCA vs. 3.1% CABG, P = NS). Significantly fewer patients treated with PTCA achieved complete anatomic revascularization compared with CABG (51% PTCA vs. 88% CABG, P < 0.001).

One-Year Outcome. No significant difference was observed in 1-year mortality (3.2% PTCA vs. 0% CABG, P = NS) or the incidence of acute myocardial infarction (3.2% PTCA vs. 1.8% CABG, P = NS) between the two study groups. The major difference between the two treatment groups was the substantially increased incidence of angina and the need for repeat revascularization procedures with PTCA treatment, which was mostly due to restenosis by 6 months (32.2% PTCA vs. 3.3% CABG, P < 0.001). However, after 6 months of follow-up, when repeat revascularizations were completed, freedom from angina was similar in both groups. Treatment with PTCA, including all repeat revascularization procedures, resulted in a significantly lower total cost at 1-year follow-up ($7,000 per patient per year PTCA vs. $12,900 per patient per year CABG, P < 0.01) (Fig. 11-5).

CONCLUSIONS

In patients with multivessel coronary artery disease, treatment with PTCA or CABG resulted in similar in-hospital complication rates and similar 1-year incidence of death and acute myocardial infarction. Treatment with PTCA was associated with a significantly higher incidence of angina and the need for repeat revascularization that was due mostly to restenosis by 6 months. Overall cost at 1 year, including all necessary repeat revascularization procedures, was significantly lower with PTCA treatment compared to CABG.

(Data from Rodriguez et al.[4]) ∎

GABI

German Angioplasty Bypass Surgery Investigation

PURPOSE

Compare the effect of percutaneous transluminal coronary angioplasty (PTCA) with coronary artery bypass graft (CABG) in relieving angina and preventing death and myocardial infarction in patients with symptomatic multivessel coronary artery disease.

STUDY DESIGN

General

- 359 patients enrolled in this prospective, randomized, multicenter trial.

- Revascularization of at least two major coronary arteries supplying different myocardial regions (the left anterior descending, circumflex, and right coronary arteries) had to be clinically necessary and technically feasible according to the judgment of local cardiologists and surgeons.

- Electrocardiograpy, echocardiography, and modified Bruce stress test were performed before the procedure, at hospital discharge, and at 3-, 6-, and 12-month follow-up.

- Coronary angiography was performed at 6 months.

Inclusion. Patients included were < 75 years of age with symptomatic multivessel coronary disease (Canadian Cardiovascular Society [CCS] class ≥ II and stenosis ≥ 70% in diameter in at least two coronary arteries).

Exclusion. The criteria for exclusion were as follows: totally occluded vessels and > 30% stenosis of the left main coronary artery or equivalent left main lesions, > 50% of the left ventricular circumference would be in jeopardy should abrupt closure occur, long lesions > 2 cm, diffuse peripheral coronary disease, aneurysms, myocardial infarction within the previous 1 month, or previous CABG or PTCA.

End Points. The criteria for end points were freedom from angina pectoris (CCS class < II) 1 year after the intervention, major cardiovas-

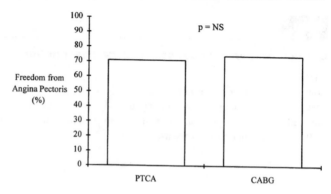

A

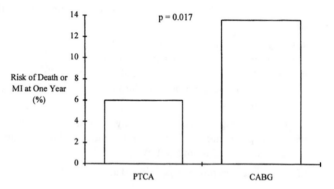

B

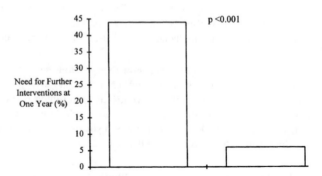

C

cular events (death or myocardial infarction), and the need for further intervention.

RESULTS

An average of 1.9 vessels per patient were dilated with PTCA compared to an average of 2.2 vessels per patient grafted with CABG. Patients treated with CABG had longer hospitalizations (19 days CABG vs. 5 days PTCA) and significantly more Q-wave myocardial infarctions related to the procedure (8.1% CABG vs. 2.3% PTCA, P = 0.022).

At 1-year follow-up, no significant difference in the percentage of patients free of angina was observed (74% CABG vs. 71% PTCA, P = not significant). The cumulative risk of death or myocardial infarction from the time of randomization was significantly higher in the CABG group compared to the PTCA group (13.6% CABG vs. 6.0% PTCA, P = 0.017). Substantially more patients required further interventions in the PTCA group (23% repeat PTCA, 18% CABG) compared to the CABG group (1% repeat CABG, 5% PTCA) (P < 0.001). Patients treated with CABG had significantly less requirement for antianginal medications (nitrates, calcium antagonists, and β-blockers) than those treated with PTCA (78% CABG vs. 88% PTCA, P = 0.04).

At 6-month angiography, 13% of vein grafts were occluded, 7% of internal thoracic artery grafts were not functional, and 16% of angioplastied vessels were occluded or restenosed (> 70% stenosis) (Fig. 11-6).

CONCLUSIONS

No significant difference in the freedom from angina was observed between PTCA and CABG at 1-year follow-up in patients with multivessel coronary artery disease. PTCA resulted in significantly less cumulative risk of death or myocardial infarction compared to CABG. CABG resulted in a significantly reduced need for repeat revascularization and use of antianginal medications.

(Data from Hamm et al.[5]) ■

Figure 11-6. *(A–C)* Major clinical events at 1 year for PTCA and CABG treatments.

Randomized Intervention Treatment of Angina

PURPOSE

Compare the long-term effect of percutaneous transluminal coronary angioplasty (PTCA) and coronary artery bypass graft (CABG) in patients with one, two, or three diseased coronary arteries.

STUDY DESIGN

General

- 1,011 patients enrolled in this prospective, randomized, multicenter trial.

- Patients with arteriographically proven coronary artery disease were considered for enrollment if myocardial revascularization was thought necessary on clinical grounds.

- Angina pectoris was not a requirement.

- PTCA was performed in a staged procedure completed within 3 months of randomization.

- Modified Bruce treadmill tests and left ventricular ejection fraction by radionuclide ventriculography were monitored.

Inclusion. For the patients included, equivalent revascularization was feasible by either CABG or PTCA according to the investigators. Each treatment vessel had ≥ 70% reduction in diameter stenosis and was judged to supply ≥ 20% of ventricular myocardium.

Exclusion. The criteria for exclusion were left main coronary artery disease, previous PTCA or CABG, hemodynamically significant valvular disease, or other serious illness.

End Points. The criteria for end points were combined end point of death and nonfatal myocardial infarction.

RESULTS

One, two, and three treatment vessels were present in 45%, 43%, and 12% of patients, respectively. At 2.5 years of follow-up, no significant difference between PTCA and CABG was observed regarding total mortality

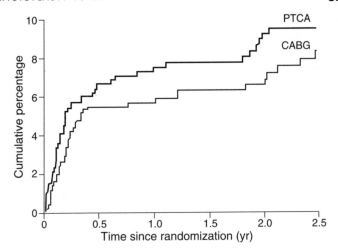

Figure 11-7. Cumulative risk of death or myocardial infarction by treatment group. (From RITA Trial Participants,[6] with permission.)

(3.1% PTCA vs. 3.6% CABG, P = NS) or combined end points (9.8% PTCA vs. 8.6% CABG, P = 0.47). The risk of death or infarction appeared unrelated to the number of treatment vessels present at randomization. Additional PTCA or CABG was required by 28.2% of patients randomized to the PTCA group compared to 2.4% of patients in the CABG group. At 2-year follow-up, 61% of patients in the PTCA group required at least one antianginal medication compared to 34% in the CABG group. PTCA resulted in shorter hospital stays after the procedure (mean 4 days with PTCA vs. mean 12 days with CABG). LVEF was not significantly changed at 6 months in either group (Fig. 11-7).

CONCLUSIONS

At 2.5-year follow-up, there was no significant difference in total mortality or combined end points (death or nonfatal myocardial infarction) between PTCA and CABG in patients with coronary artery disease regardless of the number of diseased vessels. PTCA resulted in shorter hospital stays but a substantially increased need for repeat revascularization (repeat PTCA or CABG) and antianginal medications.

(Data from RITA Trial Participants.[6]) ∎

References

1. Pocock SJ, Henderson RA, Rickards AF et al: Meta-analysis of randomized trials comparing coronary angioplasty with bypass surgery. Lancet 346:1184, 1995
2. CABRI Trial Participants: First-year results of CABRI (Coronary Angioplasty versus Bypass Revascularisation Investigation). Lancet 346:1179-84, 1995
3. King SB III, Lembo NJ, Weintraub WS et al: A randomized trial comparing coronary angioplasty with coronary bypass surgery. N Engl J Med 331:1044-50, 1994
4. Rodriguez A, Boullon F, Perez-Baliño N et al: Argentine randomized trial of percutaneous transluminal coronary angioplasty versus coronary artery bypass surgery in multivessel disease (ERACI): in-hospital results and 1-year follow-up. J Am Coll Cardiol 22:1060-7, 1993
5. Hamm CW, Reimers J, Ischinger T et al: A randomized study of coronary angioplasty compared with bypass surgery in patients with symptomatic multivessel coronary disease. N Engl J Med 331:1037-43, 1994
6. RITA Trial Participants: Coronary angioplasty versus coronary artery bypas surgery: the Randomised Intervention of Treatment of Angina (RITA) trial. Lancet 341:573-80, 1993

CHAPTER 12

New Interventional Technology Trials

OVERVIEW

Interventional cardiology has seen the development of many new devices for coronary revascularization during the past 10 years. Simpson et al. in 1986 successfully performed the first coronary atherectomy, the removal of atherosclerotic material from coronary plaques, with a device eventually named the Simpson AtheroCath. Atherosclerotic plaque, which bulges through an open cylindric window, is shaved off using a motor-driven cutter and collected in the conical end of this catheter. Other atherectomy devices were subsequently designed, including the Rotablator, a high-speed rotating diamond-tipped burr, which pulverizes atherosclerotic material, resulting in microemboli; the transluminal extraction catheter (TEC), a low-speed rotating cutting head that aspirates and removes shaved atherosclerotic material via a vacuum system; and the rotational angioplasty catheter system (ROTAC), a low-speed pulverizing bare wire device.

Xenon chloride excited-dimer (excimer) lasers have been developed to vaporize atherosclerotic plaques. Plagued by early complications, including acute thrombosis, thermal injury, and coronary perforations, laser devices have found limited success in the treatment of coronary atherosclerosis but may prove useful in the treatment of peripheral vascular disease.

A variety of endovascular stents, metallic devices used to provide endoluminal support to prevent luminal narrowing, are being deployed with exponentially increasing frequency. The most widely used intracoronary stents are the Palmaz-Schatz (PS) stent, a balloon-expanded articulated slotted stainless steel device, the Gianturco-Roubin stent, a flexible balloon expanded stainless steel coil, and the Wallstent, a self-expanding flexible woven stainless steel stent (Fig. 12-1).

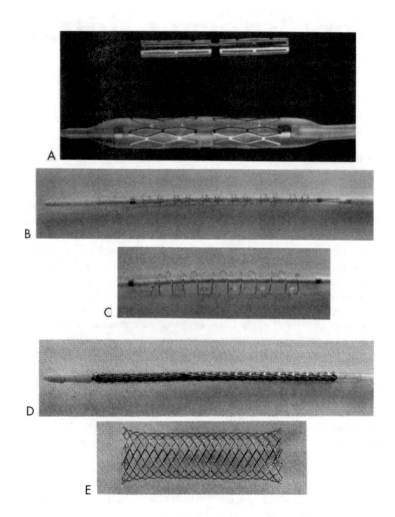

Figure 12-1. Balloon-expandable stents. *(A & B)* The Palmaz-Schatz stent. *(C)* The Gianturco Roubin stent. *(D & E)* The Wall stent. (From Anderson et al.,[1] with permission.)

Because stainless steel stents are foreign bodies, they are prone to early thrombosis and to tissue rejection, resulting in cell proliferation and inflammation. There is evidence that early thrombotic deposits may lead to late cell proliferation and restenosis. Systemic antithrombotic agents like aspirin, ticlopidine, heparin, and warfarin have provided the mainstay of therapy to prevent early stent thrombosis. These agents are given for approximately 2 to 3 months until complete endothelialization of the stent has occurred. Recent attention has focused on stent coatings, in which micron-thin layers of various materials, including heparin, hydrocarbons, and extracellular matrix, are bonded to the surface of the stent. These stent coatings may attenuate early thrombosis and subsequent tissue cell proliferation and may also obviate the need for systemic antithrombotic agents.

Completed clinical trials have compared the effects of directional atherectomy and PS stenting with standard coronary angioplasty in patients with coronary artery disease.

Directional Coronary Atherectomy Trials

The Coronary Angioplasty vs. Excisional Atherectomy Trials (CAVEATs) have compared the effects of the Simpson directional atherectomy with balloon angioplasty in native coronary arteries (CAVEAT 1) and saphenous vein bypass grafts (CAVEAT 2). CAVEAT 1 randomized 1,012 patients with symptomatic coronary artery disease to treatment with atherectomy or angioplasty. Angiographic success, defined as a residual stenosis of less than 50%, was obtained more often with atherectomy. The use of atherectomy, however, resulted in a significantly increased incidence of in-hospital myocardial infarction and an in-hospital composite end point of death, emergency CABG, acute myocardial infarction, or abrupt vessel closure. At 6-month follow-up, restenosis rates were similar, but the combined probability of death or myocardial infarction was higher with atherectomy.

CAVEAT 2 randomized 305 patients with de novo bypass vein graft stenosis to atherectomy or angioplasty. Again, atherectomy resulted in a higher angiographic success rate and a larger luminal diameter gain.

Atherectomy, however, caused more distal embolization and a trend toward more in-hospital non-Q-wave myocardial infarctions. At 6-month follow-up, the incidence of restenosis and a combined clinical end point of death, emergency CABG, acute myocardial infarction, or abrupt vessel closure were similar.

The Canadian Coronary Atherectomy Trial (CCAT) randomized 274 patients with lesions of the proximal left anterior descending (LAD) coronary artery to directional atherectomy or angioplasty. Treatment with atherectomy achieved immediate angiographic success more often than angioplasty. In-hospital adverse clinical events were similar. At 6 months, the rates of restenosis and adverse clinical events were not different between the two treatment groups. Thus, atherectomy of native coronary arteries appears to cause more in-hospital and 6-month adverse clinical outcomes. A subgroup of patients with proximal LAD artery stenosis have equivalent outcomes with the two procedures. In saphenous vein bypass grafts, atherectomy may be a viable equivalent alternative to angioplasty.

Palmaz-Schatz Stent Trials

The Stent Restenosis Study (STRESS) evaluated the effect of PS stent placement followed by 1 month of warfarin therapy vs. standard balloon angioplasty in 410 patients with symptomatic coronary artery disease. Early outcomes revealed no meaningful difference in a combined clinical end point of death, myocardial infarction, need for CABG, or repeat revascularization. Stent placement produced a trend toward more bleeding complications and longer hospital stay, which likely was due to the requirement of anticoagulation therapy. At 6-month follow-up, stent placement resulted in a significant 25% lower incidence of restenosis, a 34% reduction in the need for a repeat percutaneous revascularization procedure, and a larger luminal diameter. Stent placement produced a trend toward decreased combined clinical end points.

The Belgium Netherlands Stent Trial (BENESTENT 1) randomized 520 symptomatic patients with a single new coronary lesion to treatment with a PS stent or balloon angioplasty. In-hospital outcomes were similar, except for a high incidence of bleeding and vascular complications and longer hospital stay with stent placement. At 7-month follow-up, the most striking difference was the 42% reduction in the need for a second percutaneous revascularization procedure in the stent group. Restenosis rates were substantially reduced from 32% with angioplasty to 22% with the PS stent.

The BENESTENT 2 pilot study evaluated the effect of heparin-coated PS stents on reducing acute thrombosis and the need for systemic anticoagulation. A total of 207 patients with stable angina pectoris and a single de novo coronary artery lesion were progressively grouped into four phases. The study consisted of three initial phases in which resumption of heparin after sheath removal was delayed by 6 hours (phase 1), 12 hours (phase 2), and 36 hours (phase 3) followed by 3 months of warfarin therapy. In the fourth phase, no heparin or warfarin was given, but patients were treated with ticlopidine for 1 month and aspirin. No acute stent thrombosis occurred in any patients. Bleeding complications and hospital stay were progressively reduced from phases 1 to 4, with patients in phase 4 having no bleeding complications and an average hospital stay of 3.1 days. At 6-month follow-up, the rates of restenosis were 15%, 20%, 11%, and 6%, and the rates of freedom from clinical events (death, myocardial infarction, repeat percutaneous intervention or CABG) were 84%, 75%, 94%, and 92%, respectively, for phases 1 through 4. Two criticisms of this pilot study are that patients were not randomized and that the technique of postdeployment high-pressure inflation was used more commonly in the later phases (43% of patients in phase 1 underwent high-pressure inflation compared with 82% of patients in phase 4). Therefore, it is unclear whether actual heparin coating or deployment techniques or a combination of both resulted in the low incidence of restenosis in phase 4. A larger randomized trial comparing heparin-coated PS stents with regular PS stents using the same deployment techniques will be required to definitively evaluate the benefit of heparin coating.

The Intracoronary Stenting and Antithrombotic Regimen Trial evaluated the effect of antiplatelet therapy with aspirin and ticlopidine compared to anticoagulation therapy with phenprocoumon and aspirin on ischemic complications and stent thrombosis during 30 days after deployment of a PS stent. Patients receiving antiplatelet therapy had significant reductions in a combined cardiac end point of cardiac death, myocardial infarction, CABG, or repeat PTCA of the stented vessel compared to those receiving anticoagulation therapy. In addition, antiplatelet therapy reduced the need for transfusions and peripheral vascular complications such as serious pseudoaneurysms and arteriovenous fistula. Surprisingly, fewer occlusions in the stented vessel occurred in the antiplatelet group, suggesting that platelets play a crucial role in stent thrombosis.

Thus, treatment with PS stents provides a higher initial angiographic success rate and significantly reduced rates of restenosis and the need for a second percutaneous revascularization procedure. The coating of PS stents with heparin may reduce the need for systemic anticoagulation and restenosis rates. Treatment with ticlopidine and aspirin during the month after stent deployment considerably reduces ischemic coronary and peripheral vascular complications compared to treatment with systemic anticoagulants.

Conclusions

Interventional cardiology has made great advances during the past decade. New devices, such as atherectomy catheters, excimer lasers, and intracoronary stents, are rapidly changing the face of percutaneous revascularization. Newer diagnostic tools, including intracoronary ultrasound, flow wires, and angioscopy, are allowing a more precise understanding of the anatomy of complex lesions and the impacts of interventional techniques on these lesions. Just over the horizon are instruments like the Hemopump and synchronized coronary sinus retroperfusion, which are currently being evaluated for aiding in high-risk coronary angioplasty.

Clinical trials have shown that the Simpson atherectomy device appears to result in more early adverse clinical outcomes in saphenous vein bypass grafts and native coronary arteries, with an exception being proximal LAD artery lesions. Atherectomy has not been proven to influence 6-month restenosis or clinical outcomes. The PS stent reduces the incidence of restenosis and the need for a repeat percutaneous revascularization procedure at 6 months at the expense of initial increased bleeding complications and hospital stay. The use of heparin-coated PS stents appears to be safe and may reduce the need for systemic anticoagulation and may reduce 6-month restenosis rates. Treatment with ticlopidine and aspirin during the month after stent deployment appears to reduce ischemic coronary and peripheral vascular complications compared to treatment with systemic anticoagulants. Finally, the use of newer antithrombotic agents, such as the platelet glycoprotein IIb/IIIa receptor antagonists and direct thrombin inhibitors, may prove to reduce restenosis rates from simple angioplasty, thereby reducing the need for intracoronary stenting in the future.

BENESTENT 1

Belgium Netherlands Stent Trial 1

PURPOSE
Compare the effects of balloon-expandable intracoronary stents with balloon angioplasty on long-term angiographic and clinical outcomes in patients with coronary artery disease.

STUDY DESIGN

General
- 520 patients enrolled in this prospective, randomized, multicenter trial.
- Eligible patients were randomly assigned to treatment with a Palmaz-Schatz stent or standard balloon angioplasty.
- All patients received aspirin 250–500 mg/day and dipyridamole 75 mg PO tid starting the day before the procedure and continued for 6 months. Both treatment groups also received calcium channel antagonists until hospital discharge.
- Patients receiving a stent were given a continuous infusion of dextran and heparin 10,000-U intravenous (IV) bolus followed by a continuous heparin infusion until successful conversion to warfarin with international normalized ratio (INR) 2.5–3.5. Warfarin was continued for 3 months.
- Patients receiving balloon angioplasty were given heparin 10,000-U IV bolus with a continuous infusion used only if deemed necessary.
- Coronary arteriography was performed immediately after the procedure and at 6 months.

Inclusion. Patients included had stable angina that was due to a single new lesion in a coronary artery with the target lesion < 15 mm long located in a vessel > 3 mm diameter that supplied normally functioning myocardium. Patients have to be suitable candidates for coronary artery bypass graft (CABG) if needed.

Exclusion. The criteria for exclusion were contraindication to anticoagulation or antiplatelet therapy, ostial lesions, lesions at a bifurcation, lesions in a previously grafted vessel, or patients with a suspected intra-coronary thrombus.

End Points. The criteria for the combined clinical end point were death, cerebrovascular accidents, myocardial infarction, CABG, or a second percutaneous intervention. Angiographic end points were also a criterion.

RESULTS

In-Hospital Outcomes. No significant difference in the in-hospital combined clinical end point was observed between stent and angioplasty (6.9% stent vs. 6.2% angiography, P = NS). Specifically, there were no in-hospital deaths, one intracranial hemorrhage in the angioplasty group, similar incidence of myocardial infarction (3.4% stent vs. 3.1% angioplasty, P = NS), and similar need for CABG or repeat percutaneous intervention (3.5% stent vs. 2.7% angioplasty, P = NS). Treatment with a stent resulted in a significantly higher incidence of bleeding and vascular complications (13.5% stent vs. 3.1% angioplasty, P < 0.001) and significantly longer hospital stay (8.5 days for stent vs. 3.1 days for angioplasty, P < 0.001).

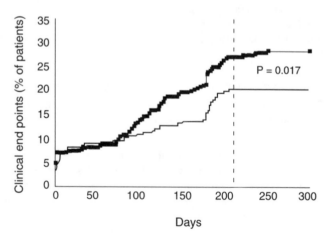

Figure 12-2. Cumulative frequency distribution curve showing the percentage of patients with clinical end points. —, stent group; ■-■-■, angioplasty group. (From Serruys et al.,[2] with permission.)

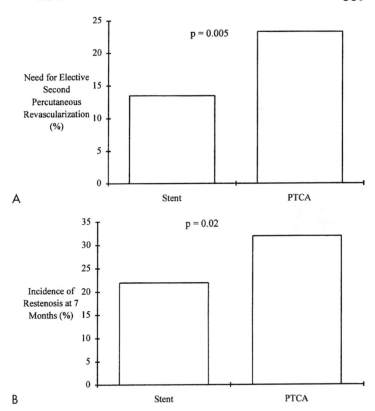

Figure 12-3. *(A)* The reduced need for a second percutaneous revascularization and *(B)* reduced restenosis at 7 months in the stent group compared to PTCA.

Seven-Month Outcomes. The use of stents resulted in significantly less combined clinical end points than angioplasty (20% stent vs. 30% angioplasty, P = 0.02). The most striking difference was the significant 42% reduction in the need for an elective second percutaneous revascularization in the stent group (13.5% stent vs. 23.3% angioplasty, P = 0.005). Stent implantation resulted in larger luminal diameter at follow-up (1.82 mm stent vs. 1.73 mm angioplasty, P = 0.09) and a significantly reduced incidence of restenosis (defined as ≥ 50% stenosis) (22% stent vs. 32% angioplasty, P = 0.02) (Figs. 12-2 and 12-3).

CONCLUSIONS

Implantation of coronary stents in patients with stable angina and a single new coronary artery lesion resulted in immediate success rates similar to those of balloon angioplasty but with higher in-hospital bleeding and vascular complications and longer hospital stay. At follow-up of 7 months, stent treatment resulted in substantially better clinical outcome, which was mainly due to less need for revascularization with a repeat percutaneous intervention and significantly less restenosis compared with balloon angioplasty.

(Data from Serruys et al.[2])   ■

BENESTENT 2

Belgium Netherlands Stent Trial 2 Pilot Study

PURPOSE

Determine the safety of reducing and eliminating anticoagulant therapy in patients receiving a heparin-coated Palmaz-Schatz stent.

STUDY DESIGN

General

- 207 Patients enrolled in this prospective pilot study.

- The study consisted of three phases in which resumption of heparin after sheath removal was delayed by 6 hr (phase 1), 12 hr (phase 2), and 36 hr (phase 3). Patients in phases 1–3 received warfarin for 3 months. Phase 4 replaced anticoagulation with ticlopidine 250 mg/day for 1 month and daily aspirin. The trial proceeded sequentially from phase 1 to phase 4.

- All patients received 250–500 mg of aspirin, beginning the day before the procedure and continued for 6 months, and diltiazem 120 mg bid until hospital discharge.

Inclusion. Patients included were scheduled to undergo angioplasty because of stable angina pectoris with a discrete (< 15-mm) de novo lesion in a coronary artery ≥ 3 mm in luminal diameter supplying normally functioning myocardium.

Exclusion. The criteria for exclusion were ostial lesions or lesions at a bifurcation, previously grafted vessels, or contraindications to the study medications.

End Points. The criteria for end points were incidence of early stent thrombosis, bleeding complications, and event-free survival.

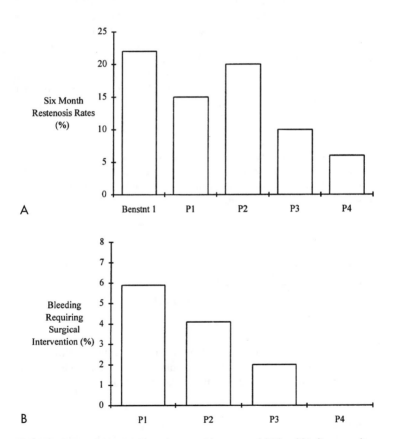

Figure 12-4. *(A)* Lower 6-month restenosis rates and *(B)* low bleeding complications with heparin-coated Palmaz-Schatz stents compared with regular Palmaz-Schatz stents.

RESULTS

Implantation of a heparin-coated stent resulted in an average residual stenosis of 18% and an overall clinical success rate at discharge of 99%. No acute stent thrombosis occurred. Bleeding complications requiring vascular surgery showed a graded reduction from phases 1–4 with successively later use and no use of anticoagulants, respectively (5.9% in phase 1, 4.1% in phase 2, 2.0% in phase 3, and 0.0% in phase 4). In-hospital stay was dramatically shortened to 3 days in phase 4 with no use of anticoagulants. Six-month follow-up revealed a very low incidence of angiographic restenosis, defined as > 50% diameter reduction (15% in phase 1, 20% in phase 2, 10% in phase 3, and 6% in phase 4) and a very high 6-month event-free survival (84% in phase 1, 75% in phase 2, 94% in phase 3, and 92% in phase 4). Post-stent deployment high-pressure inflations were used with increasing frequency from phases 1–4 (43% phase 1, 71% phase 2, 67% phase 3, 82% phase 4) (Fig. 12-4).

CONCLUSIONS

Heparin-coated stents were well tolerated, were not thrombogenic even without anticoagulation, and resulted in low bleeding complications and shortened hospital stay. Follow-up at 6 months revealed very low restenosis rates and high event-free survival.

(Data from Serruys et al.[3]) ∎

CAVEAT 1

Coronary Angioplasty vs. Excisional Atherectomy Trial

PURPOSE

Compare the effects of directional coronary atherectomy with balloon angioplasty on initial angiographic results, restenosis, and clinical outcome in patients with symptomatic ischemic heart disease.

STUDY DESIGN

General

- 1,012 patients enrolled in this prospective, randomized, multicenter trial.

- Operators were required to have performed > 400 angioplasty procedures with > 85% success rate and > 50 atherectomy procedures with > 80% success rate.

- Aspirin 160–325 mg/day and at least one calcium channel blocker were given before the procedure and were continued for 1 month after the procedure.

- Heparin 10,000-U intravenous bolus and additional boluses to keep activated clotting time > 350 sec during the procedure.

- The angiographic goal was residual stenosis < 20%, although residual stenosis < 50% was considered a success.

- Repeat angiography was performed at 6 months.

Inclusion. Patients included had symptomatic ischemic heart disease with diseased native vessels that had not undergone previous coronary intervention with ≥ 60% stenosis of ≤ 12-mm length suitable for ≥ 6-French cutter or ≥ 3-mm balloon. Patients with multivessel coronary artery disease were eligible as long as a single vessel was specified as the target lesion before the intervention began. All lesions in the target artery had to be amenable to both interventional procedures.

End Points. The criterion for end point was angiographic restenosis defined as > 50% stenosis 6 months after an initially successful procedure. The criteria for the combined clinical end point were death, acute myocardial infarction, or procedural-related complication.

RESULTS
Angiographic success was achieved significantly more often with atherectomy compared to angioplasty (89% atherectomy vs. 80% angioplasty, P < 0.001). Atherectomy, however, resulted in a substantially higher rate of in-hospital myocardial infarction (6% atherectomy vs. 3% angioplasty, P = 0.035) and in-hospital composite end point of death, emergency coronary artery bypass graft (CABG), acute myocardial infarction, or abrupt vessel closure (11% atherectomy vs. 5% angioplasty, P < 0.001) compared to angioplasty.

At 6-month follow-up, the rate of restenosis was not significantly different between the two groups (50% atherectomy vs. 57% angioplasty, P = 0.06). The combined probability of death or myocardial infarction was significantly higher with atherectomy than with angioplasty at 6-month follow-up (8.6% atherectomy vs. 4.6% angioplasty, P = 0.007). At 1-year follow-up, treatment with atherectomy resulted in a significant excess of deaths (2.2% atherectomy vs. 0.6% angioplasty, P = 0.035) and reinfarction rates (8.9% atherectomy vs. 4.4% angioplasty, P = 0.005) compared to angioplasty (Figs. 12-5 and 12-6).

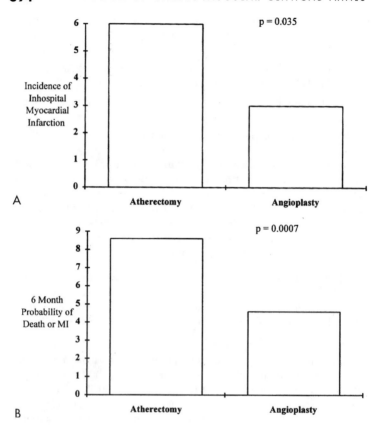

Figure 12-5. The higher incidence of (A) myocardial infarction and (B) 6-month probability of death or myocardial infarction with atherectomy compared to angioplasty.

CONCLUSIONS

Directional atherectomy resulted in a significantly higher initial success rate compared to angioplasty in patients with symptomatic ischemic heart disease. The use of atherectomy, however, also resulted in substantially higher rates of in-hospital myocardial infarction and composite end points (death, emergency CABG, acute myocardial infarction, or abrupt vessel closure). Six-month follow-up revealed no significant difference in

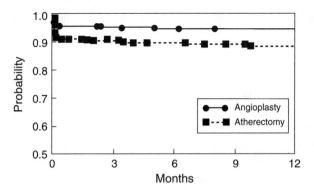

Figure 12-6. Kaplan-Meier survival curves for the combined end point of death or myocardial infarction during the first 12 months. (From Elliott et al.,[5] with permission.)

the restenosis rate between the two treatments. Atherectomy, however, resulted in significantly higher probability of death or myocardial infarction compared to angioplasty. At 1-year follow-up, atherectomy resulted in a significant excess of both death and reinfarction rate compared to angioplasty.

(6-month follow-up data from Topol et al.[4]; 1-year follow-up data from Elliott et al.[5]) ■

CAVEAT 2

Coronary Angioplasty vs. Excision Atherectomy Trial

PURPOSE

Compare the benefit of directional coronary atherectomy (DCA) with balloon angioplasty in patients with de novo bypass vein graft stenosis.

STUDY DESIGN

General

- 305 patients enrolled in this prospective, randomized, multicenter trial.

- Operators were required to have performed > 400 angioplasty procedures with > 85% success rate and > 50 atherectomy procedures with > 80% success rate.

- Aspirin 160–325 mg/day and at least one calcium channel blocker were given before the procedure and were continued for 1 month after the procedure.

- Heparin 10,000-U intravenous bolus and additional boluses to keep activated clotting time > 350 sec during the procedure.

- The angiographic goal was residual stenosis < 20%, although residual stenosis < 50% was considered a success.

- Repeat angiography was performed at 6 months.

Inclusion. Patients included had previous coronary artery bypass graft surgery (CABG) and de novo graft lesions and required revascularization suitable for DCA or angioplasty. The angiographic criteria included a vein graft suitable for a 6F atherectomy catheter, diameter stenosis of 60%–99%, and lesion length ≤ 12 mm.

Exclusion. The criteria for exclusion were myocardial infarction within the previous 5 days, all graft lesions not suitable for either DCA or percutaneous transluminal coronary angioplasty (PTCA), or restenotic lesions.

End Points. The criteria for the combined clinical end point were death, myocardial infarction, emergency CABG, or abrupt closure. Restenosis rates at 6 months were also noted.

RESULTS

DCA resulted in a significantly higher initial angiographic success rate (89.2% DCA vs. 79.0% PTCA, P = 0.019) and larger luminal gain (1.45 mm DCA vs. 1.12 mm PTCA, P < 0.001) compared to PTCA. However, the use of DCA caused significantly more distal embolization (13.4% DCA vs. 5.1% PTCA, P = 0.012) and a trend toward more non-Q-wave myocardial infarctions (16.1% DCA vs. 9.6% PTCA, P = 0.09) and combined clinical end points (20.1% DCA vs. 12.2% PTCA, P = 0.059). The in-hospital mortality rate was approximately 2% for both treatment groups. At 6-month follow-up, no significant difference was observed in restenosis rates (> 50% stenosis after an initially successful procedure) (45.6% DCA vs. 50.5% PTCA, P = 0.49), mean diameter stenosis (31.5% DCA vs. 37.6% PTCA, P = 0.10), or combined clinical end points (Fig. 12-7).

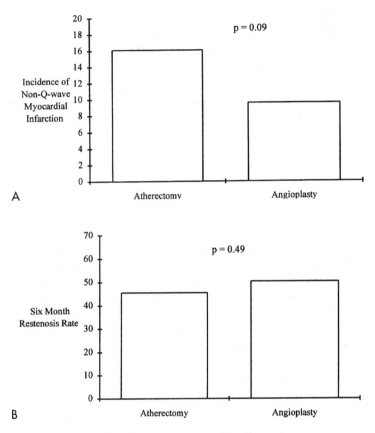

Figure 12-7. *(A & B)* Major clinical outcomes.

CONCLUSIONS

In patients with de novo saphenous vein bypass graft lesion, DCA resulted in a significantly higher initial angiographic success rate and larger luminal gain at the expense of more distal embolization and more non-Q-wave myocardial infarction compared to angioplasty. At 6-month follow-up, the two procedures were similar with respect to angiographic and clinical end points.

(Data from Holmes et al.[6]) ■

Canadian Coronary Atherectomy Trial

PURPOSE
Compare the effect of directional coronary atherectomy with balloon angioplasty on restenosis of lesions involving the left anterior descending (LAD) coronary artery.

STUDY DESIGN

General

- 274 patients enrolled in this prospective, randomized, multicenter trial.

- Operators had > 2 years experience with angioplasty and had used the Simpson atherectomy device at least 4 months for > 20 procedures with a success rate > 80% and complication rate < 10%.

- All patients received aspirin, a calcium channel blocker, and nitrates beginning at least 12 hr before the procedure and continued for at least 24 hr after the procedure. Intracoronary nitroglycerin was injected just before angiography.

- Heparin was given just after sheath insertion and administered to keep activated clotting time > 300 sec.

- After hospital discharge, antianginal medications were discontinued unless specifically indicated.

- Ω-3 fatty acids were prohibited.

- The angiographic goal was to achieve a final lesion diameter close to the normal vessel size. Angiographic success was defined as stenosis of ≤ 50% after the procedure.

- Angiography was repeated at 6 months.

Inclusion. Patients included had angina or objective evidence of myocardial ischemia and a stenosis of ≥ 60% in the proximal third of the LAD coronary artery that was suitable for either procedure.

Exclusion. The criteria for exclusion were as follows: a restenosed lesion from prior intravascular procedure, length > 10 mm; involvement of the ostium or of a branch vessel ≥ 2.5-mm diameter; total occlusion, vessel size < 3 mm; heavy calcification or severe tortuosity; acute myocardial infarction within 1 week of the procedure; severe left ventricular dysfunction; cardiogenic shock; or other serious illness.

End Points. The criterion for end point was restenosis defined as stenosis of > 50% diameter at 6-month follow-up.

RESULTS

Angiographic success was achieved significantly more often with atherectomy than with angioplasty (98% atherectomy vs. 91% angioplasty, P = 0.017). There was no difference in the composite incidence of in-hospital complications (death, myocardial infarction, coronary artery bypass graft, or abrupt vessel closure) between both procedures (5% atherectomy vs. 6% angioplasty, P = 0.98). At an average of 6-month follow-up, restenosis was observed in 46% of the atherectomy group compared to 43% of the angioplasty group (P = 0.71). No significant difference in clinical events (death, myocardial infarction, severity of angina, or repeat procedure) was observed between the two groups at 6 months (Fig. 12-8).

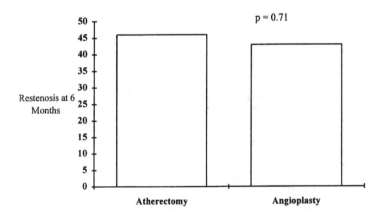

Figure 12-8. No significant difference in 6-month restenosis rate between atherectomy and angioplasty in patients with stenosis of the proximal LAD coronary artery.

CONCLUSIONS

Athrectomy resulted in higher initial procedural success rates in patients with lesions of the proximal LAD coronary artery compared with angioplasty with no difference in in-hospital complications. At 6-month follow-up, restenosis and clinical outcome were not significantly different between the two treatments.

(Data from Adelman et al.[7]) ■

STENTING ANTITHROMBOTIC REGIMEN TRIAL

Intracoronary Stenting and Antithrombotic Regimen Trial

PURPOSE

Determine the early effects of antiplatelet therapy with aspirin and ticlopidine compared to anticoagulation therapy with phenprocoumon and aspirin in patients after the placement of intracoronary Palmaz-Schatz stents.

STUDY DESIGN

General

- 517 patients enrolled in this prospective, randomized, single-center trial.
- Eligible patients were randomized to one of two treatment groups:
    1. Antiplatelet therapy: ticlopidine 250 mg PO bid for 4 weeks and aspirin 100 mg PO bid
    2. Anticoagulation therapy: phenprocoumon titrated to maintain an international normalized ratio of 3.5–4.5 for 4 weeks and aspirin 100 mg PO bid
- All patients received intravenous heparin 15,000 U and aspirin 500 mg before the procedure.
- Arterial sheaths were removed when the prothrombin time was < 60 sec, typically within 3 hr after the procedure.
- Postdeployment high-pressure inflations to an average pressure of 16 atm were used in most of the patients.

Inclusion. Patients included had successfully placed intracoronary stents. The indications for stenting were extensive dissection after percutaneous transluminal coronary angioplasty (PTCA), complete vessel closure, residual stenosis of $\geq$ 30% after PTCA, and lesions in venous bypass grafts.

Exclusion. The criteria for exclusion were patients in whom stenting was used primarily as a bridge to coronary artery bypass graft (CABG); cardiogenic shock; mechanical ventilation before PTCA; contraindications to aspirin, ticlopidine, or phenprocoumon; or absolute indications for anticoagulant therapy.

End Points. The criteria for the combined cardiac end point at 30 days were cardiac death, myocardial infarction, CABG, or repeat PTCA of the stented vessel. The criteria for the combined noncardiac end point were noncardiac death, cerebrovascular accident, or severe peripheral vascular or hemorrhagic event.

RESULTS

The target vessels stented were native coronary arteries in 95% and venous bypass grafts in 5% of patients. Characteristics of the target vessel included dissection before stenting in 58%, thrombus in the stented area in 20%, restenotic lesions in 12%, and a mean reference diameter before stenting of 3.03 mm. During the first 30 days, there was a significant reduction of combined cardiac end points in the antiplatelet therapy group (1.6% antiplatelet vs. 6.2% anticoagulation, P = 0.01). Specifically, there were substantial reductions in the incidence of myocardial infarction (0.8% antiplatelet vs. 4.2% anticoagulation, P = 0.02) and the incidence of reintervention with CABG or repeat PTCA (1.2% antiplatelet vs. 5.4% anticoagulation, P = 0.01). Combined noncardiac end points were also significantly reduced with antiplatelet therapy (1.2% antiplatelet vs. 12.3% anticoagulation, P < 0.001), mostly as a result of reductions in the need for transfusions (0.0% antiplatelet vs. 4.6% anticoagulation, P = 0.001) and peripheral vascular events (pseudoaneurysms or arteriovenous fistula requiring surgery or prolonged compression) (0.8% antiplatelet vs. 6.2% anticoagulation, P = 0.001). The occurrence of an occlusion in the stented vessel was also meaningfully reduced with antiplatelet therapy (0.8% antiplatelet vs. 5.4% anticoagulation, P = 0.004) (Fig. 12-9).

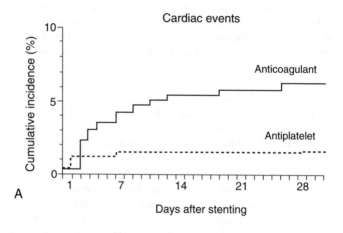

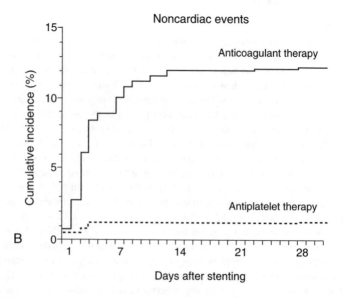

Figure 12-9. Cumulative incidence of *(A)* cardiac and *(B)* noncardiac events in the study groups. (From Schömig et al.,[8] with permission.)

CONCLUSIONS

Antiplatelet therapy with ticlopidine and aspirin in patients after place-ment of intracoronary Palmaz-Schatz stents significantly reduced the inci-dences of myocardial infarction, repeat revascularization of the stented vessel, blood transfusions, peripheral vascular complications, and target vessel occlusion compared to anticoagulation therapy with phenpro-coumon and aspirin during 30-day follow-up.

(Data from Schömig et al.[8]) ■

STRESS

Stent Restenosis Study

PURPOSE

Compare the effects of stent placement with balloon angioplasty on angiographically detected restenosis and clinical outcome in patients with symptomatic coronary artery disease.

STUDY DESIGN

General

- 410 patients enrolled in this prospective, randomized, multicenter trial.
- Eligible patients were randomly assigned to treatment with a Palmaz-Schatz stent or standard balloon angioplasty as follows:
- Patients assigned to stent placement received:
  1. Nonenteric aspirin 325 mg per day starting 1 day before the pro-cedure and continued indefinitely
  2. Dipyridamole 75 mg PO tid and a calcium antagonist starting 1 day before the procedure and continued for 1 month
  3. Dextran 40 infusion 2 hr before and for 16 hr after the procedure
  4. Heparin 10,000–15,000-U intravenous bolus, supplemented to maintain activated clotting time > 300 sec
  5. Warfarin to keep the international normalized ratio 2.0–3.5 contin-ued for 1 month
- Patients assigned to angioplasty received aspirin 325 mg per day con-tinued indefinitely.

- Repeat angiogram was performed at 6 months.

Inclusion. Patients included had symptomatic ischemic heart disease, new lesions of the native coronary circulation, and stenosis $\geq$ 70% with a length $\leq$ 15 mm in a vessel $\geq$ 3.0 mm.

Exclusion. The criteria for exclusion were myocardial infarction within 7 days; contraindication to aspirin, dipyridamole, or warfarin; left ventricular ejection fraction $\leq$ 40%; evidence of coronary thrombosis; multiple focal or diffuse coronary lesions; significant left main disease; ostial lesions; or severe vessel tortuosity.

End Points. The criteria for end points were angiographic evidence of restenosis defined as $\geq$ 50% stenosis on follow-up angiograms or clinical evidence of procedural success. The criteria for the combined clinical end point were death, myocardial infarction, coronary artery bypass graft, or repeat intervention.

RESULTS

Early Outcome (14 Days). Placement of an intracoronary stent resulted in a significantly higher rate of procedural success compared to angioplasty (96.1% stent vs. 89.6% angioplasty, $P = 0.011$). No significant difference in combined clinical end points was observed (5.9% stent vs. 7.9% angioplasty, $P = 0.41$). Bleeding and vascular complications occurred more frequently in the stent group, although the difference was not statistically significant (7.3% stent vs. 4.0% angioplasty, $P = 0.14$). Hospital stay was substantially longer with stent placement (5.8 days with a stent vs. 2.8 days with angioplasty, $P < 0.001$).

Late Outcome (6 Months). Placement of an intracoronary stent resulted in a significantly lower rate of restenosis (31.6% stent vs. 42.1% angioplasty, $P = 0.046$) and significantly less need for repeat interventions of the target vessel (10.2% stent vs. 15.4% angioplasty, $P = 0.06$) compared to angioplasty. Stent placement resulted in a significantly larger luminal diameter immediately after the procedure (2.49 mm with a stent vs. 1.99 mm with angioplasty, $P < 0.001$) and at 6-month follow-up (1.74 mm with a stent vs. 1.56 mm with angioplasty, $P = 0.007$). No significant difference in combined clinical end point was observed at 6-month follow-up (19.5% stent vs. 23.8% angioplasty, $P = 0.16$) (Figs. 12-10 and 12-11).

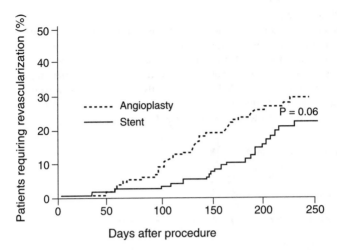

Figure 12-10. Kaplan-Meier curves for revascularization of the target lesion. (From Fischman et al.,[9] with permission.)

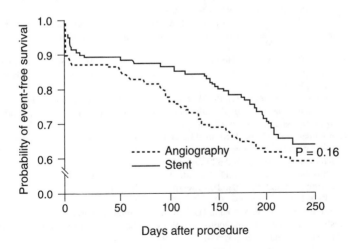

Figure 12-11. Kaplan-Meier survival curves for major cardiac events (death, myocardial infarction, coronary artery bypass graft, and repeated angioplasty). (From Fischman et al.,[9] with permission.)

CONCLUSIONS

Placement of an intracoronary stent, as compared with balloon angioplasty, in patients with symptomatic coronary artery disease resulted in a significantly improved rate of procedural success but with increased rates of bleeding and vascular complications and longer hospital stay. Six-month outcome revealed a significantly lower rate of restenosis and larger luminal diameter with stent placement but no substantial difference in clinical outcome between the two procedures.

(Data from Fischman et al.[9]) ■

References

1. Anderson HV, Smalling RW, Serruys PW: Mechanical devices. pp. 617–52. In Willerson JT, Cohn JN: Cardiovascular Medicine. Churchill Livingstone, New York, 1995

2. Serruys PW, deJaegere P, Kiemeneij F et al: A comparison of balloon-expandable-stent implantation with balloon angioplasty in patients with coronary artery disease. N Engl J Med 331:489–95, 1994

3. Serruys PW, Emanuelsson H, van der Giessen W et al: Heparin-coated Palmaz-Schatz stents in human coronary arteries: early outcome of the Benestent-II Pilot Study. Circulation 93:412–22, 1996

4. Topol EJ, Leya F, Pinkerton CA et al: A comparison of directional atherectomy with coronary angioplasty in patients with coronary artery disease. N Engl J Med 329:221–7, 1993

5. Elliott JM, Berdan LG, Holmes DR et al: One-year follow-up in the Coronary Angioplasty Versus Excisional Atherectomy Trial (CAVEAT I). Circulation 91:2158–66, 1995

6. Holmes DR, Topol EJ, Califf RM et al: A multicenter, randomized trial of coronary angioplasty versus directional atherectomy for patients with saphenous vein bypass graft lesions. Circulation 91:1966–74, 1995

7. Adelman AG, Cohen EA, Kimball BP et al: A comparison of directional atherectomy with balloon angioplasty for lesions of the left anterior descending coronary artery. N Engl J Med 329:228–33, 1993

8. Schömig A, Neumann FJ, Kastrati A et al: A randomized comparison of antiplatelet and anticoagulant therapy after the placement of coronary-artery stents. N Engl J Med 334:1084–9, 1996

9. Fischman DL, Leon MB, Baim DS et al: A randomized comparison of coronary-stent placement and balloon angioplasty in the treatment of coronary artery disease. N Engl J Med 331:496–501, 1994

Index

Page numbers followed by f indicate figures; those followed by t indicate tables.

U